Manual of Drug and Alcohol Abuse

Guidelines for Teaching in Medical and Health Institutions

Manual of Drug and Alcohol Abuse

Guidelines for Teaching in Medical and Health Institutions

Edited by

Awni Arif, M.D.

Formerly of the World Health Organization
Geneva, Switzerland

and

Joseph Westermeyer, M.D., Ph.D.

University of Minnesota Hospital and Clinics
Minneapolis, Minnesota

Plenum Medical Book Company • New York and London

Library of Congress Cataloging in Publication Data

Manual of drug and alcohol abuse.

Includes bibliographies and index.
1. Substance abuse. 2. Alcoholism. I. Arif, A. E. II. Westermeyer, Joseph, 1937–
[DNLM: 1. Alcoholism. 2. Substance Abuse. WM 270 M2938]
RC564.M26 1988 616.86 88-22414
ISBN 0-306-42890-3

233 Spring Street, New York, N.Y. 10013

Plenum Medical Book Company is an imprint of Plenum Publishing Corporation

Printed in the United States of America

Acknowledgments

We wish to thank those who have contributed extensive time and materials in the development of this work. Most have contributed in more than one way, including attending the original planning meetings, preparing the first draft, commenting and contributing sections, corrections, or references, participating in a final review meeting, critiquing and evaluating the individual chapters, and finally reviewing and proofing the entire volume.

Our principal collaborators, listed alphabetically by their names and affiliations, are as follows:

R. Arredondo, E.D.
Texas Tech University
Lubbock, Texas

M. Bean, M.D.
Harvard Medical School
Cambridge, Massachusetts

S. B. Blume, M.D.
National Council on Alcoholism
New York, New York

P. Bourne, M.D.
Global Waters
Washington, D.C.

J. Chappel, M.D.
University of Nevada
Reno, Nevada

J. Fisher, M.D.
Medical University of South Carolina
Charleston, South Carolina

M. Galanter, M.D.
Albert Einstein College of Medicine
Bronx, New York

D. Gallant, M.D.
Tulane University School of Medicine
New Orleans, Louisiana

P. K. Gessner, Ph.D.
State University of New York
Buffalo, New York

J. B. Griffin, M.D.
Emory University School of Medicine
Atlanta, Georgia

J. Kincannon, Ph.D.
University of Minnesota
Minneapolis, Minnesota

R. S. Krug, Ph.D.
University of Oklahoma
Oklahoma City, Oklahoma

G. Litman, Ph.D.
Institute of Psychiatry
London, England

J. Morgan, M.D., Ph.D.
City College of New York
New York, New York

R. Niven, M.D.
National Institute of Alcohol Abuse and Alcoholism
Rockville, Maryland

A. Pokorny, M.D.
Baylor College of Medicine
Houston, Texas

S. Schnoll, M.D., Ph.D.
Northwestern University
Chicago, Illinois

E. Senay, M.D.
University of Chicago
Chicago, Illinois

C. Suwanwela, M.D.
Chulalongkorn University
Bangkok, Thailand

F. Tennant, M.D., D.P.H.
Community Health Projects, Inc.
West Covina, California

A. Uchtenhagen, M.D.
University of Zurich
Zurich, Switzerland

R. L. Weddige, M.D.
Texas Tech University School of Medicine
Lubbock, Texas

Others who contributed collaborative expertise in the original planning or writing, offered critical comments, or participated directly in the rewriting process are listed alphabetically by their names and affiliations as follows:

T. Baasher, M.D.
World Health Organization
Alexandria, Egypt

B. G. Burton Bradley, M.D.
Mental Health Services
Papua, New Guinea

J. Calahan, Ph.D.
National Institutes of Drug Abuse
Rockville, Maryland

J. Chi'en, M.S.W.
Society for the Aid and Rehabilitation of Drug Abusers
Hong Kong

S. Cohen, M.D.
University of California
Los Angeles, California

J. Cooper, M.D.
National Institute of Drug Abuse
Rockville, Maryland

E. M. Corrigan, D.S.W.
Rutgers University
New Brunswick, New Jersey

M. Gerald, Ph.D.
Ohio State University
Columbus, Ohio

H. Ghodse, M.D.
St. George's Hospital
London, England

M. Grant, Ph.D.
The Maudsley Hospital
London, England

Z. Hasan, M.D.
Jenah Postgraduate Medical Center
Karachi, Pakistan

D. Hawkes, Ph.D.
Whitchurch Hospital
Whitchurch, Cardiff, Wales, United Kingdom

E. Heinemann, M.A. FAAN
University of Washington
Seattle, Washington

V. Hudolin, M.D.
Dr. Mladen Stojanovic University Hospital
Zagreb, Vinogradska, Yugoslavia

J. Hughes, M.D.
University of Vermont
Burlington, Vermont

P. Hughes, M.D.
Veterans Administration Medical Center
Bay Pines, Florida

F. Iber, M.D.
University of Maryland Hospital
Veterans Administration Medical Center
Baltimore, Maryland

W. Jilek, M.D.
University of British Columbia
Vancouver, British Columbia, Canada

L. Jilek-Aall, M.D.
University of British Columbia
Vancouver, British Columbia, Canada

E. Larkin, M.D.
Addiction Research Foundation
Toronto, Ontario, Canada

J. Makanjola, M.D.
ARO Neuropsychiatric Hospital
Abeokuta, Ogun State, Nigeria

G. Martin, M.D.
Addiction Research Foundation
Toronto, Ontario, Canada

R. Masaroni, M.D.
World Health Organization
Geneva, Switzerland

D. Mohan, M.D.
All India Institute of Medical Sciences
New Delhi, India

M. H. Mubbasher, M.D., D.P.M.
Rawalpindi, Pakistan

C. A. Naranjo, M.D.
Addiction Research Foundation
Toronto, Ontario, Canada

J. C. Negrete, M.D.
Montreal General Hospital
Montreal, Quebec, Canada

E. D. Nelson, Pharm. D.
University of Cincinnati
Cincinnati, Ohio

P. O'Gorman, Ph.D.
Berkshire Farm Center and Services for Youth
Canaan, New York

E. M. Pattison, M.D.
Medical College of Georgia
Augusta, Georgia

R. E. Popham, M.D.
Addiction Research Foundation
Toronto, Ontario, Canada

N. Sartorius, M.D.
World Health Organization
Geneva, Switzerland

R. Segal, Pharm. D.
Addiction Research Foundation
Toronto, Ontario, Canada

H. Sell, M.D.
World Health Organization
New Delhi, India

J. Severinghaus, M.D.
Dartmouth Medical School
Veterans Administration Hospital
White River Junction, Vermont

A. Showanasai, M.D.
Phra Mongkutlao Army General Hospital
Bangkok, Thailand

R. Smart, Ph.D.
Addiction Research Foundation
Toronto, Ontario, Canada

M. I. Soueif, M.D.
Cairo, Egypt

S. Sparber, Ph.D.
University of Minnesota
Minneapolis, Minnesota

J. T. Ungeleider, M.D.
University of California
Los Angeles, California

A. Zweben, M.D.
Addiction Research Foundation
Toronto, Ontario, Canada

Finally, we thank most graciously our final reviewers, who read and critiqued the entire book prior to publishing:

S. Blume, M.D.
National Council on Alcoholism
New York, New York

J. Fisher, M.D.
Medical University of South Carolina
Charleston, South Carolina

J. F. Maddux, M.D.
University of Texas Health Science Center
San Antonio, Texas

A. Pokorny, M.D.
Baylor College of Medicine
Houston, Texas

F. Seixas, M.D.
Harvard Medical School
Belmont, Massachusetts

Several WHO Collaborating Centers have also participated in the development of this volume, as follows:

Addiction Research Foundation
Toronto, Ontario, Canada

Drug Dependence Research Center
Universiti Sains
Penang, Malaysia

Health Research Institute
Bangkok, Thailand

Institute of Psychiatry
Mexico City, Mexico

National Institute of Alcohol Abuse and Alcoholism
Rockville, Maryland

National Institute of Drug Abuse
Rockville, Maryland

Numerous others have provided critical assistance at many points along the way in the development of this manual. These include colleagues who have commented and assisted on technical points, medical educators and educators in other fields (nursing, social work, psychology, public health), house officers, residents, and medical students. We cannot cite each of them by name, but wish to acknowledge the value of their efforts.

A. Arif, M.D.
Geneva, Switzerland

J. Westermeyer, M.D., Ph.D.
Minneapolis, Minnesota

Foreword

During the last few centuries, and particularly in recent decades, problems resulting from the excessive use of drugs and alcohol have spread virtually as an epidemic to every country in the world and to almost every community. Abuse of alcohol and drugs is related to numerous other health problems, such as the spread of acquired immune deficiency syndrome (AIDS) on all continents. Health and social services today cannot afford to ignore this crisis since it affects all levels of society and manifests itself in diverse health and social problems.

In recent years, the World Health Organization has received numerous requests for training material for physicians in this field. This manual therefore meets an urgent need. The availability of new data and the dearth of suitable textbooks have made its preparation mandatory.

The influence of sociocultural factors on drug dependence and alcohol-related problems—on their cause, development, and consequences as well as on their treatment and prevention—has been taken into account in the preparation of this manual in order to ensure that its usefulness is not limited to one country or region. It has been prepared primarily for the teaching of physicians and medical students, although much of it is relevant to the training of nurses, midwives, health educators, primary-care workers, medical social workers, counselors, and psychologists. In fact, suggestions have been included for adapting the manual for use in the training of such varied groups of students. An entire chapter has been devoted to providing guidelines for the training of clinicians in drug–alcohol dependence, paying particular attention to the clinician's attitude toward the patient.

The authors are to be commended for the preparation of this valuable guide for health workers in combating this major health problem.

Dr. T. A. Lambo
Deputy Director-General
World Health Organization
Geneva, Switzerland

Contents

1

Introduction and Definitions

Awni Arif and Joseph Westermeyer

1. Background

This manual has been prepared in response to numerous requests to the World Health Organization (WHO) for educational materials concerning drug dependence and alcohol-related problems. Over the last few decades, WHO has addressed issues of diagnostic criteria, definitions, epidemiology, treatment approaches, and evaluation of treatment. However, WHO publications on these topics have been primarily technical in nature, meant for the specialist in the drug–alcohol dependence field, as well as for the researcher. They have not been designed for the generalist or for the medical educator training the generalist.

Pressing public health problems involve the issue of alcohol and drug abuse. For example, the spread of acquired immune deficiency syndrome (AIDS) has been linked directly to intravenous drug use. Abuse of alcohol and nitrite drugs has facilitated the spread of AIDS by producing inhibition, loss of judgment, and casual sexuality. Damage to unborn infants has resulted from alcohol, cannabis, cocaine, solvent–inhalant, and tobacco use.

As many areas of the world have been experiencing a virtual pandemic of drug dependence and alcohol-related problems in recent decades, the voices calling for such materials as in this manual have become louder and more widespread. It is evident that this problem is too broad merely for the specialist's concerns. Medical facilities, health services centers, and ministries of health therefore perceive an increasing need for educational materials designed for the generalist and, more specifically, for the teacher of generalists in medical facilities and training centers. This manual has been designed to meet those needs.

2. Organization and Structure of the Manual

The manual has five major sections: Part I deals with the guidelines for teaching and training. This has deliberately been placed at the beginning of the manual so that the educator can go through it before studying the material in the other chapters. The guidelines address the pedagogical and curricular issues and provide a concept and suggestions for designing and implementing a curriculum in drug dependence.

Part II contains four chapters that cover the historical background, epidemiological assessment, etiological factors, and natural course and psychosocial manifestations of drug–alcohol dependence.

Part III deals with the pharmacology of commonly abused drugs.

Part IV covers the medical aspects of management in five chapters on clinical diagnosis and assessment, management of medical emergencies, medical complications, psychosocial management, and pharmacotherapy.

Part V deals with the public health aspects of alcohol and drug problems. It contains chapters on public health planning and prevention strategy for these problems.

A predominantly clinical orientation has been adopted in the organizing theme. That is, the subject is covered from the standpoint of history, epidemiology, etiology, course, medical complications, diagnosis, management, and prevention.

This organization should not be interpreted as meaning that drug and alcohol dependence should only be taught in the clinical years. On the contrary, the contributors and the authors of this text are strongly of the opinion that material should be included during the basic science years of clinical education. These basic materals should reflect the normal or phenomonological aspects of drug and alcohol use, rather than its pathological aspects. Basic science aspects of drug and alcohol dependence should be presented, with special reference to such topics as epidemiology, genetics, pharmacology, pathology, and psychopathology. These basic science aspects of the problems can be gleaned from this text by referring to the index. In particular, the teacher of behavioral science, clinical interviewing, pharmacology, epidemiology, pathology, and neurophysiology will find much of value in this text, specifically as these topics relate to alcohol and drug problems.

Like many of the chronic illnesses and behaviorally related disorders not affecting the world's health, the curriculum in drug–alcohol dependence presents special pedagogical dilemmas. We have devoted an entire chapter to these problems. This chapter should serve as a guideline to the medical educator. Further, it is anticipated that this volume will be widely used by those responsible for educating health workers from other disciplines besides medicine. These disciplines include nursing, social work, counseling or psychology, pharmacy, and primary health care workers. Materials are included here to guide the educator in adapting this volume to the curricular needs of these various health disciplines. It is hoped that eventually each of the other disciplines will have similar materials at their behest for designing curricula. In the meantime, we trust to the ingenuity of these educators to adapt the materials contained herein.

3. Purpose and Aim

This manual has been designed primarily for the medical school educator. We anticipate that readers will include both basic science and clinical educators in the 4000 medical schools around the globe. This has been our primary target audience as the volume has been prepared. It is also anticipated that other audiences will find the book equally valuable. In particular, educators in hospitals and health centers concerned with postgraduate medical education, as well as continuing medical education, will find it helpful. Selected chapters and sections will also prove valuable to educators in the other health-related disciplines.

The volume was not designed for direct use by the medical student, since economics will prevent its distribution to individual medical students. Nevertheless, it is anticipated that the volume will serve as a library resource for medical students. A glossary has been added to be of help to the medical student; this glossary should also prove useful to many readers not familiar with medical terminology.

Residents and physicians in practice will also want access to this volume in their hospital libraries. There is much useful information regarding diagnosis and immediate clinical management (e.g., for overdose, withdrawal, certain medical complications); these may be encountered infrequently in some settings. We have included specific drug regimens and other modes of intervention in sufficient detail to permit their ready application.

The contents of this volume, in their entirety, may be too complex for other community health workers. A separate abridged version has been prepared for those designing training for these workers.[6] Still, trainers may wish to use this text for reference materials.

4. Methodology—How Was This Manual Produced?

This volume was prepared over a 3-year period by approximately 20 primary contributors and 80 collaborators from around the world. It began with a survey conducted by WHO in all of its major regional offices ascertaining the need for and interest in such a volume. The initial outline for the volume was based on the expressed needs of member countries. This outline was then sent to WHO regional offices and to medical educators for their comment and further development.

Once a final outline was produced, identified clinician–educators and investigator–educators around the world were asked to prepare and write material needed for the various chapters. These included designated primary contributors, each of whom had three or four collaborating authors from other countries. The primary contributor, along with an equal number of international collaborating authors, participated in a WHO Workshop in Berkeley, California, in November 1982. Following intensive discussion from this meeting, the second draft was prepared. The two coeditors have subjected the second draft to preliminary testing by health sciences students and educators at the University of Minnesota. Following their consultation and guidance, the coeditors then prepared a third draft. A WHO advisory group meeting met on October 24–30, 1983, and reviewed the entire manual. Following the deliberations and advice of this group, the fourth draft was prepared in 1984, taking into consideration the comments and advice of the advisory group meeting. This fourth draft was then sent to an international panel of educators for further comment and critique. Specific supplementary sections and additions were assigned in order to round out the volume for international applicability.

In writing this volume we have sought to avoid including untested approaches, especially those which may have some popularity at the moment but whose longevity is in question. The contributors and reviewers to this volume have demonstrated considerable consensus toward the materials contained herein. Much in this volume will probably remain relevant and current through the remainder of this century. However, the last few decades have taught us that, in this rapidly advancing field, there is no way of knowing how and when new breakthroughs in our knowledge will occur. The medical educator must keep abreast of these changes in order that such texts may prove a key to useful information, rather than a millstone from the obsolete past. It is likely that WHO, with its demonstrated commitment to this field, will continue to prepare updated materials as they are needed.

5. Special Aspects of This Volume

This volume differs from existing publications in the field in several ways, as follows:

1. This manual and guidelines were not solely produced by the two coeditors. The book is the result of collective collaboration, including contributions from more than 100 international educators and experts from developing and developed countries. Experience and knowledge were gathered from six WHO Collaborating Centers in the field of training and research.

2. This volume marks several notable milestones in medical education. It defines more clearly the role of the general physician and other primary health care workers in the prevention, early recognition, and treatment of drug dependence.[1] This is both a clinical and a public health role. This combined clinical–

public health task in drug dependence reflects that which we increasingly encounter in several areas of medicine: an overlapping, often complex admixture of individual and societal morbidity. Health care workers of the future must be able to address the often difficult social, ethical, and doctor–patient problems that result from drug dependence and similar social health problems. This manual may thus serve the general purpose of sensitizing medical teachers and practitioners to the behavioral and social dimensions of clinical work.

3. This book focuses on a problem that has traditionally not been viewed as a medical or health problem. In the past, societies (as well as their physicians) have considered drug problems to be in the province of legislation, law enforcement, social welfare, and religion, but not in the province of health services and public health. Complex social health problems like drug dependence must receive broad-based consideration from legislators, law enforcement personnel, social workers, and others, including teachers, mass media specialists, and family members. Health care workers alone cannot solve broad-based social health problems. Nevertheless, physicians can and must assume responsibility for diagnosing and treating drug dependence. Drug dependence follows a long list of disorders once seen as nonmedical, immoral, or incurable, including leprosy, tuberculosis, venereal disease, malaria, and malnutrition.

4. This volume demonstrates that our knowledge regarding drug dependence has progressed to the point where it can be addressed like other medical disorders. Principles of etiology, pharmacological pathophysiology, course, diagnosis, treatment, and prevention bear many similarities to the major health problems in this last quarter of the twentieth century, from cancer to cardiovascular disease, malnutrition to depression.

5. This book has been written for a particular reader: the educator of the general physician. The need for clinical skills and therapeutic attitude, as requisite complements to knowledge, has been emphasized. It is likely that students and practitioners will also find much useful information in these pages. By addressing the educator, however, the authors have sought to gain access to a wide audience: the next generation of medical practitioners. Educators of other health professionals—nurses and midwives, psychologists, and public health specialists—will no doubt find valuable content in various chapters.

6. Finally, this book has a guideline for teaching and training in the field of drug dependence. Very few existing publications have such an advantage of guidelines. It provides concepts as well as suggestions for designing and implementing a curriculum in this important field.

6. Definitions and Terminology

In this manual the authors use the term *drug dependence* as equivalent to the term *substance abuse,* alcohol being considered one of the drugs of dependence.

In 1964 a WHO Expert Committee[5] recommended that the term *drug de-*

pendence replace the previous terms *addiction* and *habituation*. Drug dependence was defined as a state ensuing from repeated administration of a drug on a periodic or continuous basis and with characteristics that varied according to the agent involved. With this concept, it was also necessary to designate the particular type of drug dependence under consultation.

The first attempt by WHO to define alcoholism is to be found in the Expert Committee Report of 1951,[4] when the dependence formulation was promulgated. Alcohol took its place as one of the family of drugs capable of producing a dependence picture, but in 1977 a WHO group of investigators suggested the idea of dependence syndrome.[3]

In August 1981 a WHO working group[2] reviewed earlier work on definition and terminology and presented a concept and terminology in detail. The group proposed the term *neuroadaptive state* as an alternative to *physical dependence,* and a profile was given of the elements that constitute a "drug-dependence syndrome."

WHO updated its definitions of psychoactive substance use disorders in preparation for the tenth *International Classification of Disease* (ICD-10), which were tested in field trials in 1987. The classification and definitions must be approved by WHO. Clinical descriptions and diagnostic guidelines for field trials are categorized under "Mental and Behavioral Disorders due to Psychoactive Substance Use." This category includes disorders due to alcohol, tobacco, opioids, cannabinoids, sedatives or hypnotics, cocaine, other stimulants, including caffeine, hallucinogens, multiple drug use, and other (including volatile solvents) and unidentified substances. Within each category, the patient's clinical condition would be specified as follows: acute intoxication, use, harmful use, dependence syndrome, withdrawal state with delerium, psychotic disorder, drug- or alcohol-induced amnestic (Korsakoff) syndrome, drug- or alcohol-induced residual and late-onset psychotic disorder, such as flashbacks, and unspecified mental or behavioral disorder induced by drugs or alcohol.

References

1. Edwards G, Arif A: *Drug Problems in a Socio-cultural Context*. World Health Organization Public Health Paper, no. 73. Geneva, WHO, 1980.
2. Edwards G, Arif A, Hodgson R: Memorandum on nomenclature and classification of drug and alcohol related problems. *Bull WHO* 1981; 59(2):225–242.
3. Edwards, G, Gross MM, Keller M, Moser J. Room R (eds): *Alcohol Related Disabilities*. World Health Organization Offset Publication, no. 32. Geneva, WHO, 1977.
4. *World Health Organization Technical Report Series,* no. 42. Geneva, WHO, 1951.
5. *World Health Organization Technical Report Series,* no. 273. Thirteenth report of the WHO Expert Committee on Drug Dependence. Geneva, WHO, 1964.
6. World Health Organization: *Drug Dependence and Alcohol Related Problems: A Manual for Community Health Workers, with Guidelines for Trainers*. Geneva, WHO, 1986.

I

Teaching Approaches

2

Guidelines for Teaching and Training

1. Introduction

No one discipline can completely cover all aspects of drug dependence. All basic and clinical departments of a medical college are involved to some extent. In particular, departments of pharmacology, behavioral science, pathology, community medicine, family medicine, internal medicine, psychiatry, and public health typically share the teaching responsibility for drug dependence. Leadership—whether by a dean or a curriculum committee—is a key factor in assigning and coordinating the teaching task.

This chapter provides concepts as well as suggestions for designing and implementing a curriculum in drug dependence.

2. Curriculum Design

2.1. Statement of the Problem: Sociomedical Crises Today

Societies everywhere are experiencing a growing number of major sociomedical problems, of which drug dependence is a model disorder. The traditional response of communities to drug dependence in times past was to regard this problem as the responsibility or misfortune of those afflicted. That view has been changing. Communities now increasingly perceive that drug–alcohol dependence demands societal responses and that the medical profession should participate in the development and delivery of these responses. As a result, health science centers have been challenged to educate and train clinicians who are more responsive to demographic, social, and economic changes which have deep implications for health care.

Every individual entering a clinical career cannot acquire sufficient training and experience to deal with all aspects of drug dependence. At the same time, all clinicians should have certain basic skills and information. Translating such concerns into meaningful curricular changes poses a major challenge for medical educators. The curriculum is invariably well filled already. Yet several alternatives are available to deal with this problem. Subject material of an interdisciplinary nature can be incorporated into existing disciplinary courses. Or drug dependence can be introduced as a selective topic in survey courses dealing with a range of sociomedical problems (including nutrition, cancer, and maternal–child health). Students may profit more from in-depth instruction in one or a few areas than from a course that attempts to deal superficially with them all. An in-depth course on drug dependence can be offered as an elective for those with special interest in the field.

Medical students are often overwhelmed by problems in the sociomedical arena, and this can lead to negative attitudes. Focus on individual patients and the benefits to be derived from treatment can overcome these obstacles. Panel discussions or pedagogical interviews with recovered drug-dependent patients are instructive and can help change negative attitudes toward these patients. These interviews also can serve as a warning for the future professional regarding the dangers of personal substance use, especially if the patient is a physician. Of course, interviews alone cannot substitute for a rigorous, data-oriented exploration of the field.

2.2. Approaches to Curriculum Design

Medical education in drug dependence, its etiology, diagnosis, and treatment, should be no less scientific, critical, and rigorous than education in cancer or infectious disease. Certain aspects of substance abuse should be introduced early in medical education. For instance, in biochemistry the manner in which the ratio of adenosine diphosphate and phosphate to adenosine triphosphate regulates the rate of oxygen utilization can be used to illustrate the effects of chronic alcohol consumption on this ratio and thereby on the rate of oxygen utilization by the hepatocyte. In the second phase of medical education, the study of the modification of normal biology by disease and other agents, medical educators can emphasize the tissue, psychological, behavioral, and social changes induced by pathological drug use. In the third phase of the educational process, clinical instruction, each patient with drug dependence can become the vehicle for in-depth study and instruction on this disorder. In most areas of the world today this instruction can take place on all clinical services, but especially in internal medicine, psychiatry, family medicine, obstetrics and gynecology, primary care, public health or community medicine, ambulatory care, pathology, and radiology. Attention can thus be given to drug-dependence problems in all medical school courses and clinical assignments. The frequent practice of restricting clinical instruction in drug dependence to one department, such as pharmacology or psychiatry, is questionable since this disorder concerns all basic medical and clinical sciences to some extent. Since the problems of drug dependence are significantly lessened by early treatment, its timely diagnosis must also be the concern of all clinicians.

Often an outside expert consultant can help to develop a curriculum in this field. This can contribute greatly when local expertise is lacking, or when competing departments cannot agree on the distribution of assignments or curriculum time. This approach can be particularly valuable in developing areas where resources are limited.

A curriculum committee whose members are appointed by the heads of the individual departments is likely to be unsympathetic to the emergence of interdepartmental curricular time specifically identified with drug or alcohol abuse. Thus, those interested in the introduction or expansion of drug-dependence instruction should become familiar with the table of organization of their institution and the lines of responsibility within it.

One effective mechanism for enhancing the instructional attention given to drug dependence is to convene a task force of students and faculty interested in the subject. Such a group can identity the existing strengths of the curriculum in drug dependence and can consider how to influence the formal educational offerings of the school, by bringing appropriate materials and presentations into established courses or by organizing a specific course that addresses drug dependence. The next proper concern for such a group consists of enhancing the interests and strengths already existing among the faculty and stimulating such interest where it is currently lacking. The seriousness of drug dependence will be transmitted most effectively to the students if it is apparent that many of the school's faculty have knowledge and concern in this area. The display of widespread interest regarding drug dependence will convey the importance of the problem more effectively than if only one or two faculty members, however well informed, address the students on this subject.

A group of interested members of a medical school faculty can exert influence by passing resolutions, issuing position papers, making requests, and appearing at conferences. It is highly desirable that the group enlist student members.

When proposing a drug-dependence course, it is well to recruit some allies from other disciplines or departments who can speak up favorably. This helps in supporting an educational program on its merits, whereas one faculty member doing all the talking may seem self-serving. In proposing changes to a curriculum committee, it is well to line up some supporters and allies in advance. A person who wants to bring about a change should be sure to become a valued, useful, and responsible member of committees such as the curriculum committee. One thereby earns the influence and capacity to bring about favorable change.

Bringing about curriculum changes in drug dependence may take several years. A useful procedure is first to offer a drug dependence course as an elective. Another useful procedure is to have interested faculty incorporate drug dependence material into their own courses.

In order to direct the attention of educators to drug dependence, it is useful to include items on this topic in certifying examinations.

2.3. Problems in Curriculum Development

Drug and alcohol content cuts across all departments and all phases of medical training. It is not feasible for one person or department to implement a total curriculum in this field. The committee in charge of curriculum at each medical school must be responsible for developing a curriculum in drugs and alcohol. In order to accomplish this, the curriculum committee collaborates with individual departments as well as the dean of curriculum.

Instruction in drug dependence can and should be made stimulating and intellectually rewarding. This can be accomplished by the following proven strategies in medical pedagogy: courses in which specific issues of drug dependence are considered in depth; courses in which students meet with instructors knowledgeable in drug dependence and have an opportunity to join in discussion of the clinical issues; contact with drug-dependent patients successfully recovering from their disorder; and involvement in drug-dependence research.

A major problem is the shortage of time due to an ever-increasing body of knowledge that students must acquire. Teaching some students in depth about this disorder on an elective or selective basis can be useful since it will necessarily result in transmission of some of the acquired knowledge to the other students. The nature and extent of drug dependence vary widely in different societies. Whether all students need to be exposed in depth to all aspects of this problem must be dictated by local conditions.

Inclusion of drug dependence in the curriculum requires regular reevaluation of the material presented. Drug-use patterns in any society can change dramatically, according to the relative availability of a given substance, perceptions of its potential toxicity, and the status or symbolic value of its use. In recent years this changing pattern has occurred with cocaine in many countries, as cocaine has become less expensive, more available, less feared, and used by younger people. As use patterns change, so does the incidence of medical consequences. Social views regarding the role of the physician in treating drug dependence also continue to evolve, and these views impinge on the medical curriculum.

3. Curriculum Development

3.1. Instructional Tasks

Several instructional tasks are involved in training clinicians in drug dependence. These include conceptual, attitudinal, perceptual, interpersonal, nosological, dynamic, and therapeutic tasks.

3.1.1. The Conceptual Task

This is concerned with the basic concepts the health care professional brings to the physician–patient relationship. Typically the beginning student brings moralistic stereotypes that prevail in society at large to the student–patient interaction. Moral condemnation may lead to a rejection of the patient and refusal of health care. Thus, students must acquire new concepts that will form the basis for care of drug-dependent patients.

3.1.2. The Attitudinal Task

Clinicians bring their personal attitudes to the patient encounter. They must address the question "Why am I treating this patient?" Sometimes clinicians do not like patients who have drug-dependence problems. Consequently they may be harsh and punitive with them. If the patient then abandons treatment, this may reinforce the clinician's attitude that drug-dependent patients are hopeless.

3.1.3. The Perceptual Task

This task covers that which the practitioner sees, hears, smells, and feels when encountering the patient. It requires that the clinician establish rapport with and obtain pertinent information from the patient and describe this information correctly. This description requires accuracy of perception that is not filtered through distorted concepts or unproductive attitudes toward drug dependence.

3.1.4. The Interpersonal Task

This consists of the clinician's behavior toward and relationship with the drug-dependent patient. It involves verbal and nonverbal behavior. Eliciting relevant information and gaining the patient's collaboration in treatment strongly influence the clinician's success in this task.

3.1.5. The Nosological Task

Nosology is concerned with the classification of disease and making a differential diagnosis. Since drug dependence (like most chronic disorders) is a pathoplastic phenomenon with many manifestations and courses, the nosological task is not easy. Ideally, the established diagnosis should include a constellation of signs and symptoms, a pathological process or course, an etiology or etiologies, a treatment plan, and a prognosis. Since laboratory diagnosis of drug dependence is in its infancy,[15] the nosological task relies strongly on the traditional clinical skills of history taking and physical examination. Skill in this sophisticated activity must be acquired under the guidance of experienced mentors.

3.1.6. The Dynamic Task

The dynamic task entails understanding the pathogenesis of drug dependence in the particular patient. This disorder has certain common expressions, but with different physiological, psychological, and sociological causes for each individual. Simply positing one etiological understanding for all persons with drug dependence (e.g., a neurotransmitter deficiency) will not be therapeutically efficacious.

3.1.7. The Therapeutic Task

After each of the previous tasks has been successfully addressed, the clinician is ready to begin the therapeutic task. This presumes that:

1. The patient is a cooperative partner in treatment.
2. The interpersonal interaction is not simply a friendly social event.
3. Treatment is more than common sense; in fact, commonsense approaches may be detrimental to the patient's successful recovery.

If the curriculum in drug dependence is organized along these task lines, students readily become sensitive to the issues involved in the complex phenomenon of drug dependence. They can then effectively address the patient's needs.

3.2. Faculty and Students

3.2.1. Faculty as Specialist and Generalist

A patient who has two problems from more than one clinical field (e.g., acquired immune deficiency syndrome and opioid dependence, or hypertension and cocaine abuse) tends not to fit the usual pedagogical mold. Students trained in only one specific subject will not know how to address the other issue. This is exemplified by the orthopedic surgeon who treats the fractured mandible and clavicle of the drug-dependent person involved in an auto accident. The surgeon may not address the etiology of the orthopedic problem. This is analogous to treating a localized problem (such as an abscess) while ignoring the systemic problem that caused it (such as septicemia). In order to overcome tunnel vision of this sort, medical educators must teach students to recognize and treat more than one disorder concomitantly. Despite the popularity of specialized medicine in recent decades, all practitioners must have certain general skills. This is especially true of medical educators in clinical settings.

3.2.2. Discipline of the Student

Medical students are often oriented more toward doing things *to* patients than doing things *with* patients to achieve the goal of better patient health. This can present problems in working with drug-dependence rehabilitation. On the other hand, medical students are clearly service oriented and assume major personal responsibility for the health of patients. This can be an asset in the early treatment of drug-dependent patients.

Nursing students expect to interact with patients more intensively or for longer periods of time than do other professionals. This can lead to an overly solicitous approach or one engendering too much reliance on professionals by the drug-dependent patient. Nursing emphasizes education of patient and families in caring for themselves and assuming personal responsibility for health. These latter characteristics can benefit such patients considerably.

Social work students providing service to patients are usually ill prepared to understand drug dependence from pharmacological and biomedical perspectives. Their orientation is toward working with the socioenvironmental milieu so the individual is not locked into a situation that may encourage maladaptive behavior. The latter is frequently a major consideration in working with drug-dependent patients. They are likely to have contact with clients who express concern about excessive drug use by others in the family.

In contrast to the service orientation of nursing, medicine, and social work professionals, persons trained at a Ph.D. level—such as psychologists or pharmacologists—have greater interest in research and special investigative techniques. They usually do not have strong backgrounds in basic medical sciences which would help them appreciate drug dependence and its complications from a more holistic biopsychosocial perspective.

3.2.3. Educational Level of Students

Preclinical students often are expected to memorize and reproduce information. Teaching about drug dependence is most readily accepted by students at this level if the instructor is conversant with both clinical and basic science data and can integrate these data into a coherent picture for the student.

During clinical years teaching is oriented toward assisting students to interact with patients, make clinical judgments, and choose relevant intervention procedures. The instructor who attempts to teach basic science information alone to clinical-level students will predictably lose them and have information rejected.

3.3. Course Content

Drug dependence, like mental illness and tuberculosis, makes the individual appear or behave abnormally. Historically, people suffering these stigmatized conditions have been viewed by the public as being immoral, weak-willed, sinful, or incurable. Removal from society, or quarantine, has been the preferred disposition for the supposedly hopeless sufferer. These attitudes and beliefs are not based on medical fact, but nevertheless many students possess them as they encounter education about drug dependence. Course content cannot ignore these historical prejudices and ignorance.

3.3.1. Knowledge

In the field of drug dependence, research over the last decade has markedly increased knowledge. The instructor's task is not presenting all available data, but rather choosing the relevant information that students must have at their particular level of development.

3.3.2. Attitudes

Attitudes stem from beliefs which, in the drug-dependence field, may be supportive or detrimental to treatment. Since there is an emotional component to an attitude, the emotional aspect may override even accurate information and be counterproductive. Perhaps the most important goal of medical education in drug dependence is to address this attitudinal component so that students may deal more effectively with what they perceive as a stigmatic disease.

A critical factor involves shaping students' attitudes toward those which are the most productive in the care of drug-dependent persons. An accepting attitude toward a drug-dependent patient is desirable to circumvent the pejorative stance that many people take toward the illness. While accepting the patient is important, condoning the patient's behavior at times may be counterproductive. For example, the physician may need to set limits on, or at least not collude in, self-destructive behavior. It is important to assist students in (1) understanding their own attitudes and (2) recognizing those attitudes which are productive in the treatment of drug-dependent patients.

The attitudes that appear to be the most productive are those which are positive toward drug-dependence treatment and the outcome of various interventions.[3] Students may still maintain a belief that use of illegal substances, or diversion of legal substances to illegal use, is morally wrong. Furthermore, identifying an individual as ill does not absolve that person from any responsibility for his or her actions. It only removes the presumption that the illness itself (e.g., being an alcoholic) is a purposeful act.

3.3.3. Skills

The skills most important for clinicians include (1) ability in acquiring and integrating information from the patient to make an appropriate diagnosis, and (2) facility in implementing primary, secondary, and tertiary prevention of drug dependence. Primary prevention involves preventing substance abuse from ever developing, such as reducing risk factors before the person initiates drug use. Secondary prevention consists of early intervention in drug dependence and returning the person to the level of functioning that existed previously. These skills include diagnosis, detoxification, treatment, and rehabilitation. Skills in tertiary prevention consist of treating drug dependence so that further deterioration does not ensue. These skills involve (but are not limited to) assessment, utilization of laboratory tests, detoxification and stabilization, knowledge of rehabilitation resources in the community, and ability to make an effective referral.

3.3.4. Training Objectives

Training objectives are observable, measurable end points in the educational process. They are a mechanism by which both the educator and the student can be clear about content.[10]

The training objectives contain the elements of behavior that must be mastered. For example, if the goal is to teach students to evaluate the effect of drug use on a patient's mental status, the following might be training objectives:

1. Observe and describe the patient's behavior.
2. Examine the patient's orientation to person, place, time, and situation.
3. Test the patient's immediate, recent, and remote memory.
4. Examine the patient's attention span and concentration.

This method of formulating behavioral tasks to be mastered assists the faculty in organizing course material and students' experiences at specific points rather than allowing education to proceed in a haphazard manner. It also has the advantage of allowing evaluation to proceed logically from the objectives. That is, if the instructor clearly indicates in training objectives what is expected of the students, then examination tasks or questions can be formulated that reflect those objectives. If a particular student does not perform well on certain items, then clearly the student is deficient in acquisition of the requisite knowledge or skill, or there are attitudinal deterrents. However, if an examination task or question is missed by many students, then either the examination or the instruction may be faulty.

3.4. Timing and Location of Teaching Drug Dependence

If the training in drug dependence is delayed until postgraduate years, considerable difficulty can be anticipated along several lines. For example, there will be disagreement regarding which clinical specialty should address drug dependence. The debate will inevitably lead to numerous narrow foci in the field, such as emphasis on physiological effect in laboratory medicine, tissue damage in pathology, short-term detoxification in internal medicine, or long-term rehabilitation in psychiatry.

A drug-dependence curriculum woven throughout all courses across the entire course of study is the ideal situation. For example, during basic science education, biochemistry can emphasize aspects of metabolism related to drug dependence, physiology can cover the effects of abused substances on basic physiological processes, and behavioral sciences can present the psychological and sociological concomitants of drug use and abuse. When persons who have substance-abuse problems are encountered on each of the clinical specialty rotations, students should observe that the patient's drug dependence is assessed and treated.

Providing drug-dependence information to students in a classroom setting has the potential for being sterile and uninteresting or, worse, reinforcing counterproductive attitudes. Teaching from clinical case examples, while emphasizing clinical significance and pointing out general principles and concepts, can be effective in stimulating interest and facilitating therapeutic attitudes.

Teaching on hospital units has the clear advantage for students of learning medical management of persons with substance-abuse problems. There are also disadvantages. One danger of observing only inpatient management is that students will learn erroneously that the clinician's role in treating patients is simply detoxification. Consequently students may not appreciate the continuity of care necessary for effective rehabilitation. Supervising teachers may be unsympathetic to patients who have drug-dependence disorders. If this occurs, the students will learn an inappropriate role by identification with an inadequate role model. Teaching in the outpatient department facilitates the development of diagnostic and early-intervention skills, but does not permit training in detoxification or rehabilitation.

Education in special substance abuse units and clinics offers the advantage of observing ongoing treatment of drug dependence. Students can be involved in the initial intake and detoxification of patients, as well as later treatment and rehabilitation. They can observe the beneficial outcomes in recovered persons and their families, note the effectiveness in continuity of care, and have role models experienced in managing the disorder. Conversely, the disadvantages to confining education to units and clinics specializing in drug dependence include the fact that only limited numbers of students may be accommodated. It may also isolate patients with substance-abuse problems into quarantined areas, giving the impression that treatment must be effected in this format alone, and that only specialty physicians have a role in treating this disorder. This setting also does not lend itself to teaching early diagnosis and referral skills. Perhaps most effective for students is a curriculum that involves supervised clinical experience, focused on drug dependence, in both primary care and specialty settings.

3.5. Education Methods

A major key is the organizational ability and skill of the instructor. When students are dealing with a stigmatized disorder, they frequently experience anxiety and anger about the topic. They may feel that, in dealing with such patients, they too will become stigmatized. This tension can lead to hostility if students do not receive adequate preparation for their future responsibilities or do not have role models with whom they can identify. This same tension can also mobilize student curiosity and attention. The instructor can help students deal with their tension by providing well-integrated, thoughtful, detailed outlines of material and by providing clear behavioral objectives. Simply providing these materials for students is ineffective if the instructor does not serve as a role model and guide the student in the mastery of the subject.

Small-group discussion is an effective medium for presenting drug-dependence materials while allowing students to discuss and integrate them. Seminar-style discussions facilitate an exchange of ideas and perceptions so areas of misunderstanding can be corrected. Instructors can observe each student's interaction in this setting. Reluctant students almost always become involved in the instructional process. A personal relationship can be formed between the student and the instructor so the students view the instructor as a mentor who is able to demonstrate empathic, humanitarian, ethical care.

Teaching on ward rounds can also be productive. Bedside teaching permits the clinical tutor to demonstrate respect for the patient while eliciting information.

Instructors often invite patients to appear in class in order to discuss their disorder and their recovery. As with other pedagogical methods, the use of recovered persons is both advantageous and problematic. Since drug dependence is a pathoplastic phenomenon with multiple origins, its treatment and rehabilitation also have multiple courses. Effective treatment for one person may not be effective for another. Some recovered persons may proselytize their own method of recovery while denigrating other methods. Instructors should take care to minimize the amount of preaching or testimonials in which former patients sometimes indulge, while actively guiding the discussion into the clinical phenomenon. For example, topics of interest include the impact of the drug dependence on the family and occupation, the means of getting the patient into treatment, and methods the patient uses to sustain the recovery and prevent relapse.

An effective antidote to negative feelings toward drug dependence lies in linking the disease to positive concepts. This is the rationale behind having recovered movie stars and prominent government officials make public statements about their recovery. The instructor can do this by always referring to the patient as a person who has a drug-dependence problem or an alcohol problem. By continuously referring to the person with a drug problem, the human being is placed first and the drug dependence is secondary. However, if the individual is labeled as a substance-abuse problem or an addict or an alcoholic, the label confuses the person with the disease—a confusion that interferes with clear thinking and with effective treatment.

Audiovisual techniques can effectively hold the students' attention and enhance the educational experience. Self-instructional slide/audio tape and computer-assisted learning packages on drug dependence are available for self-learning exercises.

In some countries the history of drug dependence has been rich with drug-related songs, films, theater, and books. Since students are usually familiar with popular music or films of the day, this can hold their attention and interest while simultaneously stressing underlying clinical principles.

Videotapes or films can be used to record a particular clinical phenomenon that cannot be readily presented at a scheduled lecture or at morning rounds. For instance, if the instructor is talking about alcohol amnestic disorder (Korsakoff's disease) then a videotape or film of a patient demonstrating perseveration, confabulation, and other memory problems can help the student appreciate the disorder. Videotaped materials can be replayed until the educational point is clear; this is an advantage over film. Both tapes and films can also be used to stimulate thought and discussion between students and teacher.

3.6. Local Resources

Local resources must be assessed, mobilized, and integrated into the educational effort. If there is no clinical program, then a possible first step is to establish one or to affiliate with one that is located near enough for use in teaching. Once drug-dependence treatment is established within the medical school's affiliated clinical facilities, and once faculty are skillful at this work and enjoy doing it, this will create interest among medical students and residents. Ultimately, competent faculty will recruit trainees with an interest in this work themselves.

4. Teaching Diagnostic Skills in Drug Dependence

4.1. Importance of Early Diagnosis

The ability of health professionals to identify alcohol- and drug-related problems can be seriously impaired by their lack of training. As a result of this absence of knowledge, alcohol and other drug use may not be considered the cause or even a contributing factor in many of the complaints presented. Skill in the early recognition of drug dependence requires the ability to ask routine questions about the use of drugs. The examiner must be able to follow these queries with other, more probing questions.

Of course, it is usually possible for professionals to diagnose a problem when a patient exhibits the obvious and severe consequences. It is at the point when disabling symptomatology has already appeared that most professionals recognize a drug-dependent patient. They are then frequently discouraged by the recalcitrance of the patient, by the massive denial, and by the patient's reluctance to enter a treatment program despite what seems to be overwhelming evidence that such a regimen is required.

4.2. The Clinical Context

Drug-dependent patients present to the attention of the medical practitioner in various ways, including the following:

1. Those who identify themselves as drug or alcohol dependent and are seeking assistance voluntarily.
2. Patients who are referred without the subject's willing participation in that decision.
3. Cases detected by skilled physicians in the course of their routine clinical work.

Medical students must be taught how to deal with patients presenting in these different circumstances as well as others. Different skills are required in each different context. Attitudinal factors on the part of the patient and the therapist often vary widely as a function of the context; these may influence the clinical intervention.

Most clinicians are familiar with the negative pictures that drug-dependent patients present to personnel in the emergency room and medical units of large general hospitals. These patients are either treatment failures or have never sought help voluntarily for drug dependence. With only this exposure, students often develop a pessimistic, negative attitude toward this patient group. Working with recovering outpatients is the key in overcoming these negative stereotypes.

4.3. Elements of the Physician–Patient Relationship

Trust is the essence of the physician–patient relationship as well as other human relationships. Without this trust, the most intense efforts of a physician may be useless when it comes to helping a patient. As distrust enters the relationship, patient noncompliance increases, as does the dropout rate from treatment.

Three important elements of a therapeutic relationship have been described by Truax and Carkhuff,[17] as follows:

1. Nonpossessive warmth: the ability to show the patient that you care without being overly parental.
2. Accurate empathy: the ability to convey to patients that you understand their feelings.
3. Genuineness: conveying honesty to the patient and being able to admit your mistakes in an appropriate manner.

These comprise the foundation for conveying an attitude of professional competence to the patient. Once the clinician is able to incorporate these elements into the relationship with the patient, a bond of trust is established and treatment begins.

A reciprocal beneficial relationship results when the instructor conducts an interview with the patient and any family members who are available. As the students learn from active participation during the process of asking questions, drug-dependent patients and their families appreciate the attention and concern devoted to them. This learning process gives impetus to the development of future therapeutic relationships between the student and the drug-dependent patient. Personal exchange between student and patient helps the student develop a more sensitive approach to the patient's feelings. Exchange with the patient humanizes the subject of drug dependence.

If the patient's spouse or family is available for interview, this may be an even more meaningful experience for students. Listening to a wife or husband explain that the children are no longer tense or resentful and that warmth now exists where previously there had been only rebellious or sullen anger can have a dramatic impact on the students. This type of learning experience gives the students a more positive and optimistic attitude toward clinical work with drug dependence. It also enhances students' ability to form more positive relationships with such families in future treatment settings.

4.4. Teaching the Interview Process

Teaching medical students to interview patients in a sensitive manner in order to obtain a reliable history is one of the most important goals in medical school. The instructor should beware of using unnecessarily complex interview models for the student, as this may create resistant attitudes in a student.[19]

The drug use history should begin with questions about the least threatening subjects. Thus, the faculty member should instruct the student to begin by inquiring about substances that are legal or culturally acceptable, such as the number of cups of caffeinated beverages per day, the number of cigarettes, and then other drugs. After each specific drug is discussed, the patient should be asked a question about the effects of the drug-related behavior on other people: "Does your husband or do your fellow employees ever comment that you may be drinking too much?" If the answer is yes, a subsequent question should be "How many drinks does it take to elicit these comments?" These same questions can be asked about other drugs as each substance is reviewed in the history. An introduction to these subjects such as "Some of these drugs can cause changes in a person's behavior or affect the action of other drugs" may help to smoothe the path. These questions must be asked in a nonjudgmental manner, and labels with negative connotations, such as alcoholic or addict or drug abuser, should be avoided. Attention to type, amount, and pattern of drug usage will result in more reliable and valuable information.

At the beginning of a therapeutic relationship, one should not attack the patient's denial of drugs as a source of the clinical problems. Instead, one works around it without allowing the denial to preclude a reliable history. When the interview is skillfully conducted, it enables the patient to start taking an honest look at the problems related to drug usage.

It should be emphasized to the students that a screening drug use history is an essential part of all complete medical examinations and that a methodical but concerned approach will decrease the number of undiagnosed cases. Carefully worded questions about chemical use in other family members may yield additional information. The appropriate setting to initiate the teaching of the interview process could be either during the human behavior course or during the history-taking course.

Use of written questionnaires or clinical rating scales may help the student to gain a more complete understanding of the interview as well as the diagnostic approach. After an initial relationship with the patient has been established, use of these scales may enable the patient to take a more honest look at himself or herself without being offended by the interviewer. Students themselves can be asked anonymously to complete these scales as a source exercise, and the results can be tabulated and reviewed in the next class session. Change from a passive to an active participation in this way stimulates the interest of the class.

4.5. Teaching Assessment and Diagnostic Skills

Students must be trained to recognize different patterns of drug use, especially when dealing with cases referred by nonmedical third parties (e.g., legal agencies, employers, school authorities, parents). They should also be able to identify different degrees of dependence and to recognize patients also are nondependent, abusive, or occasional users. Students must be able to conduct independent evaluations and to form their own diagnostic assessments on the basis of available information. Mistaken labels which the referring person may have attached to the case must not be simply endorsed in an unquestioning fashion.

Students should be taught to include drug dependence in their differential diagnosis. For example, they must be aware that withdrawal symptoms can appear in patients hospitalized for causes other than substance abuse. Drug dependence can also be manifested by high tolerance for anesthetics in surgical patients, or by absenteeism or frequent sick leave requests from work. Unless students consider the many facets of drug dependence, they will not be able to intervene therapeutically.

Students should be trained to detect subtle evidence of drug dependence as well as such gross findings as hepatomegaly, splenomegaly, proximal myopathies, or peripheral neuropathies. Evidence of acne rosacea, palmar erythema, spider nevi, cigarette burns, cheilosis, injection scars, multiple trauma, and poor nutrition may all suggest heavy drug or alcohol intake and thus contribute toward establishing a diagnosis.

Teaching differential diagnosis of intoxicated mental states is essential. When a patient arrives in a physician's office or an emergency room with symptoms of slurred speech, difficulty with coordination, ataxia, loquaciousness, and difficulty with attention, there may be a natural tendency by the physician to attribute the patient's symptoms to drug intoxication. Similar symptoms may be caused by neurological diseases such as multiple sclerosis or cerebellar dysfunction, or by metabolic diseases such as diabetes mellitus. Even if the diagnostic impression is supported by a relatively high blood level of alcohol, it would be wise to teach the student to follow the patient carefully. Intoxication can mask underlying physical sequelae such as subdural hematoma.

In medical, health, and social science training, the trainees should learn the techniques of early intervention therapy with drug-dependent patients. In many cases this may save years of hardship for the family and friends as well as for the patient. Early intervention is a therapeutic maneuver to help the patient now rather than wait interminably for the patient to lose or destroy family, health, or job.

5. Attitude Assessment and Change

Relatively little has been done about the transmission and acquisition of attitudes in health sciences. Attitudes are difficult to define, measure, and influence. Developing and achieving attitudinal objectives in medical education challenges both teachers and clinicians. The nature of this challenge and ways in which it can be met are described here.

The concept of attitudes has arisen from attempts to account for observed regularities in the behavior of individuals. When asked to account for these regularities, people make evaluative responses that have cognitive, affective, experiential, and even physiological components. Describing attitudes is difficult because they involve value systems and life experience that are often not in current awareness. To add to the complexity, people often have attitudes that are mutually inconsistent or even contradictory. For example, physicians with strong positive attitudes toward preserving life may apply their lifesaving skills selectively when they encounter patients or situations toward which they hold strong negative attitudes.

Complex problems of drug dependence require high levels of knowledge and skill if they are to be successfully treated. When negative attitudes interfere with either the acquisition or the application of professional knowledge and skills, then patient care suffers and the cost to society increases.

5.1. Attitudinal Problems

If attitudes are so important, then why have they been so neglected in medical education? In one medical school less than 1% of preclinical objectives were defined as affective (i.e., related to the student's feelings) whereas in the clinical years affective objectives increased to 24%.[7] These affective objectives primarily involved understanding the physician–patient relationship and getting along well with clinical staff and supervisors. Since attitudes are connected to our personal values and beliefs, they have an importance similar to that of politics or religion. Students may view any attempt to change attitudes, or even to examine them, as an invasion of privacy. However, from an historic point of view, we are emerging from a time when drug dependence has been viewed as a moral and legal problem, not medical. Medical students can and must be expected to develop attitudes that are therapeutic vis-à-vis their effects on patient care.

Attitudes toward patients with alcohol problems become increasingly negative through medical school and residency training.[5] Physicians working in hospital settings have been found to have a derelict stereotype regarding alcoholism.[1] A disparity between the attitudes of alcoholic patients and the psychiatrists and psychologists treating them has been observed: the patients believed that individual sessions would help, but the mental health professionals were pessimistic about the outcome of treatment and unwilling to devote much of their own time and effort to such activity.[8] In the emergency room, alcoholic or drug-abusing patients have been defined as management problems rather than medical cases to be diagnosed and treated.[11]

Change in medical attitudes toward drug dependence is occurring. Health disciplines in many regions have recognized the need for medical school education on drug dependence.

5.2. Origins and Determinants of Attitudes

The origins and determinants of attitudes need to be understood before designing educational approaches that have attitudinal impact. It is generally agreed that attitudes have three components[9]:

1. Cognitive—involves belief, knowledge.
2. Affective—involves feeling, emotion.
3. Conative—involves decision, behavior.

The cognitive component is the most conscious and consists of knowledge and information. This is a logical place to start the educational attempt to influence attitudes, but is not sufficient. The affective component is emotional, less conscious and associated with physiological change. It has the most impact in shaping and changing attitudes but, since it is viewed as subjective, the affective component is less likely to be valued or expressed by health science students. Direct experience and role modeling influence the affective component. The conative component has to do with the will and motivation to act. We know least about this component, but actual practice of the desired behaviors (i.e., establishing habit patterns) is a useful way to influence it.

Favorable attitudes are positive in all three components. Unfavorable attitudes are negative in all three components. However, both positive and negative components can coexist.

Acquisition and application of attitudes are most apparent in adolescence. Medical students, having just emerged from adolescence, can be expected to have well-established attitudes on many aspects of drug dependence. They do not come to the classroom or clinic as a *tabula rasa* upon which the teacher can inscribe the desired attitudes. Questioning students' established attitudes can create strong feelings, such as anxiety or hostility. This is typically resolved as new attitudes emerge. Resistance and conflict can be reduced if we first attend to the attitudes already held, respecting their origins and illustrating their impact on the diagnosis and treatment of alcohol and drug dependence.

Communication, both verbal and nonverbal, plays a major role in the development of religious, political, cultural, racial, and other attitudes. Nonverbal communication, through body movement and facial expression, is most influential when it comes from significant people, such as parents or teachers who serve as role models. Art, music, film, and television can also have attitudinal influence. Verbal communication, used in persuasion and propaganda, impacts most on the cognitive component. Medical students encounter many powerful role models among their clinical teachers who have negative attitudes toward drug dependence. If these negative influences are to be countered, the role models chosen to communicate positive attitudes must be carefully selected.

Direct experience plays a powerful role in determining attitudes. Repeated, continued involvement and communication, in family and community settings, results in shared attitudes which are accepted as natural and rarely questioned. It is only after repeated experience and active involvement that attitudinal change occurs. Occasionally a single salient encounter results in a dramatic attitudinal change (e.g., love at first sight, religious conversion, or phobic terror), but this is uncommon. Medical schools, hospitals, and organized medicine also exert powerful influences on the professionalization of medical students, residents, and practicing physicians. While these influences are generally positive, they can be negative, as in the case of drug dependence.[13] Altering institutional attitudes is even more difficult than altering individual attitudes. While individuals may be moved by logic, institutions respond more to economic, management, and political pressures.

Altered physiological states also influence attitudes. Drugs, disease, hormones, biogenic amines, blood supply, hunger, thirst, fatigue, and other factors altering physiological function can all have a marked, although often temporary, effect on attitudes. They usually alter the affective and conative components, which makes their influence more difficult to describe or measure.

5.3. Attitudinal Measurement and Educational Goals

The complexity of attitudes makes them difficult to measure accurately. Self-reports have the virtue of being easy to obtain, but suffer from a validity problem. Self-reports are most likely to be accurate about the cognitive component of attitudes. If the affective and conative components are incongruent with the cognitive, then the self-reported attitude may have little resemblance to the behavior of the individual.

Observed behavior in specified situations more accurately reflects the conative component of attitudes. Obtaining such data is more expensive in time and energy than is self-reporting.

Investigators have identified two general sources of attitudinal bias among physicians. The first occurs when the patient is so similar to the student that the student loses objectivity. The second prevails when the patient is so different from the student that the student fails to identify problems.[12]

Educational interest in attitudes should not be hidden from students. Clear identification of the attitudes and behaviors targeted for reassessment reassures students that their personal values are not being attacked. Clarity of educational focus makes it easier for students to adopt therapeutic attitudes and behavior as part of their professional approach to patients, even though they may retain negative or conflicting attitudes in their personal lives. In this way a two-stage process is established. Initially the students adapt to the expectations of faculty with a minimum of personal or interpersonal conflict. Later, at their leisure, the students can make whatever adjustments they wish, to reconcile the differences between their own professional and personal attitudes.

Upon completion of a drug-dependence course, students might be expected to demonstrate the following objectives which involve attitudes:

1. Interest and curiosity in approaching and maintaining contact with drug-dependent patients.
2. Persistence in obtaining the information necessary for assessment of patient's drug use.
3. A positive approach to the spectrum of treatment resources and community services (e.g., treatment intervention).
4. Optimism about treatment outcomes.

5.4. Teaching for Attitude Change

The first problem encountered in medical schools is that every student brings already formed attitudes into the classroom. These reflect the family and culture from which the student comes. Students need to understand the importance of separating personal values from the professional values being emphasized in the course. Attempts to change students' personal values directly will always be resisted. Failure to make this separation between personal and professional values probably accounts for the difficulty experienced in achieving attitudinal objectives.[14] The purpose is to help our students become more tolerant and open to patients who behave differently and hold values different from themselves. These different behaviors and values can be understood and appreciated in the context of medical problem solving and patient care, without having to give up one's own personal values.

5.5. The Process of Attitude Change

A message has more attitudinal impact if its source has credibility and perceived expertise. Including information on both sides of a question or issue is more likely to influence attitudes than presenting only one side.[9]

Student attention and comprehension, critical steps, are enhanced by a dynamic delivery.[18] Presenting early on the conclusions that will be reached and providing written material that complements the presentation are also important educational tactics.

Yielding is a little-understood step in which the recipient agrees with the presented attitude. Cognitive yielding probably precedes affective and conative yielding in most situations. However, if affective and conative yielding occur, then cognitive yielding is more likely to follow. Mothers, sports coaches, army sergeants, and political leaders have long recognized this. Humor facilitates this yielding process by ameliorating its uncomfortable aspects.

Retention is enhanced by repetitions over time. Long or intermittent courses on drug dependence have an advantage over brief or concentrated courses. A review of the literature on attitude change during medical school has indicated that the positive attitudinal effect of one course on attitudes does not persist; at least 2 years of exposure are needed.[14] An attempt to get medical residents to adopt a psychosocial perspective led to the observation that despite 6 months of training, only one-third of the residents demonstrated retention of the new approach.[16] Active participation in the learning experience contributes to persistence of such changes.[20] An even more important factor in the persistence of attitude change is the presence of a supportive group of peers and faculty.[6]

Overt behavior reflecting the new positive attitudes is the final stage. Available data suggest that requiring the desired behavior in conjunction with close supervision helps maintain behavioral change. The behavior itself may have a strong influence on attitudinal change, especially if the behavior is accompanied by favorable results such as positive treatment outcome. Improvisation by the learner also appears to be important in establishing new behaviors.

6. Evaluation and Testing

Student performance should be assessed in the areas of knowledge, skills, and attitudes.[4] In dealing with subject matter as complicated as drug dependence, the most thorough evaluation should include a combination of both objective and subjective methods. Direct observation of students as they undertake clinical assessments and function within the treatment team is especially important during later clinical training.

6.1. Examination of the Student

The field of drug dependence covers an assortment of areas some of which are better tested by objective means and others by subjective methods. Objective testing is particularly valuable for areas in which there are considerable consensus and firm data. Such areas in the drug dependence field include pathology, pharmacology, epidemiology, and certain aspects of diagnosis and treatment.

Areas that cover data in which there are differing opinions among authorities in the field are better covered by subjective methods of evaluation. Such areas include ethical, legal, cultural, sociological, and some psychological concepts. Specific research data are better covered with objective testing, while theories based on research often can be better evaluated in a subjective format.

If the teaching program is built around objectives, the questions should adequately sample all the major areas described in the objectives. A subject grid should be developed to ensure adequate representation of all important areas. For example, the National Board of Medical Examiners in one country developed such a subject grid for preparing questions on drug dependence. (See Table I.) This grid had three axes based on the type of drug, content area, and type of clinical or social presentation. Every question represented a topical area within each of the three axes. The percentage of questions within each axis was assigned so that the total was 100% within the axis. The decision concerning the percentage of questions for each area was based on the experience of the authors, although they tried to represent the general importance of each topic.

6.2. Teacher Evaluation

If students are clearly demonstrating that they have learned effectively, the teacher's prime objective has been accomplished. Nevertheless, direct monitoring of teacher performance is of value. Such monitoring can produce continuing

Table I
Drug Dependence Examination Grid

Substance	Content area	Clinical presentation
Alcohol	Research, theory, epidemiology	Acute intoxication, overdose, withdrawal
Sedatives		Chronic dependence
Opioids	History, legal, ethics, sociocultural	Associated medical problems and complications
Stimulants		
Cannabinoids	Psychological, pharmacological, pathological	
PCP/hallucinogens	Clinical, diagnosis, treatment, rehabilitation	Social dysfunction: family, employer, finance, law, community
Tobacco		
Volatiles		
Belladonna/other	Miscellaneous, multiple areas content	Miscellaneous: multiple clinical problems
Miscellaneous, multiple drugs		

feedback to help teachers improve their skills and can be invaluable in locating areas of difficulty.

Assessment of teacher performance is typically done with a combination of subjective and objective ratings. When rating scales are mailed or distributed to students to be turned in later, the return rates are usually between 50 and 70%. Conclusions drawn from such a sample are clearly questionable. One technique for ensuring full response from students is to provide time for the rating scale to be completed at the time that the students take their final examination. If students turn in the final examination without the rating scale, they can be asked to return to complete the rating scale. When full participation is obtained, these rating scales can give information of great value concerning faculty performance. Program directors, however, should be careful to avoid the trap of causing faculty to feel themselves to be participants in a popularity contest. Student opinion concerning faculty is important but should not be the single controlling factor in faculty evaluation. Although effective teachers are often popular with students, this is not invariably the case.

Direct observation of faculty performance by other faculty members is one of the most useful ways of measuring effectiveness. Such observation should be coupled with feedback to the instructors so that they can correct deficits in their teaching.

Evaluation of program effectiveness usually requires open administrative channels to allow free communication with other programs that relate to the drug- and alcohol-dependence curriculum. An effective program must provide skillful instructors who should coordinate teaching across various medical school departments. A mechanism for providing continuing program review is formation of a drug-dependence education committee composed of representatives of each department having responsibility for substance abuse teaching. Regularly scheduled review of the substance abuse curriculum by this committee can be very useful both in avoiding duplication and in assuring adequate coverage of the field of drug dependence. Energetic leadership is a critical component in this process.

It is desirable, whenever feasible, to have both intramural (e.g., within the medical school) and extramural program evaluation. Visiting professors giving presentations related to drug dependence can consult regarding the drug-dependence teaching program. Program evaluation should include attention to cost-effectiveness both in teaching and in patient care.

One of the difficulties in the evaluation of drug-dependence curricula relates to lack of an extramural instrument for evaluation of student performance, such as a national board examination. In many traditional fields, such as internal medicine, psychiatry, and surgery, a school can obtain accurate data concerning the performance of their students. This is usually not the case in drug dependence. In order to provide help in this deficit area, some countries have appointed a task force to work in the development of evaluation materials for national examinations.

7. Summary

In setting forth course objectives the instructor must attend to the various instructional tasks; the discipline and educational level of students; the knowledge, attitudes, and skills to be developed; the sequencing of materials over the instructional time available; the location in which training is to take place; and the technique of instruction to be used.

Throughout the educational process, behavioral objectives are a useful mechanism around which to organize the instructional material. Evaluation can then be tied to the behavioral objectives, allowing for a more accurate assessment of both the student's performance and the teacher's success.

Special pedagogical problems attend the teaching of drug dependence in medical schools. These include the fact that patients present with an extremely wide diversity of problems and are variously motivated to treatment. Students encounter special problems related to drug-dependent patients, such as special interviewing techniques and assessing the severity of the problem.

Attempts have been made to influence medical students' attitudes toward drug dependence. Preliminary results indicate that attitudinal objectives can be set and that significant positive changes can be obtained.[2] Experience indicates that attitudes may change more in response to a spaced curriculum of several months than to a block or compressed curriculum of several days.

Thorough evaluation of student knowledge, skills, and attitudes in substance abuse involves use of both objective and subjective methods. Objective methods are particularly useful for areas in which there is considerable consensus and firm data in drug dependence, such as pathology, pharmacology, epidemiology, and certain aspects of treatment and diagnosis. Subjective evaluation such as oral examinations and essay questions gives the examiner an opportunity to observe the student's reasoning ability. Subjective testing is especially valuable in evaluating ethical, legal, sociological, and some psychological concepts. Use of a subject grid in the construction of examinations in substance abuse ensures adequate representation of all important areas.

The performance of teachers in substance abuse should also be evaluated. Usual methods for evaluation of teachers include student ratings and direct observation by other faculty members. Extramural program evaluation can be obtained by use of visiting consultants and examination instruments prepared by agencies outside the medical school.

References

1. Chafetz ME: Research in the alcohol clinic and around the clock psychiatric service of the Massachusetts General Hospital. *Am J Psychiatry* 1968; 124:1674–1679.
2. Chappel JN, Jordan RD, Treadway BJ, Miller PN: Substance abuse attitude changes in medical students. *Am J Psychiatry* 1977; 134:379–384.

3. Chappel JN, Krug RS: Substance abuse attitudes: Their role and assessment in medical education and treatment. In *Alcohol and Drug Abuse in Medical Education.* National Institute on Drug Abuse Monograph. Rockville, Maryland: NIDA, 1980.
4. Charvat J, McGuire C, and Parsons V: A review of the nature and uses of examinations in medical education, in *World Health Organization Bulletin,* Chapter 4. Geneva, WHO, 1968, pp 25–49.
5. Fisher JC, Mason RL, Keeley KA, Fisher JV: Physicians and alcoholics: The effects of medical training on attitudes toward alcoholics. *J Stud Alcohol* 1975; 36:949–955.
6. Frank JD: *Persuasion and Healing: A Comparative Study of Psychotherapy.* Baltimore, Johns Hopkins University Press, 1973.
7. Gjerde CL: The domains and cognitive processes in medical school objectives. *J Med Educ* 1978; 53:352–355.
8. Knox WJ: Attitudes of psychiatrists and psychologists toward alcoholism. *Am J Psychiatry* 1971; 127:1675–1679.
9. McGuire WJ: The nature of attitudes and attitude change, in Lindzey G, Aronson E (eds): *Handbook of Social Psychology,* ed. 2, vol 3. Reading, Massachusetts: Addison-Wesley, 1969.
10. Mager RF: *Preparing Educational Objectives.* Belmont, CA, Fearon, 1962.
11. Mannon JM: Defining and treating "problem patients" in a hospital emergency room. *Med Care* 1976; 14:1004–1013.
12. Marcotte DB, Held JP: A conceptual model for attitude assessment in all areas of medical education. *J Med Educ* 1978; 53:310–314.
13. Mendelson JH, Wexler D, Kubzansky PE, Harrison R, Leiderman G, Solomon P: Physicians' attitudes toward alcoholic patients. *Arch Gen Psychiatry* 1964; 11:392–399.
14. Rezler AG: Attitude changes during medical school: A review of the literature. *J Med Educ* 1974; 49:1023–1030.
15. Ryback RS, Eckardt MJ, Pautler CP: Biochemical and hematologic correlates of alcoholism. *Res Commun Chem Pathol Pharmacol* 1980; 27:533–550.
16. Schildkrout E: Medical residents' difficulty in learning and utilizing a psychosocial perspective. *J Med Educ* 1980; 55:962–964.
17. Truax CB, Carkhuff RR: *Toward Effective Counseling and Psychotherapy: Training and Practice.* Chicago, Aldine, 1967.
18. Ware JE, Williams RG: The Dr. Fox effect: A study in lecture effectiveness and ratings of instruction. *J Med Educ* 1975; 50:149–156.
19. Waring EM: An interpersonal model for teaching psychiatry to medical students. *Psychosomatics* 1980; 21:998–1005.
20. Watts W: Relative persistence of opinion change induced by active compared to passive participation. *J Person Soc Psychol* 1967; 5:4–15.

Further Reading

Cohen S: *The Substance Abuse Problems.* New York, Haworth Press, 1981.

Gallant DS: *Alcohol and Drug Abuse Curriculum for Psychiatry Faculty.* Rockville, MD, National Institute of Alcohol Abuse and Alcoholism, 1982.

Hostelter V: *Alcohol and Drug Abuse Teaching Methodology Guide for Medical Faculty.* Rockville, MD, National Institute of Alcohol Abuse and Alcoholism, 1982.

Kissin B, Begleiter H (eds): *Biology of Alcoholism: Treatment and Rehabilitation of the Chronic Alcoholic.* New York, Plenum Press, 1977.

Lowinson JH, Ruiz P (eds): *Substance Abuse Clinical Problems and Perspectives.* Baltimore, Williams & Wilkins, 1981.

Pattison EM, Kaufman E: *Encyclopedic Handbook of Alcoholism.* New York, Garden Press, 1982.

II

The Problem and Its Assessment

3

Historical Background

1. Introduction

Those unfamiliar with the past are likely to repeat its errors. Opium, cannabis, coca leaves, betel-areca, and alcohol use for nonmedical purposes has been known since the beginning of historical times, and drug dependence has been reported for over 2000 years. Religions, cultures, and governments have struggled with drug problems over this period, sometimes successfully and other times unsuccessfully. Innovations in drug types, routes of administration, production, and commerce have greatly complicated the issues surrounding drug use. Physicians should be aware of these historical trends in order to understand their patients' drug use, as well as drug-related problems facing human society today.

2. Drugs and Their Uses

2.1. Drug Discovery, Production, and Spread

People have shown as much diversity in developing medicinal as well as recreational drug use as they have in developing social organization, religion, dress, and food production over the centuries. Variations have included developing methods of producing a particular drug, discovering new substances with psychoactive properties, or employing new routes of administration with old compounds.

Over the Eurasian land mass and Africa as well as in North and South America numerous means have evolved for producing a single drug: alcohol. Sources of carbohydrate to make ethanol have included camel and mare's milk, rice, millet, barley, wheat, cactus, sugar cane, grapes, apples, honey, and tubers such as the potato. Pulque, a fermented drink from a fleshy agave plant, is still popular in Mexico. Production methods have varied from beer making over days or weeks, to making wines over months or years, to the distillation process for whiskies.

Opium poppy was used as a medication in early Mesopotamian and Egyptian cultures. Poppy seed in Turkish archaeological sites goes back several thousand years. Cannabis probably originated somewhere in Asia, although its current distribution is worldwide. Its use is recorded in Hindu literature from 1400 B.C., where it is described as a sacred grass. The origin of betel-areca is not clear, but its continued, widespread use from South Asia, to Southeast Asia, to the Malay Archipelago, to Oceania suggests its possible origin somewhere in that region.[3,19,22]

Africa has a long history of beer production, widespread cannabis use, and some opium consumption. Many plant stimulants and mild stimulant–hallucinogens also originated there. Khat* and cocoa bean are a few examples.[10] The tribes as well as the highly civilized societies of the Americas refined literally hundreds of plant stimulants and hallucinogens. Many are still consumed but only by small, isolated tribes, or in particular regions or countries; coca leaf and peyote are examples. Other drugs, such as tobacco, have been exported and are now used around the world.[7]

In the past five centuries diffusion of drug use technology around the world has greatly accelerated. In part this has been due to more sophisticated transportation, with increased travel and commerce. Tobacco and later cocaine from the American continents spread to Europe and then throughout the world. Opium and cannabis spread in the opposite direction from Europe to the Americas. While alcohol from fermentation was indigenous in some areas of the Americas, the distillation process was imported from Europe.

Some industrial products and drugs, never meant to yield a psychotropic effect, have been used for this purpose. These have included gasoline, kerosene, aerosols, cleaning solvents, paint compounds, and even smelling salts. Widely available and inexpensive, they add to the environmental factors that must be considered in assessing drug-dependence problems.

2.2. Drug Uses

The decision to use a drug may be made by the individual, or others, such as healers, may make the decision for the individual. Some uses are based on the

*"Khat" is also spelled "chat" or "qat."

traditions of society. For example, American Indian groups have used tobacco and peyote as sacramental drugs, just as wine is sacramental in certain Christian rituals. Certain Asian and Caribbean peoples consume cannabis during ritual meals and religious ceremonies. Over the centuries drugs used as aphrodisiacs have included yohimbine, cannabis, opium, and alcohol.

2.2.1. Medical Use

Archaeological evidence and field studies of tribal people indicate that mankind has had the concept of medication from prehistoric times. Therapeutic compounds have been taken to preserve health and to treat illness. Most medications have had plant origins (e.g., roots, bark). Some have come from animals (e.g., bile, testicles) or from inanimate objects (e.g., certain stones, iron).

Pharmacologically active medications developed over centuries have usually had plant origins. These include digitalis, belladonna, reserpine, and opium. Several drugs discovered in the last several decades have come from animals; these include thyroid, insulin, antiserum, and vitamin B_{12}. Even the antibiotic discoveries of the last half-century were derived from microorganisms. Earlier plant compounds have been modified chemically to produce more powerful and concentrated substances, such as heroin and morphine from opium, and cocaine from coca leaf. It has only been during the last few decades that biochemists have begun to target synthetic compounds in the laboratory for specific therapeutic purposes. Some synthetic compounds have the potential for abuse, including the barbiturates, phencyclidine (PCP), amphetamines, and opioid drugs such as methadone, meperidine (pethidine), and fentanyl.

Many older drugs of abuse have long been used for medicinal purposes, including opium, cannabis, alcohol, coca leaf, and mescaline. Newer drugs of abuse have often first been sold as medications, such as the barbiturates, heroin, meperidine, methadone, and PCP. Both older and newer drugs have provided relief for cough, diarrhea, pain, nausea, vomiting, asthma or other respiratory problems, insomnia, agitation, anxiety, and melancholia. They have been of great benefit for the sufferings that befall us. Often these newer drugs have initially been sold as nonaddicting substitutes for known dependence-producing drugs; this occurred with morphine as well as heroin soon after their discoveries. It was 15 years after the original synthesis of heroin that the first cases of heroin dependence were reported in the medical literature.

An individual may use drugs for their desirable effects, and not for a disease or disorder. Farmers or laborers may take analgesics for relief from aches resulting from episodic hard work, or office workers may take mild stimulants to relieve fatigue or boredom. Opium use by laborers and hill tribe villagers in Asia may be for relief of such discomfort. Cannabis preparations and other stimulants are used to combat fatigue in many parts of the world. Coca leaf is chewed to overcome hunger as well as fatigue in the Andes region. Truck drivers, factory workers, nighttime workers, and students may use amphetamines and other stimulants to keep awake in order to perform their tasks. In parts of rural South Asia some nursing women give opium solution to their infants to keep them quiet while the mothers work.

2.2.2. Recreational Use

Drugs can be taken to enhance life, to provide relief from anxiety and inhibition, or to escape from unpleasant reality. This can be undertaken in isolation by a single individual or socially in a group. Group use can be in the mainstream of the culture, or it can be a deviant activity practiced by only a small number.

Recreational use differs around the world according to the availability of drugs and the sociocultural setting. Alcohol and tobacco in various forms are used on all continents. Dependence on both these substances is a major public health problem in many countries. Opium, which earlier was a medicinal preparation in the Middle East, India, and China, later became a drug for recreation. This led to a high level of use which spread in India and China during the sixteenth and seventeenth centuries. Recurrent widespread use of opiates has occurred in China, Asia, Europe, and North America during the twentieth century.

2.2.3. Sociocultural Use

Certain psychoactive substances with mild effects, or stronger substances used infrequently in moderate amounts, are socially accepted as a means to enhance social interactions, sometimes by relaxing and sometimes by stimulating the user. For example, alcohol drinking is a part of the social life of many cultures throughout the world. Earlier civilizations in India, China, Central America, Egypt, Greece, and Rome all approved the use of alcohol, although approval was suspended at times when excessive use was recognized. In their teachings Buddhism and the Islam religion both prohibit the use of alcohol.[1] Use of beer, wine, and spirit in social gatherings is acceptable in many societies today so long as there is no undesirable behavior.

Tobacco smoking has also been widespread. Smoking in public places has been widely tolerated, but possible harm inflicted on nonsmokers has been increasingly recognized. This change in social norms and attitude has accelerated in recent years, although smoking prohibitions have occurred in China, Japan, Russia, Turkey, and other places since the seventeenth century.

Coca leaf chewing by South American peasants, khat chewing in East Africa and Yemen, opium smoking by hill tribe villagers in Southeast Asia, and betel-areca chewing in Oceania and South Asia follow a similar pattern as an acceptable practice. These substances are offered to guests in the home and are used during intervals between work. Coffee and tea are also socially acceptable in many societies (although this has not always been true). Cannabis use in some countries is also of a social nature. Some psychoactive substances are taken to enhance the taste of food, such as specific wines with certain dishes, or cannabis sprinkled on soup, curry, or mixed in a pastry.

Some forms of social use have a strong ritual component in family, community, and religious activities. Intoxicants may assist ritual performers to go into a trance. Alcohol has been a part of social rituals through the ages. Cannabis serves this purpose in South and Southeast Asia and some Caribbean islands. High priests of the Middle and South American societies took stimulant–hallucinogen drugs at ritual times to commune with the gods. Some North American Indians did curing, performed spiritual cleansing, and celebrated tribal reunions by tobacco smoking or peyote chewing.

Certain drugs have attained near-sacramental aura. Wine used during some Christian rituals and the hallucinogen peyote consumed during Native American Church rituals are typical examples. Alcohol or cannabis use often accompanies ritual feasting.[12,25]

Oral ingestion is probably the oldest route of administration for psychoactive substances. Certainly it remains the most widely used method for most substances. Cannabis cakes in the Middle East, opium spherules in South Asia, and tea, coffee, or alcohol almost everywhere are taken *per os*. This method has several advantages: ease of administration, no need of special paraphernalia, and general medical safety as compared to other routes. It also has several disadvantages. Some drugs are either poorly absorbed in the gut or are modified by gastric juice. Oral administration may be desirable from a medical perspective in order to reduce side effects or stave off intoxication. However, drug- or alcohol-dependent persons often seek rapid onset of drug effect, which is more enjoyable to them than slow or gradual onset.

Chewing has long been used for such substances as coca leaf, tobacco, betel-areca, and tea. Absorption occurs across the oral mucosa. Certain drugs that produce gastrointestinal irritation (e.g., tobacco, khat, or betel-areca) can be better tolerated by chewing. While virtually absent in some areas of the world, chewing is highly prevalent in other areas.

Nasal insufflation (also called snuffing, nasal inhalation, or snorting) relies on absorption through the nasal mucosa. More sophisticated methods involve blowpipes in the Amazon areas of South America. This method evolved in South America, where it is still used today among tribal groups for ritual hallucinogen use. Snuffing may be done with tobacco, dried and powdered opium, cocaine, and heroin. Sniffing of amyl nitrate and similar volatile compounds has appeared in several areas of the world for the purpose of stimulation and sustaining sexual excitement. Nasal insufflation has changed in popularity over time. Where it is not widespread or well known, myths sometimes appear regarding it. For example, the notion that heroin snuffing cannot lead to heroin dependence has been a popular misconception in some areas.

Smoking seems to have first appeared in the New World, although there are reports of it in the Middle East and Africa around the fifteenth and sixteenth centuries.[19] Special preparation or paraphernalia are needed for pipes or other means of smoking, and fire must be applied to initiate combustion. While originally only North American drugs such as tobacco were smoked, smoking was soon adapted in the post-Columbian era to opium and cannabis, and more recently to barbitone, heroin, coca paste, cocaine free base, "crack" cocaine, PCP, and various mixtures of these and other drugs.

Rectal administration also developed in the New World. Administration of drugs by rectum is recorded in Middle American art prior to contact with Europe.[9] This approach to drug administration was subsequently adopted by medical practitioners throughout the world. It has not proven popular among those who abuse drugs or become dependent on them.

Parenteral administration appeared in the midnineteenth century. Morphine users soon employed it for self-administration. Since none of the drug is lost, this is an efficient use of the entire dose—an important factor if the drug is expensive. This method has led to widespread health problems when employed by drug users.

3. Evolution of Drug-Related Problems

3.1. Changing Concepts and Awareness

In the mass media, the spread of drug problems is often ascribed to modern technology or current-day civilization. They note changes from a traditional to a secular society, the undermining of family and clan, and the socioeconomic pressures of urban life. While these factors have indeed been associated with some recent drug epidemics, their role in the genesis of drug problems is not a simple etiological one. Such problems long predate the Industrial Revolution.

Early written accounts indicate that the acute and chronic effects of psychoactive drugs were known over 2000 years ago. Medical and religious treatises from Mediterranean countries, the Middle East, and South and East Asia describe drug problems with excessive use of opiates and alcohol.

Modern observations of some tribal people have shown high prevalence rates of drug dependence. Among rural poppy farmers in South and Southeast Asia, as many as one in three adults is addicted to opium.[22,27] Similar rates of alcoholism have been noted among rural North American Indian tribes.[24] These rates exceed any of those recorded thus far among industrialized or urban people.

While sporadic cases of substance abuse have been known throughout historical times, widespread or epidemic drug dependence is a comparatively recent event. In the seventeenth century, governments began to express alarm at the increasing use of one or another substance, including not just alcohol and opium, but also tobacco, tea, and coffee. By the eighteenth century evidence of widespread drug problems became stronger. China and the Philippines passed laws against production or import of certain psychoactive substances (e.g., coffee, tea, tobacco, and later opium). European and North American nations put taxes on their importation (e.g., tea). By the end of the eighteenth century European and American alcoholics were being treated in the asylums of the day. The Gin Epidemic in England became a national scandal.

During the nineteenth century drug dependence spread despite earlier attempts to contain it. Efforts in China were no longer directed merely at tobacco use, but were aimed at the increasing opium addiction. Opiate addiction became so widespread in the United Kingdom and the United States that medical organizations as well as governmental bodies became alarmed.[13]

Recognition of drug and alcohol dependence as a problem evolved through the ages. Religious teachings prohibiting the use of alcohol appeared due to socially undesirable behavior. Awareness of economic loss, health problems, and social cost contributed to the political awareness of the problem in this century.

Definitions of drug dependence vary both within and across cultures. Unlike cancer or pregnancy (all-or-none phenomena), drug dependence varies over a spectrum—more like hypertension or depression. Psychoactive substance abuse overlaps with socially acceptable use and behavior, so that the setting of specific definitional criteria is difficult. Such definitional problems are usually resolved in medicine by setting criteria consistent with moderately severe disorder, so that milder or early cases may not be included in the definition. Recognition of and attention to these earlier cases can be useful in preventing later full-blown cases; for example, early intervention of incipient hypertension can prevent later cardiovascular complications.

The harmful effects on health, such as the occurrence of cirrhosis and neurological disability from alcohol, and cancer of the lungs and cardiovascular diseases from tobacco smoking, have been recognized only in recent decades. This link between certain drugs and health problems was not made until medical evidence demonstrated the association. Physicians and society in general have been reluctant to accept the relation of certain drugs to health problems.

3.2. Transportation and Commerce

Although the Sumerians in Mesopotamia knew the medical values of opium six or seven thousand years ago, spread of opium use by land trade route from the eastern Mediterranean region to India and China took several centuries. Emergence of Arab sea trade led to an accelerated spread. Improvement of ship design by Europeans (Portuguese in the late sixteenth century, and the Dutch and English in the seventeenth century) further increased the volume of sea trade. Opium from India, well established since the sixth century A.D., was exchanged for products from China. Alarming increases in opium use led to Opium Wars between China and European nations. As a result of China's defeat, there was increased importation. Subsequently, opium dependence increased to epidemic levels in China.[22]

European travel to the American continents and increasing international trade led to the spread of tobacco from America to Europe and hence to Asia. Alcohol in the form of wine and distilled liquors spread from Europe to America. Ease, speed, safety, and low cost of travel by sea, land, and air have also contributed to the spread of drug problems. This has resulted in annual transport of many thousands of tons in drugs and alcohol from one place to another.

Not only have drug technologies and drug imports spread around the world, drug subcultures have also done so. Drug subcultures have adapted cultural elements chosen from virtually every continent, including drug-focused songs or music, and even drug-related philosophies and ethics (e.g., turn on, tune in, drop out of the 1970s). Mass communication and higher education spread cultural and social values from one part of the world to the other, setting up new social norms as well as conflict between traditional and modern mores. When villagers come to town for education, urban customs of drug use may follow them back to the village. Students going to school in other countries have sometimes brought new social values as well as new attitudes toward drugs back to their home countries. Students and tourists, new to the city or a particular culture, may lack traditional barriers against drug use. Widespread cigarette smoking in recent years is a example of this phenomenon.

3.3. Technical Development

The Industrial Revolution contributed to the improvement of the economy and living conditions in many countries over the last few hundred years. Drugs also underwent changes during this period. Through extracting processes, natural drug compounds were altered to pure compounds. Examples include cocaine, morphine, and hashish oil. Chemical modifications led to some more potent substances, such as heroin. Such semisynthetic compounds have been much more potent than the naturally occurring ones. New compounds, such as PCP, barbiturates, benzodiazapines, and amphetamines, also emerged.

Medical technology also progressed. The invention of syringes and needles led to parenteral injections into skin, muscle, and vein. Refined preparations could then be injected directly into veins for therapeutic purposes. Drug-dependent persons readily adapted this method with certain drugs (e.g., heroin, amphetamines, and cocaine).

Technologies for production of chemically pure compounds and synthetic psychoactive drugs have also spread around the world. Until the last few decades these were produced only in industrial cities with access to trained chemists and industrial-grade chemicals. Now the requisite knowledge, skills, equipment, and raw materials are so widespread that illicit stimulants, sedatives, hallucinogens, or opiates can be produced in many places.

Technical development has also led to greater affluence. Among the options available with increased disposable income is the purpose of psychoactive substances. The increased ability to buy drugs may contribute financial support to drug production and commerce. The high retail cost of prohibited drugs, combined with the relatively low cost of production, has resulted in high profits for those conducting illicit drug traffic. Entrepreneurs are usually available to meet an increased social appetite for drugs if the profit is attractively high and the risks are sufficiently low.

Increasing affluence is often, but not always, associated with increased use of psychoactive compounds. Certain religious groups have realized extraordinary economic progress while maintaining their control over or stricture against psychoactive substances. Some nations have been able to eliminate certain forms of drug abuse while increasing their per capita income. An example is the elimination of widespread opium addiction in China during the 1950s.[16]

4. Social Controls over Drug Use and Abuse

Through the ages, societies have reacted in diverse ways to problems related to drugs. At times, use of certain substances has not been considered a problem, whereas at other times drug use has been considered a problem.

Beginning in the eighteenth century and continuing into the twentieth century, social interventions to deal with drug epidemics intensified. These efforts included the following: special laws regarding producing, importing, and prescribing psychoactive drugs; special governmental commissions or police agencies to deal with drug production and commerce; private and public treatment for drug-dependent persons; campaigns by the mass media and by concerned citizens' groups to change social attitudes toward and patterns of drug use; government-franchised or -supervised distribution of opiates to registered addicts; new treatment approaches for drug-dependent persons; and antidrug law enforcement efforts. International treaties against opium trade began in the late nineteenth century, and they increased greatly during the first half of the twentieth century. At times these treaties had detrimental effects on weaker or smaller countries, especially in Asia, where government actions to comply with the treaties unexpectedly led to a change from traditional opium use to heroin use.[26]

Along with expanded efforts against drug dependence, two new developments have further complicated the situation. One of these has been the development of new psychoactive substances synthesized in chemical laboratories. The other has been the appearance of drug subcultures; these consist of people whose unifying feature is the consumption of psychoactive substances.

4.1. Restrictions on Production and Import

Today every country in the world has laws regarding such drugs as alcohol, cannabis, sedatives, stimulants, and opioids. Laws governing the amount and frequency of alcohol use go back several centuries.[18] These laws are most effective when the governed concur with the right of the government to pass such laws. Illicit production, smuggling, or sale of psychoactive substances can result if law enforcement is not effective. Corruption and anarchy have favored illicit opium, cocaine, and cannabis production and trafficking.

Laws can play a useful preventive role before widespread drug dependence has appeared. After drug dependence has spread, laws alone are rarely successful without concomitant antidrug efforts by police, health officials, educators, welfare officials, and religious and political leaders. In public health terms, laws alone can have a preventive effect vis-à-vis drug dependence, but they rarely have a curative effect once widespread drug dependence has appeared.

4.2. Control of Therapeutic Drugs through Prescribing Laws

Production and importation of certain drugs cannot be completely prohibited because they are useful for therapeutic and other purposes. Registration of persons allowed to handle and prescribe these drugs does help in the control of drugs necessary for medical practice. Several levels of control depending on the abuse potential of specific drugs are also used.

Pharmaceutical drugs in many areas of the world can be obtained without a physician's prescription. Even in countries that require a prescription, pharmacy records may be incomplete and enforcement may be lax. Some physicians prescribe psychoactive substances too readily, or for chronic conditions in which drug dependence may be an imminent risk. Prescriptions can be easily forged in some locales. In some areas the most common means of obtaining illicit stimulants, sedatives, or opiates is through the diversion of licit pharmaceutical drugs into illicit channels. Both governmental policy and professional ethics are necessary to minimize this danger. Health professionals are themselves at special risk to drug dependence due to their increased access to drugs.

4.3. Taxation and Revenue

Import taxes on tea, coffee, and distilled alcohol go back over 200 years.[11] Originally these taxes were meant only to raise funds for government expenditures. While this original purpose remains important, a second purpose has evolved in recent years. Increased taxation can also limit the public consumption of a recreational intoxicant, such as tobacco or alcohol.[2] Drug taxation—especially on tobacco and alcohol—has led to government dependence on such taxation for public funds in several countries. Ministries of finance, in need of funds, can then be at odds with ministries of public health and social welfare and justice which are trying to reduce drug-related problems.

There are boundaries to the limiting effect of taxes on licit psychoactive substances. If the tax becomes too burdensome, people may begin to produce their own drug—such as home-brewed alcohol beverages[5]—or purchase it through illicit channels. This not only loses revenue for the government, it also undermines public respect for the law. In addition, quality control by the government is prevented by illicit production, so that various toxic epidemics (e.g., methanol and lead poisoning from illicit alcohol) have resulted. These toxic epidemics have led to widespread permanent disability from blindness or paralysis.

Increasing profit from illicit drug trafficking can result in well-financed and organized crime. This in turn can lead to corruption through bribes to police, judges, and governmental officials.

Revenue from psychoactive substances can become so important to the economics of a society that governments may act to stimulate and increase production and use. This has occurred in numerous areas that produce tobacco, opium, wine, whiskey, and coca leaf.

4.4. Prohibition

A psychoactive substance may be totally prohibited from a society for any use. Of course this presents little or no problem if the substance is not used or is used only by a few. Prohibition becomes much more difficult if many people traditionally use the substance.

Prohibition against specific substances has been tried many times during the last half-century. At times it has succeeded, as with the laws during the 1940s and 1950s against opium in China and Korea and against amphetamines in Japan and Scandinavia. At other times it has been a mixed success, such as the prohibition against alcohol in the United States in the 1920s. Although the latter law had some limited success against alcohol-related problems (such as reducing cirrhosis deaths), it led to increasing illicit sale of beer and liquor, organized criminal gangs, police corruption, and disrespect for the law. Eventually this prohibition law in the United States was repealed.

A side effect from prohibition is that the drug-dependent person may be labeled as a criminal, which can further complicate treatment efforts. Some countries with prohibition laws have managed this problem by making production, sale, or possession of a drug against the law, while not making drug dependence an illegal status.

Certain interventions intended to reduce or eliminate widespread drug abuse can instead stimulate even more social problems, including poorly planned antidrug laws and treatment programs unrelated to social goals. For example, antiopium laws have stimulated heroin epidemics in several areas, including Hong Kong, Thailand, Laos, and Pakistan. These laws have often been instituted due to pressures from other countries or international organizations.[26]

4.5. Other Sociocultural Approaches

A number of other methods have been employed to stem widespread drug abuse. One approach consists of campaigns through the mass media to change peoples' attitudes against heavy drug use. This type of intervention was effective almost two centuries ago in the English Gin Epidemic. Recently advertisements to use such psychoactive substances as tobacco and alcohol have become widespread. These have been directed especially toward youth. Advertising may likewise help to stem drug abuse.

Some religious groups have convinced people to abstain from recreational drug use. These groups have also been active in helping people substitute religious affiliation for dypsomania or narcotomania.[15] Self-help groups or drug rehabilitation groups often hold their meetings in Buddhist temples, Islamic mosques, Christian churches, and Jewish synagogues. Islam has been forceful in prohibiting alcohol and drug use.[1]

Peer and family support for sobriety can be critical in preventing drug abuse or intervening early if it appears. For this to occur, a population must recognize drug abuse as a problem, have knowledge about the early signs of drug-related problems, and possess skills to confront the person firmly but supportively. Peer and family support can be powerful means to reduce the prevalence of drug abuse.[23]

4.6. Provision of Treatment Facilities

Simple application of law and law enforcement measures can create certain problems. Some dependent persons cannot immediately cope with drug-free life if treatment is not provided. Without treatment, they seek other drugs which are available in the licit market or drugs from illicit sources.

Provision of treatment applied simultaneously with an antidrug law is an important measure. At times limited provision of the problematic drug under strict control can aid in rehabilitation. Legal opioid distribution has been used in the management of opioid dependence for over a century. Government-run opium franchises were administered by Thailand, the Malay States, Straits Settlements, and Indochina in the 1930s and 1940s. The United States had morphine clinics during the 1920s, and England has had heroin clinics in recent decades. Methadone, a long-acting opioid, has been used for the same purpose in parts of

North America, Europe, and Asia in recent years.[6] This approach has been ideologically disagreeable to some religious, social, and political leaders.

Other pharmacological interventions have become available in recent years. For example, disulfiram has been used with good effect as an adjunctive treatment in some cases of alcoholism. Naltrexone, an opioid antagonist, has been successfully combined with contingency contracting in the care of former opioid-dependent patients. Tricyclic antidepressants are useful in selected cases of drug dependence.

Governments have organized treatment systems in diverse ways. Facilities may be under the jurisdiction of health, education, welfare, finance, justice, or interior ministries. Often the distribution of social responsibility has been assigned according to ministry resources and function. For example, health may be under Finance; prevention, under Education; early detection, under Interior; and drug-related crime, under Justice. Coordination at the highest level is essential when the responsibilities are thus divided. A special coordinating body, with its own budget and resources, often resides in the prime minister's office. Private, charitable, or voluntary groups usually establish liaison relationships with a central coordinating group. Legislation has at times been necessary to protect the populace from unsuitable programs in the private sector. Some governments have facilitated the efforts of local communities in overcoming their local drug problems.

Elimination of drug use can take a long time. When Prophet Mohammed prohibited the use of alcohol, he allowed 11 years as a transitional period to accomplish this policy even among his faithful followers.[1]

5. Drug-Abuse Problems Today

The drug-abuse patterns that occur today are the result of evolution in many locations in the world. These patterns also result from concomitant social, economic, and political evolution. A number of patterns overlap each other. For example, worldwide alcohol-related problems are remarkably similar, albeit with some variation in extent and societal reaction.[20] In addition to the alcohol problem, other drug problems are specific to certain locations. Opium, cannabis, coca leaf, khat, and betel-areca produce different problems due to diverse pharmacological effect and modes of consumption. In the past two decades, multiple or polydrug abuse has become prominent. It is characterized by the use of multiple drugs, including alcohol, opiates, cannabis, and synthetic compounds. It has especially affected adolescents and young adults in many areas.

Today there are many of the same alcohol problems which Galen described in Rome 15 centuries ago. Opiate epidemics exist today. In addition, new drug problems appear as new drugs are created and unpredictable social changes occur. Modern technology has also complicated the picture. When oxcarts or horses were the only means of transportation, an intoxicated driver or rider could do only limited damage. Now an automobile driver going 80 kilometers an hour, a boatman on a crowded river, or an airline pilot flying with 200 passengers can do considerable harm if impaired by a psychoactive substance. High-speed industrial and farm machines, electrical appliances, and effective surgical techniques also put the worker, the housekeeper, and the surgeon's patient at risk if judgment and perceptuomotor coordination are impaired.

One dilemma is the rapidity with which drugs can be transported. Recent surveys of university students in India show that methaqualone and diazepam are used more frequently than India's traditionally used drugs, alcohol and cannabis.[17] Volatile inhalant sniffing epidemics have occurred among children on all continents.[8,14] Elimination of traditional opium abuse has frequently been followed by epidemic heroin, alcohol, and tobacco abuse.[21]

Multidrug abuse is not a new or urban phenomenon. Chopra[4] described it in India several decades ago. Nonetheless, it presents with two modern innovations. First, there is the matter of mixing potent synthetic or purified drugs with unpredictable effects. And second, as law enforcement officials eliminate a particular drug of choice from a region, local drug-dependent persons flexibly adapt to other available substances, including available weeds or flowers, volatile industrial hydrocarbons, proprietary over-the-counter drugs for cough or asthma, and various mixtures of these. The results can be even more entrenched drug abuse, with increased medical and psychiatric casualties from drug abuse.

Effective law enforcement usually leads to increased cost of illicit drugs, which can in turn lead to more effective means for route of drug administration. Increased parenteral use inevitably causes greater morbidity and mortality and greater societal cost for health services as compared to smoking or ingesting a drug.

As treatment for drug abuse has expanded around the world in the last few decades, the chronic patient with repeated treatment failure has become a noteworthy problem. Large amounts of medical and welfare funds are devoted to such patients, but often without demonstrable benefit. These chronic patients go from facility to facility—so-called institutionalization on the installment plan. This difficult patient subgroup presents ethical and legal dilemmas for society. These dilemmas include such matters as involuntary treatment, long-term state guardianship, or denial of treatment to those not able to benefit from it.

Another difficult problem is the person whose drug dependence is accompanied by a psychiatric disorder. These disorders include depression, organic impairment, and various drug-precipitated psychoses. Certain drugs cause specific types of psychopathology. For example, alcohol may produce delirium tremens, alcohol amnestic disorder (Korsakoff's disease), and alcoholic dementia. Amphetamine psychosis can mimic confusional, hallucinatory, or delusional states. Opium, one of the most addicting drugs, produces minimal psychopathology as a direct effect, although it can produce psychopathology indirectly through nutritional deficiencies and through various social concomitants of addiction (such as family problems, theft, deteriorating social status).

As more difficult patients are encountered, physicians typically search more deeply among their therapeutic alternatives to provide relief. One treatment approach consists of long-term medication for selected patients (e.g., methadone for opiate dependence, disulfiram for alcohol dependence). Long-term medication creates problems for governments which regulate the practice of medicine. Public officials may have difficulty understanding that a person who abuses drugs may benefit from drug treatment. Sometimes an example of the victim of vehicular or wartime trauma, who benefits from additional surgical trauma to reverse the underlying pathophysiological process, can facilitate their understanding.

Physicians and other social leaders may understand pathological dependence on purified or synthetic stimulants, opioids, sedatives, and alcohol. The social and economic cost of complications from drugs such as tobacco, cannabis, or betel-areca may not be so immediately evident, however. These drugs may even relieve minor ailments or facilitate social interchange. Serious tobacco effects, for example, do not appear until after decades of use. Until recently, cigarette smoking has been viewed primarily as an individual rather than a societal problem despite widespread respiratory and cardiac problems, cancer, and oral pathologies. As people live longer, however, these chronic diseases have become more manifest. Since medical and welfare services are increasing and are underwritten by government funds, former social perspectives are changing. Dependence on tobacco and other drugs is now seen as having economic and public health implications.

References

1. Baasher T: The use of drugs in the Islamic world. *Br J Addiction* 1981; 76:233–243.
2. Brunne K: *Alcohol Control Policies in Public Health Perspective*. Helsinki, Finnish Foundation of Alcohol Studies, 1975.
3. Burton-Bradley BG: Some implications of betel chewing. *Med J Aust* 1977; 2:744–746.
4. Chopra RN: The present position of the opium habit in India. *Indian J Med Res* 1928; 16:389–439.
5. Connell KH: Illicit distillation: An Irish peasant industry. *Historical Stud Ireland* 1961; 3:58–91.
6. Dole VP, Nyswander ME: The use of methadone for narcotic blockade. *Br J Addict* 1968; 63:35–57.
7. DuToit BM: *Drugs, Rituals and Altered States of Consciousness*. Rotterdam, Balkema, 1977.
8. Eastwell HD: Petrol-inhalation in Aboriginal towns. *Med J Aust* 1979; 2:221–224.
9. Furst PT, Coe MD: Ritual enemas. *Natural History* 1977; 86:88–91.
10. Getahun A, Krikorias AD: Chat: Coffee's rival from Harar, Ethiopia. *Economic Botany* 1973; 27:353–389.
11. Greden J: The tea controversy in colonial America. *JAMA* 1976; 236:63–65.

12. Klausner SZ: Sacred and profane meaning of blood and alcohol. *J Social Psychol* 1964; 64:27–43.
13. Kramer JC: Opium rampant: Medical use, misuse and abuse in Britain and the west in the 17th and 18th centuries. *Br J Addict* 1979; 74:377–389.
14. Kaufman A: Gasoline sniffing among children in a Pueblo Indian village. *Pediatrics* 1975; 51:1060–1064.
15. Kearny M: Drunkenness and religious conversion in a Mexican village. *Q J Stud Alcohol* 1970; 31:248–249.
16. Lowinger P: The solution to narcotic addiction in the People's Republic of China. *Am J Drug Alcohol Abuse* 1977; 4:165–178.
17. Mohan D, Setthi HS, Tongue E: *Current Research in Drug Abuse in India.* Delhi, Gemini Printers, 1981.
18. Paredes A: Social control of drinking among the Aztec Indians of Mesoamerica. *J Stud Alcohol* 1975; 36:1139–1153.
19. Rubin V (ed): *Cannabis and Culture.* Hague, Mouton, 1975.
20. Sargent MJ: Changes in Japanese drinking patterns. *Q J Stud Alcohol* 1967; 28:709–722.
21. Singer K: Drinking patterns and alcoholism in the Chinese. *Br J Addict* 1972; 67:3–14.
22. Suwanwela C: *The History of Opium in Asia.* Bangkok, Institute of Health Research, 1979.
23. Swed JF: Gossip, drinking and social control: Consensus and communication in a Newfoundland parish. *Ethnology* 1966; 5:434–441.
24. Shore J, Kinzie JD, Hampson JL, Pattison EM: Psychiatric epidemiology of an Indian village. *Psychiatry* 1973; 36:70–81.
25. Washburne C: Primitive religion and alcohol. *Int J Comp Sociol* 1968; 9:97–105.
26. Westermeyer J: The pro-heroin effects of anti-opium laws in Asia. *Arch Gen Psychiatry* 1974; 33:1135–1139.
27. Westermeyer J: *Poppies, Pipes and People: Opium and Its Use in Laos.* Berkeley, University of California Press, 1983.

Further Reading

Arif A: *Adverse Health Consequences of Cocaine Misuse.* World Health Organization Offset Publication. Geneva, WHO, 1987.

Edwards G, Arif A: *Drug Problems in Socio-cultural Context.* Geneva, World Health Organization, 1980.

4

Epidemiological Assessment

1. Introduction

Abuse of drugs in most societies resembles an iceberg. That which is visible on the surface is measured by police arrest, medical problems, admissions to drug dependence treatment programs, surveys, and other methods. These indicators reach a part of the problem that lies beneath. Risk of job loss, stigma associated with excessive use, or other urges to deny the problem make data acquisition difficult.

The search for epidemiological data is further frustrated by the problem of defining drug dependence. To one person it may mean any use of an illegal substance, to another it may imply physical or psychological dependence. For some, dependence on sedative or stimulant drugs, as long as they are prescribed by a physician, would not be considered drug dependence. Clinicians in a society where heavy social drinking is the norm might define alcohol abuse differently from clinicians in a Moslem country where any alcohol use is prohibited.

Thus, collecting incidence and prevalence data on drug dependence poses quite different obstacles from collecting data on measles or cholera, where cases can be easily counted and cultural or religious factors are largely irrelevant. (Some infectious diseases, such as gonorrhea and leprosy, do present reporting obstacles similar to drug dependence.) Assessment of drug dependence problems often originates from secondary data sources (e.g., arrests, mortality statistics), which may be influenced by subjective factors resulting from individual differences in perception. Any attempt to produce uniform data for regional or national comparisons must take these biases into account.

Drug abuse and dependence are dynamic phenomena which can change appreciably over short time spans. Large expensive studies, while valuable in establishing the nature and extent of drug-related problems, are not practical for following these changes over time. Consequently, less expensive monitoring systems must supplement more definitive, yet episodic studies.

Despite the difficulties, an effective epidemiological assessment of drug dependence underlies any successful program to reduce its incidence or prevalence. First, programming for controlling drug dependence whether at the community, regional, or national level depends on an estimate of the extent and nature of the problem. Targeting the population groups at high risk, geographic placement, and even the choice of treatment modality should be determined by epidemiological studies. Second, and most important, repeated monitoring or epidemiological studies are the key to monitoring changes in drug dependence statistics. This permits modifications in treatment approaches as well as better public education, law enforcement, and similar activities.[11,18]

A key step in any epidemiological study is the definition of criteria for drug dependence. This subject is covered in Chapter 1.

Epidemiology originated from the study of infectious diseases, although today it is also used to study noninfectious disorders. Epidemiology was defined by the World Health Organization (WHO) in 1973 as the study of the distribution of a disease or a condition in a population and of the factors that influence that distribution. Epidemiological studies of drug taking began over a century ago, but have become especially important over the last 30 years.[30]

Case definition is much easier when the investigation is of diseases such as cholera or peptic ulcer than when focus is on conditions such as drug-related problems. These conditions often involve behavior (e.g., accidents, falls, overdose, social disability) rather than specific and objective pathology of tissues and organs.

Prior to the 1940s, drug dependence was confined to relatively circumscribed areas of the world, according to the drug type. With rapid transportation and high mobility, cultural diffusion, and the development of a worldwide cosmopolitan youth culture, all forms of drug abuse have spread to cover much of the globe. Heroin use and opium use, once limited primarily to Asia and North America, are now prevalent throughout Europe and in many developing countries. Cocaine use, once restricted to a few countries of Latin America in the form of coca leaf chewing and to a limited population in North America in the pure extracted form, has spread widely in the United States and to a certain extent in Europe. Cannabis, with a long history of use in China, India, the Middle East, and Africa, has spread to Europe, North America, and other parts of the world. Barbiturates, other sedatives, and benzodiazepine tranquilizers have become perhaps the most widely abused drugs in the world, affecting both industrialized and developing nations. Epidemic use of amphetamines has appeared from time to time in various countries, including Asia, Europe, and the

Americas. Alcohol abuse has grown steadily in recent years as populations throughout the world have become more affluent and traditional cultural constraints against its use have dissolved. Tobacco dependence is producing virtual epidemics of heart disease and lung cancer on every continent.

While men have traditionally used drugs more heavily than women, this is now changing as women everywhere move toward social equality. Similarly, drug abuse, traditionally involving only adult populations, is more often affecting youth. Initially drugs may first be used in a culture by the more affluent, but generally all substances of abuse spread across the socioeconomic scale. In addition, certain populations, such as physicians and other health workers with special access to drugs, are particularly at risk.

2. Sources of Data

Various methods have been developed to assess the incidence and prevalence of drug dependence. These methods have varying degrees of accuracy. Some indicators are applicable to all forms of substance abuse, while others are relevant only to certain routes of administration—such as serum hepatitis and intravenous administration. Other indicators, such as alcoholic cirrhosis of the liver or tobacco-induced lung cancer, correlate with specific substances.

Counting the total number of users directly or surveying a representative or random sample has been undertaken. Some investigators have measured causally connected events to estimate the number of users by inference (such as combining register data and morgue data).

2.1. Sales and Seizures

Legal sales of psychoactive substances provide a crude measure of consumption levels. In nations where there is relatively little nonindustrial manufacture of alcohol, figures for beer, wine, and spirits sales provide a per capita measure of consumption levels for the population as a whole.[29] The utility of such figures is largely for comparisons over time and with other populations, since the per capita figure alone does not directly indicate individual variation and abuse levels. Prescription data for psychoactive drugs similarly provide a general measure of consumption levels in the society. With the increasing use of computerized data systems, it is becoming possible to know the total quantity of a drug prescribed. In countries where pharmaceutical products are imported largely or wholly from abroad, the quantities of each drug imported can provide a useful measure of consumption levels even where the drugs are sold over the counter or where no prescription register exists.

Seizures of illicit drugs by law enforcement agencies can provide a similar crude measure of production and distribution levels, although drugs seized may merely be en route through a region.

2.2. Registers

Several countries have developed registers for drug-dependent persons, especially those addicted to opioids. Most notably in Hong Kong, Singapore, Iran, Britain, Malaysia, and New York City, registration of addicts has at times provided a useful measure. Such systems are most effective when the addict population is relatively small and stable, and when there is some inducement for addicts to register. Inducements include provision of treatment or access to freely dispensed drugs for opioid addicts. In epidemic situations where the number of addicts is rapidly expanding, where there is little perceived benefit in registering, or where the number of addicts is large, registers are of limited value. They do provide incidence data when the addict population is relatively stable. National registers, for all practical purposes, have been effective only for opiate addiction. Those dependent on other drugs have little incentive to register.[4]

2.3. Surveys of Special Populations

Some drug-dependent persons come to the attention of prisons, courts, general hospitals, mental health centers, and drug treatment facilities. Careful interviewing of patients can reveal extensive demographic data and the history of their drug use prior to seeking treatment. Especially where patients are seeking treatment on a voluntary basis, the variation in the number of patients seeking treatment, the dropout rate, and the reentry rate can indicate drug availability and styles of drug use.

Drug-dependence treatment facilities may offer the greatest volume of data. There may be either much or little overlap with drug users encountered in other institutions. General hospitals see drug- and alcohol-abusing individuals for medical conditions, such as drug overdose, hepatitis, endocarditis, thrombophlebitis, or bronchitis, which are secondary to their drug use; many may not have sought treatment for their drug use. Especially where urban heroin use is widespread, large numbers of drug users may be identified through the court system. Urine screening and health alcohol analysis have been used as a method of identification in hospitals, clinics, and jails. Similar screening procedures have been used on populations such as students and military personnel for both epidemiological and disciplinary/treatment purposes. It should be kept in mind that each of these special populations of drug users is a selected subgroup and may not reflect the epidemiological profile of the drug-using segment of the general population.

Key informants can provide valuable information, especially when initiating a study. This approach has been employed in field studies of villages, drug subcultures, taverns, and opium dens or vends.

2.4. Surveys of General Populations

Social scientists have studied drug use with questionnaires, especially among school populations. If the students are guaranteed anonymity, this method of data collection has certain advantages. Useful instruments for conducting surveys of students and of nonstudent youth have been developed by WHO.[26,27]

Surveys offer the opportunity to study a sample unbiased by the need for treatment or involvement with the criminal justice system. A survey can ascertain the level of all substances of abuse at one time. The data can be rapidly collected. WHO, in collaboration with member states, has developed instruments for conducting surveys of students.[27]

The survey method has certain inherent problems. It presumes the honesty of the respondents, who may be fearful of reporting their use accurately. Bravado may make some individuals claim excessive use that is not true. Some heavy drug users may form an isolated subculture, which may not be included within random samples of the population. Drug-dependent adolescents may drop out from school, so that school surveys may underreport drug-dependence problems among school-age children.

Despite the limitations in self-report, studies of the reliability and validity of survey self-report have shown that most respondents truthfully report their use of licit and illicit drugs.[24] This is especially true if the data provided are anonymous or confidential and do not have adverse consequences for the individual (such as discharge from medical care or loss of civil liberties).

2.5. Death Rates

The number of annual overdose deaths from drugs can serve as a rough guide to the level of drug dependence in a community. Especially when a potent drug has recently appeared in a community, overdose morbidity or mortality may be high. The number of deaths is significantly altered by the type of drug, fluctuations in the purity of the drug, the number of new or naive drug users, and the frequency with which detoxified persons are dropping out of treatment and returning to use with significantly lowered tolerance. Nevertheless the overdose death rate can provide a rough indication of the magnitude of the drug problem. There is a relationship between blood alcohol concentration and the probability of a fatal automobile crash. (See Figure 1.)

Deliberate overdose with drugs also occurs, since suicide is more common among drug-dependent persons than among the general population. Those who use a drug for suicide may not be chronic abusers.

2.6. Other Indicators

Although an indirect measure of drug abuse in a community, serum hepatitis (type B) is caused by a virus entering the body through a break in the skin.

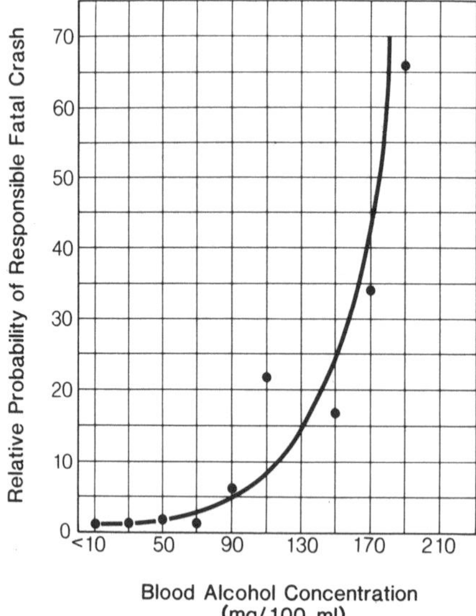

Figure 1. Effect of blood alcohol level on relative risk of fatal crash. (From Ref. 25. Reprinted with permission.)

Intravenous-drug users commonly share needles, so that the incidence of this disease is significantly higher among drug abusers than among the general population. There is no reliable formula by which the incidence of hepatitis can be translated into a specific figure for the number of intravenous-drug users.

A number of other sources of information are indirectly related to the level of drug use. None offers complete reliability, but each provides an additional source of empirical data. As with all sources of data on this subject, it is the ability to come up with consistent numerical estimates from enough different indicators that provides the best hope for accuracy and not the ability to find a single, highly valid data source. These include the following data sources.

2.6.1. Prescription Records

For licit drugs, such as barbiturates, amphetamines, methaqualone, or morphine in many countries, changes in the number of prescriptions being filled can be an early indication of an increase in abuse levels of those drugs.

2.6.2. Drug Thefts

An increase in the theft of controlled substances from pharmacies, drugstores, hospitals, and doctors' offices can signal a growing trend in abuse of specific drugs.

2.6.3. Crime Rates

Especially in urban areas, property crime may be related to drug dependence, as some people steal to support their habits. In some countries, there is a rough correlation between the number of active drug-dependent persons in a community and the crime rate, so that an increasing crime rate might indicate a growing opioid-dependent population.

2.6.4. Price and Purity

Generally, when drugs are plentiful, prices are lower and purity is higher than when there is a shortage. Under the latter circumstance, suppliers of illicit drugs dilute the drug more with fillers or diluents and increase the price. As the price goes up, the drug-dependent person must get more money to support the drug habit; hence the crime rate rises. This model does not always apply. On occasion, the scarcity causes some individuals with low levels of addiction to cease their use entirely, at least until supplies are again adequate.

2.6.5. Arrests for Intoxication

Disorderly or dangerous conduct in public settings may parallel increases of alcohol abuse in some societies. Arrests for driving while intoxicated can similarly reflect changing rates in alcohol dependence.

2.7. The Capture–Recapture Model

Traditional survey methods for detecting drug dependence reach only a percentage of any group. The number is especially small if the drug use is illicit. In recent years a method for assessing the rate of drug dependence in a population has been developed that does not rely on the usual survey approaches. This method is referred to as the recapture method and can be best understood by considering the analogous situation of a pond full of fish. Twenty fish are caught and identified with markers before being returned to the water. Then, assuming a homogeneous mixing of marked and unmarked fish, a second catch of 20 fish is made. The number of marked fish in this second group is counted. If, for instance, they number five, or a quarter of the group, the presumption is that the original catch of 20 that were marked comprise a fourth of the total fish population in the pond. This means the total population is 4 × 20, or 80 fish. If 10 fish (or 50%) in the second catch were marked, the population is 20 × 2, or 40; if only 1 of 20 is marked, then the total is 20 × 20, or 400.

This method can be applied to counting drug dependents by obtaining from one source, such as the police, a list of such persons known to them. That list is then compared with one from another source, such as a treatment facility, and the degree of overlap is determined. As with the fish in the pond, the total drug-dependent population is calculated based on the proportion of the first list represented in the second.

Lists for the capture–recapture technique can be obtained from several different sources. These include hospital emergency rooms, morgues, jails, and mental health centers. Data may even be obtained from cooperative drug-dependent persons who are willing to write down the names of all their acquaintances who are users. A series of estimates of the total addict population can be calculated from comparing pairs of lists. An overall average can then be taken from these pairs.

2.8. Special Aspects of Alcohol-Related Problems

The imprecise distinctions between social drinking, heavy drinking, and alcohol dependence in many countries presents a special problem in the epidemiology of this disorder. If alcohol consumption is legal, certain aspects of data collection are substantially easier. Data on alcohol sales are readily available in many countries.

Random surveys using breathalyzers allow the amount of alcohol in expired breath to be measured by a small, hand-held instrument. It accurately reflects blood alcohol level. This may be used to measure the proportion of alcohol users at work, in an emergency room, or driving vehicles. Of course, these survey methods tap into special samples which may not represent the population. In countries where a high percentage of the population works or drives, the figures obtained from this source may approximate those for the adult population. Such testing can also be done in clinical facilities, such as emergency rooms. Accidents in the home as a result of alcohol use commonly involve women in many countries with high rates of alcoholism. As many as 35–50% of all accidents encountered in emergency rooms in many areas are the result of intoxication. In many countries about 50% of serious traffic accidents involve alcohol abuse.

Breathalyzer studies require that the person has recently consumed alcohol. This may be useful for assessing certain problems (e.g., accidents), but is less useful in assessing chronic alcohol abuse. Since many chronic abusers are not constantly using alcohol, other measures are needed. Recently, investigators have used certain biochemical indicators such as γ-glutamyl transferase and mean corpuscular volume of red blood cells, which are abnormal in many chronic alcohol abusers.

More than 90% of all cases of cirrhosis of the liver are associated with alcoholism in many countries with prevalent alcoholism. Of course, endemic parasites as well as abuse of solvents can also contribute to hepatic morbidity. Consequently, the interpretation of cirrhosis figures depends on local conditions.

2.9. Drug-Dependence Complications as Epidemiological Indicators

The morbidity and mortality rates of many medical conditions can be assessed fairly accurately. For example, a percentage of juvenile-onset diabetics will be registered as blind within 20 years, or a certain percentage of people with cancer of the stomach will die within 5 years of diagnosis. Such numerical precision is frequently not possible for drug dependence, for the following reasons[8]:

1. Case definition often varies greatly from one investigation to another.
2. Case recognition can differ according to the effort put into identifying cases or over time with changing medical awareness.
3. The proportion of casualities attributed to drug dependence often changes over time and between localities. For example the percentage of individuals sustaining a particular complication may fluctuate widely (e.g., rate of serum hepatitis among heroin addicts who inject themselves).
4. The relationship of an illness or death to drug use is sometimes a matter of degree rather than an absolute cause–effect relationship; the degree of relatedness is frequently difficult to determine.

3. Extent of Drug Dependence Today

During the first half of the twentieth century one could describe areas of the world where different types of drug abuse prevailed. These traditional patterns of drug use have changed. Recent youthful drug use has swept many major cities throughout the world, beginning during the 1960s and continuing to the present time. Some drugs (e.g., opiates and cannabis) are abused on virtually every continent, whereas other drugs (e.g., khat or coca leaf chewing) are confined to limited areas. Certain patterns of drug abuse are changing rapidly (e.g., stimulant and sedative abuse in some areas). Polydrug abuse has increasingly appeared as a common pattern.

3.1. Opium and Heroin

Opium has been used for many centuries in the areas where the opium poppies have been grown. Tribal groups in the highland areas of Thailand, Laos, and Burma—the Golden Triangle—have long cultivated and smoked opium. In Turkey, Iran, Afghanistan, Pakistan, and India—the Golden Crescent—opium has been grown and primarily used orally for medicinal purposes, but also smoked for recreation (except in Turkey) over many generations. Opium has been grown in India for several hundred years, although local usage has been minimal in recent decades. The primary purpose of its cultivation under the British administration was sale to the Chinese. Opium was widely smoked in China during the latter half of the nineteenth century and the first half of the twentieth century, but for all practical purposes its use has been nonexistent since 1948. Opium poppy has been grown in Turkey for sale to the international pharmaceutical industry. Turkey has also been a source, especially since World War II, for the illicit market. Opium is produced for legal purposes (but not illicit local consumption) in several other countries, including Australia, France, Soviet Union, Spain, and Yugoslavia.

During the nineteenth century, Chinese immigrants started to cultivate opium poppy in small quantities in Mexico. This remained a relatively minor activity until World War II, at which time Mexican opium became a source for the illicit heroin market in North America. During the 1970s, this source again exploded to many times its previous size, becoming the major source of illicit opiates in North America. (See Map 1 for the distribution of opium use around 1980.)

Heroin was first synthesized from morphine for medicinal purposes in 1898, but quickly became the drug of choice for opiate addicts in many areas of Europe and North America. In the 1960s and 1970s, youthful urban populations in Asia began to use heroin widely. This was a significant change from the traditional use of opium. In Bangkok, Rangoon, Saigon, and Hong Kong large heroin addict populations of 100,000 addicts or more developed in each city, and this situation still persists in several Asian cities. Prevalence of heroin use in several European countries also has been high in recent years.

Sporadic reports of heroin use have come from Africa and South America, but heroin has not yet posed a significant problem on these continents. In several Arabic countries and elsewhere in the Middle East heroin use continues as it has in the past. (See Map 2 for the distribution of heroin use.)

3.2. Coca Leaf and Cocaine

The coca bush, source of the world's cocaine supply, grows in the foothills of the Andes Mountains. Peru, Bolivia, and Ecuador are the primary source countries. In those three countries, especially in Bolivia, the indigenous population has long chewed the coca leaves to overcome fatigue at high altitudes and as an appetite suppressant. Used in this way coca seems to have produced few adverse health effects. Cocaine, extracted chemically from the coca leaves in illicit laboratories located mainly in Colombia, has been used very little in any of these producer countries and in the past was exported almost exclusively to North America. In the United States more than a million individuals use the drug regularly and many millions do so occasionally. Since 1980 increasing amounts of cocaine have flowed to Europe. Coca paste smoking has spread in epidemic proportions in some Latin American countries.[13] (See Map 3 for the worldwide prevalence of coca use.)

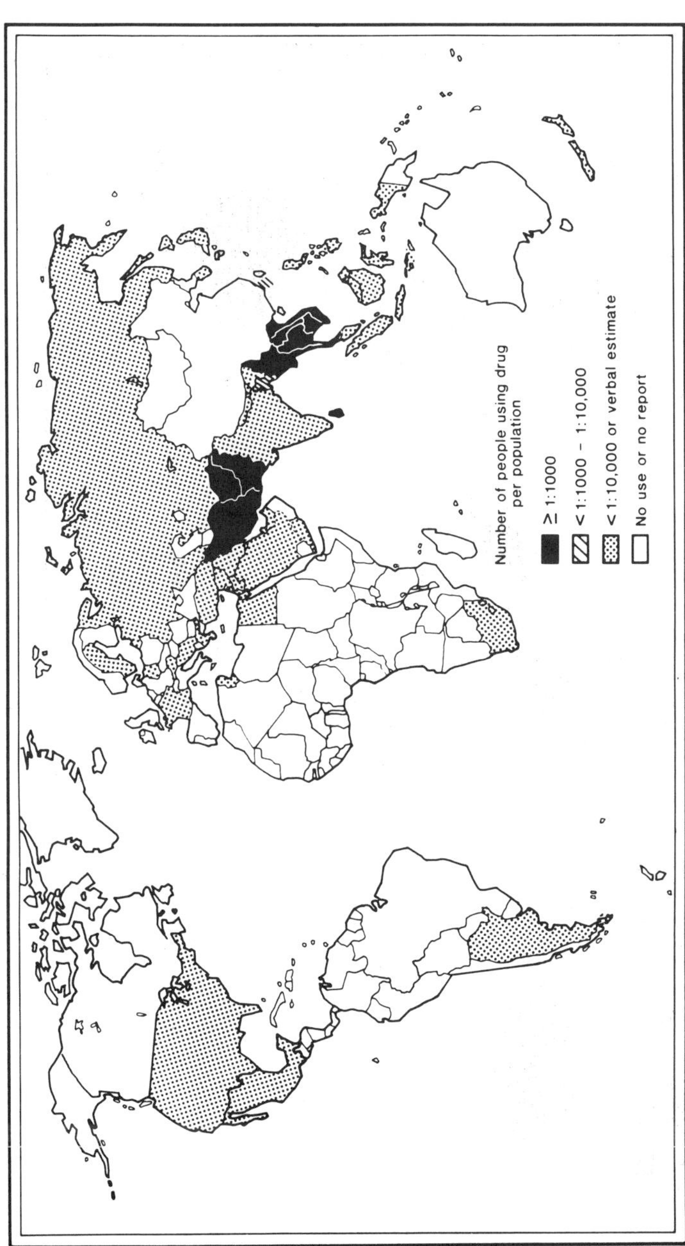

Map 1. Opium. (From Ref. 12. Reprinted with permission.)

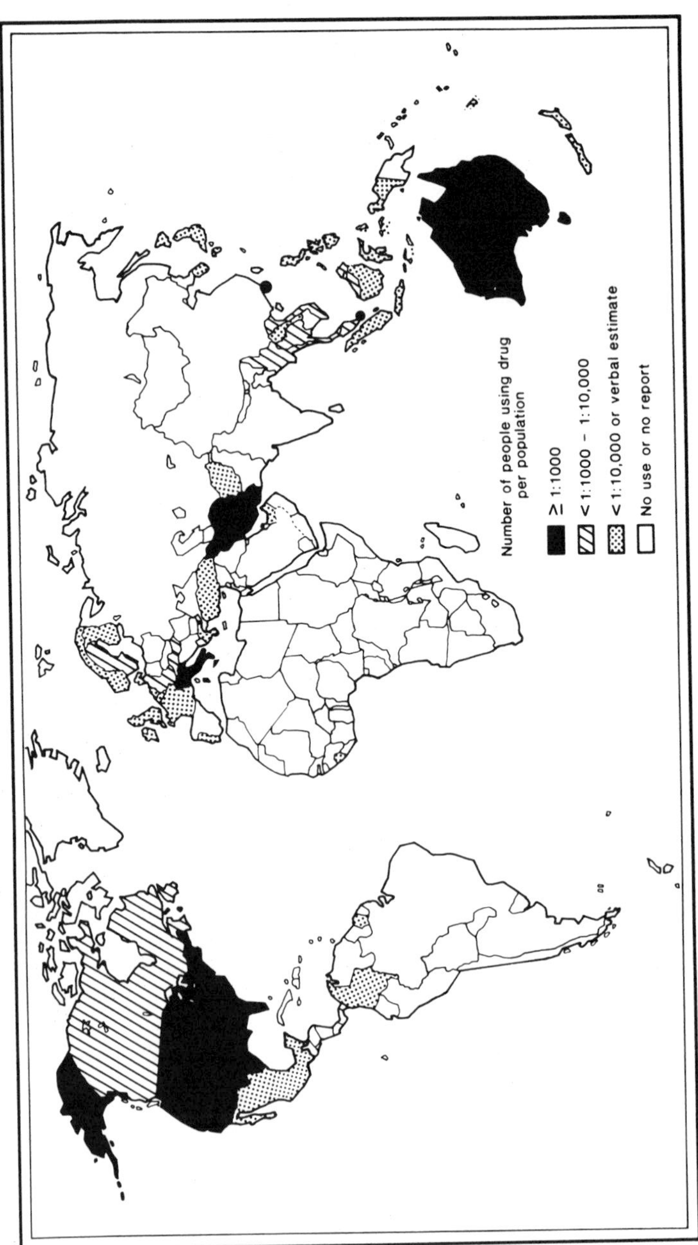

Map 2. Heroin. (From Ref. 12. Reprinted with permission.)

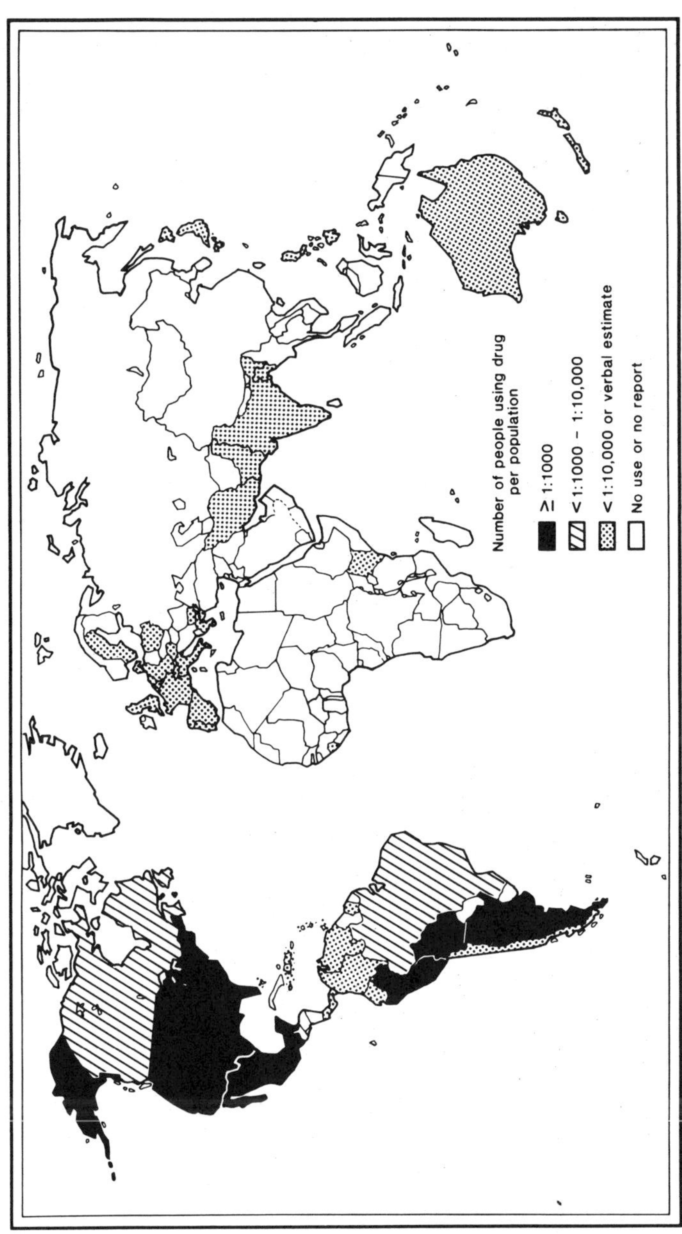

Map 3. Coca type. (From Ref. 12. Reprinted with permission.)

3.3. Cannabis

As far back as recorded history the intoxicating effects of cannabis were known in China, India, the Middle East, and Africa. In this century cannabis use has spread to the New World and Western Europe. Mexico was long the primary source for cannabis used in North America, and its indigenous use in Mexico has been long established. Since 1960 there has been an explosive spread of cannabis use through parts of North America and Europe. A high level of regular use, up to 10% of the population in some places, persists now in many areas of the world. Use, primarily in the form of hashish, also persists in the Middle East and Indian subcontinent. Cannabis use also seems to be increasing significantly in the urban centers of Africa. There is some use of cannibis in Southeast Asia and the Malay Archipelago, but it is not currently viewed as a major problem compared with use of other drugs. Cannabis use in various countries is shown in Map 4.

3.4. Sedatives

Barbiturate, sedative, and tranquilizer use is often initiated by physicians as part of a legitimate medical regimen. Patients become dependent on the drug and frequently mix it with alcohol. Aggressive marketing of pharmaceutical companies combined with relatively lax internal controls in many countries has led to a flooding of many countries with a wide variety of anxiolytics, sedatives, and other psychoactive drugs. As a result, large quantities of these substances are consumed outside of any medical or other professional supervision. This problem is particularly severe in parts of Africa, Asia, and Latin America, as shown in Map 5.

Reliance on sedatives has become an integral part of many cultures. The bulk of the consumption is under the direction of a physician, although this has not prevented excessive use of these drugs. For example, 85 million prescriptions for diazepam were filled by pharmacists in the United States during one 12-month period. In addition to the prescribed consumption of these drugs, large quantities also get into illicit channels. The benzodiazepine drugs are probably today the most widely and frequently consumed drugs in the world; more people take these drugs more often than any other pharmaceutical compound. In 1984, 33 benzodiazepine compounds have been recommended by WHO to come under the Psychotropic Substances Convention of 1971.

3.5. Amphetamines

Amphetamine use has often been of epidemic intensity, lasting a few to several years, and influenced by the availability of the drug and the rapidly progressive destructive effect it has on most heavy users. There have been several identified epidemics of amphetamine abuse since the drug was first

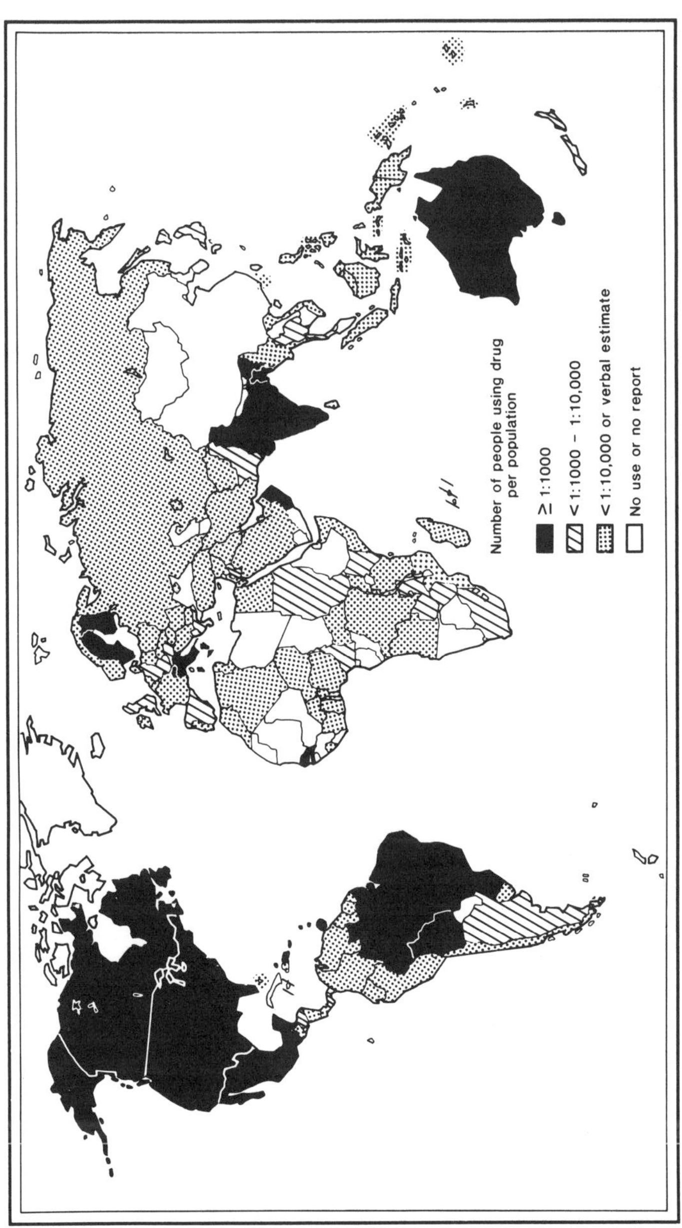

Map 4. Cannabis. (From Ref. 12. Reprinted with permission.)

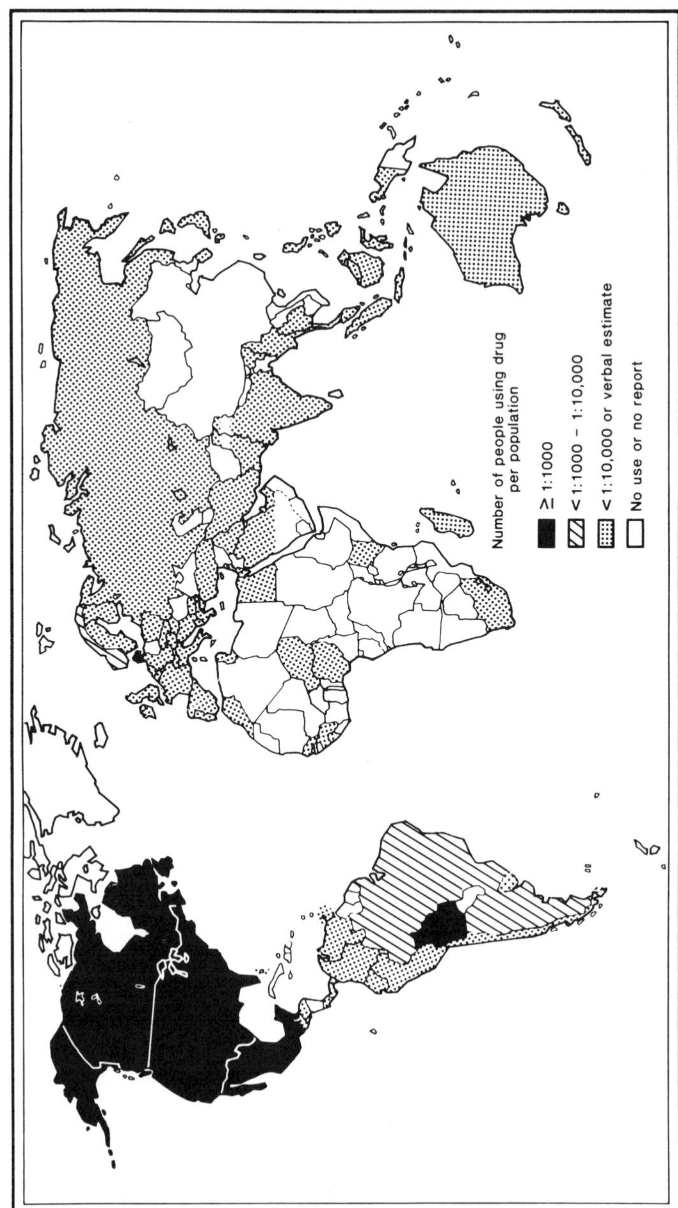

Map 5. Barbiturates, tranquilizers, other sedatives. (From Ref. 12. Reprinted with permission.)

introduced. Most notable have been those in Japan, Sweden, Northern Ireland, the United States, and Thailand. Today there is increasing use of amphetamines throughout the world. (See Map 6 for amphetamine use.)

3.6. Alcohol

Alcohol is the most widely used mind-altering substance. Financial constraints formerly limited the access of many people to alcohol, especially distilled spirits, but this is now changing. Increasing affluence in the developing world over the last few decades has been accompanied by a dramatic rise in alcohol use. Alcoholism has for centuries been a problem primarily affecting Europe and North America. It now affects people in virtually every country.

The Hindu, Moslem, and certain Christian religions that have prohibited alcohol consumption among their followers now have declining influence. Across South Asia illicitly brewed alcohol has been dramatically increasing. The problem is further aggravated by the mobility of the upper classes who are exposed to social alcohol drinking. Upon returning home, they may feel less under the sway of religious constraints.

In Figure 2, liver cirrhosis mortality is compared with alcohol consumption in 18 countries of Europe.

4. Demographic Variables

4.1. Gender

Historically, women everywhere have generally been less involved with recreational drug dependence than men. Use of certain drugs has predominated among women, however, such as belladona among nineteenth-century European women and betel-areca chewing among contemporary women in Southeast Asia. Women have become drug dependent as a result of taking medication with either inadequate or no medical supervision. Examples include morphine among nineteenth-century women, barbiturates in the first half of the twentieth century, and anxiolytics in the last half of the twentieth century.

The recreational use of certain mind-altering substances is linked with masculine identity and therefore offers less attraction to women in many cultures. This has been particularly true with regard to alcohol and intravenous injection of drugs. As more women have gained socioeconomic and political equality, this distinction has lessened. In industrialized countries the incidence of tobacco, sedative, and alcohol dependence among women has climbed dramatically.

Drugs adversely affect both the fetus and the woman whose body is already changed by pregnancy. Fetal alcohol syndrome is a condition affecting to vary-

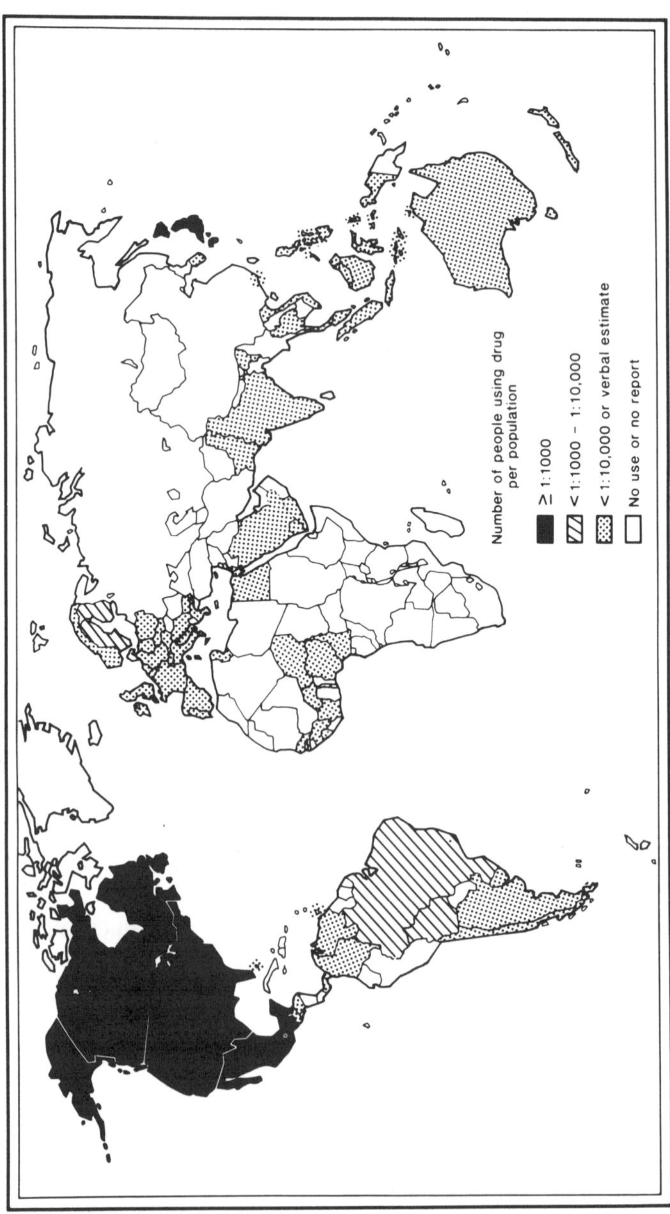

Map 6. Amphetamines. (From Ref. 12. Reprinted with permission.)

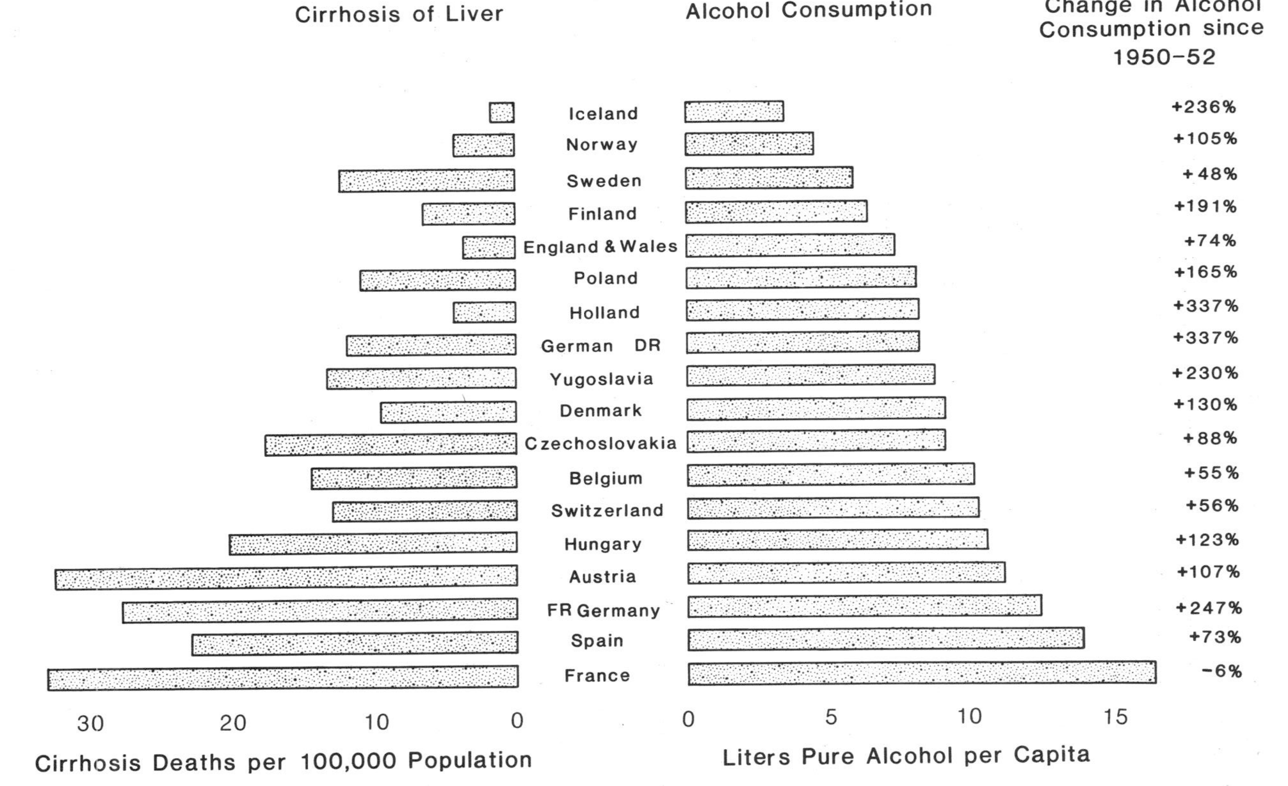

Figure 2. Liver cirrhosis mortality and alcohol consumption in selected countries mid-1970s. (From Ref. 17. Reprinted with permission.)

ing degrees the infants of alcoholic mothers, causing symptoms ranging from death to mental retardation to reduced birth weight. Pregnant women dependent on sedative or opiate drugs deliver babies who require treatment for drug withdrawal. Tobacco-dependent women deliver underweight babies.

4.2. Age

Drug dependence has mostly been restricted to adults in past centuries. In recent years a significant shift toward younger users has occurred in many countries. Especially use of heroin, cannabis, and alcohol has increased among those in their teens and early twenties. This upsurge in youthful drug use around the world over the last two decades has been closely linked with the so-called youth subculture. Consumption of cannabis, cigarettes, alcohol, and heroin has frequently occurred in part as a symbolic protest against the older generations and their mores.

Opium and alcohol dependence were once considered disorders of persons in their forties and fifties. Now younger drug-dependent persons are seen because heavy drug use is occurring at a younger age. In many places diagnoses are being made at an earlier stage in the course of drug dependence; this contributes to a younger patient population. The course of drug dependence appears to progress faster in younger people. And some of the newer drugs, such as heroin, may lead to earlier onset of problems as compared to older drugs, such as opium.

Older patients are often taking several different medications, including psychoactive compounds as well as other drugs with psychoactive effects (e.g., antihypertensives, anticholinergics). They may be confused about the correct frequency and quantities of their doses. Older people often possess an increased sensitivity to the effects of psychoactive substances. Some elderly people, especially those who live alone, may be inclined to rely heavily on drugs that relieve discomfort or depression. Physicians should be particularly alert to this problem in their care of the aged.

4.3. Social and Other Variables

The relationship between socioeconomic level and drug dependence is complex. When drugs are relatively scarce in a community or when there has been relatively little exposure to other cultures and their drug-dependent populations, those who first use drugs recreationally may be at the top of the socioeconomic scale. This can occur because wealthy people have (1) exposure to other cultures where drugs are used or (2) money to purchase drugs. Other groups who introduce drug use are international travelers, such as sailors, boatmen, truck drivers, returning students, airline personnel, and traveling technicians.

Physicians virtually everywhere have a higher incidence of drug dependence than any other professional group, closely followed by nurses, pharmacists, and other health workers who handle drugs. This is in part due to their ready access to drugs, but also because they often feel that their familiarity with psychoactive substances renders them invulnerable to the addicting effects. Most clinicians are reluctant to confront their addicted colleagues. Competent physicians must learn to overcome this reluctance.

5. Current Global Trends in Drug Abuse and Dependence and Future Trends

5.1. Current Global Trends According to the Type of Drug Abuse and Dependence

For the period 1975–1980 an international review on the extent of drug abuse has been carried out by WHO.[12] This study, which has implications for health planners, is based primarily on United Nations data obtained from standardized annual reports from countries that are party to the international drug control treaties. The study reflects the extent of drug abuse by drug type.

A high rate of opium abuse was found in the Middle East, Southeast Asia, and the Western Pacific, with a total of approximately 1.76 million opium abusers. The highest rates were found in opium-producing countries and neighboring countries, especially in rural opium poppy-growing regions. The risk of dependence was greatest among adult males. This pattern of opium abuse does not seem to have changed substantially over recent decades.

Heroin abuse is reported from many countries of the world. During recent decades extensive abuse has existed in North America and in the highly industrialized European countries. Over the last several years other countries, particularly the Southeast Asian and Middle East regions and parts of Europe not previously affected, have also become involved in heroin abuse. The target populations are mainly adolescents and young adults, with peaks in the 18–25 age group. In countries where former opium users have changed from opium to heroin use, all ages are involved.

High rates of coca/cocaine misuse, such as coca leaf chewing and coca paste smoking, are found primarily in the Americas, especially in Peru, Bolivia, Argentina, Colombia, Chile, Ecuador, and parts of Brazil. Sniffing of cocaine powder and injection of cocaine have increased, especially in North America and in various European countries. Inhaling of the free base is mainly reported from the United States. The worldwide number of coca leaf abusers has been put at 1,600,000 in the mid-1960s, while cocaine abusers have been estimated to number 4,800,000. In recent years cocaine misuse has shown the highest rate of increase internationally. Coca leaf chewing occurs among all age groups in the indigenous populations. While coca paste smoking predominates among adolescents and young adults, middle- and upper-class urban males show the highest rates of cocaine sniffing and injecting.

Amphetamine dependence has been reported from 68 countries, indicating a worldwide distribution. Over 80% of abusers, however, are in the United States. A global total of 2,300,000 abusers is mentioned, but the statistical basis for this group seems less reliable than for other drugs. No extensive changes have been reported in recent years. The WHO Expert Committee on Drug Dependence (1985) has now recommended that 17 amphetaminelike substances be controlled under the 1971 Convention of Psychotropic Substances.

A total of 29,000,000 cannabis users are reported from 120 countries. Twenty-five countries from the African, American, and European regions of WHO fall into the high-use category. The users are found in all age groups and social strata. Special target groups are adolescent smokers in rural areas of Africa, Asia, and the Middle East and the young urban or semiurban population in almost all regions of the world.

Hallucinogens are reported to be abused by 2,000,000 persons living in 15 countries, but mainly in the United States. However, abuse of these substances has shown a recent decline on an international level. The main risk groups are urban youth and indigenous peoples of North and South America.

Khat abuse in the form of khat chewing is reported from countries in the Middle East and East Africa, with abuse most prevalent among the male population. All the age groups and social classes are affected. The abuse of this stimulant, although seemingly increasing, is mostly restricted to the area now affected, unless new ways of conservation are developed. Some limited licit and illicit transportation of khat by airplane to Western Europe and North America does occur.

A large, but unknown number of abusers obtain barbiturates, sedatives, and tranquilizers from physicians or pharmacies and therefore are not reported. This has to be kept in mind in interpreting the significance of the reported global number of 3,400,000 abusers. At least some misuse of these substances was identified in 88 countries. Almost all world regions are concerned. The populations most at risk are medical and psychiatric patients. The abuse of these drugs is also reported among illegal drug abusers.

The most complete and reliable data on epidemiological trends in substance abuse have been reported from the United States and concern adolescents, young adults, and the elderly adult groups. The main finding of international surveys of drug abuse made in 1982, in comparison with a similar survey in 1972, indicates the reversal of upward trends recorded earlier. Since 1979 there has been a leveling off in the spread of cannabis abuse in the youth population as well as a significant decline in the percentage of persons who regularly abuse cannabis, alcohol, and various other drugs.

Alcohol consumption has steadily increased worldwide. Between 1950–1952 and 1970–1972 per capita consumption increased by at least 50% in Austria (+126%), Bulgaria (+436%), Czechoslovakia (+76%), Denmark (+82%), Finland (+114%), Federal Republic of Germany (+210%), German Democratic

Republic (+242%), Hungary (+95%), Iceland (+142%), Ireland (+67%), Luxembourg (+59%), the Netherlands (+210%), Norway (+75%), Poland (+80%), Switzerland (+62%), and Yugoslavia (+180%).[28] Reports from Africa, South and Central America, Asia, the Pacific Islands, and the Caribbean also suggest increasing levels of consumption.[5] Considering the close relationship between per capita alcohol consumption and the prevalence of alcohol-related health problems in the population, this trend evidences an enormous increase in the health risk and corresponding costs. Since the early 1970s this trend has continued in many countries[19]; in others a leveling off or even slight decrease in consumption has been observed. Countries with a fast-increasing alcohol consumption between 1960 and 1981 are the following: the Netherlands (+243%), Denmark (+61%), Finland (+132%), The German Democratic Republic (+125%), Hungary (+69%), Poland (+68%), Federal Republic of Germany (+93%), Austria (+25%), Canada (+95%), Japan (+169%), Mexico (+80%), and the Republic of Korea (+762%).[31]

Tobacco and nicotine abuse is reported to have leveled off or decreased in North America and several European countries, with an increasing number of ex-cigarette smokers. This trend has been reported only for male populations, whereas in females such a reverse trend has not yet become sufficiently obvious.[1] In many developing countries, however, smoking is becoming increasingly prevalent. The corresponding health risks are starting to become visible only in the form of an increase in lung cancer mortality rates.[32] A shift from developed to developing countries in the marketing policy of the tobacco industry has been observable, paralleling the increasing awareness in the developed countries of the health risks associated with a high rate of cigarette smoking.

5.2. Current Overall Global Trends

With increased life expectancy the number of elderly adults is growing considerably. Nevertheless, there is only sparse information on drug abuse and dependence risk in this age group. Some 20 years ago this risk seemed to be lower than in younger age groups.[21] In recent years the epidemiological literature has indicated an increased risk concerning alcohol[9] and sedative/hypnotics.[6,22]

The overall picture concerning the recent trends in drug abuse and dependence shows two different scenarios. The first is characterized by traditional drug use with a history of many centuries and a high degree of integration into the cultural and everyday life of the adult, mostly rural, populations. This applies to the use of opium, cannabis, coca leaves, and alcohol in certain countries. In other countries, while this scenario is partly unchanged, it has become complicated by the availability of other drugs and by an overproduction and/or suppression of traditional drugs. Together with changes in the sociocultural context, these latter factors have resulted in a destabilization of traditional drug abuse and in establishment of a new pattern of multiple drug abuse. The other scenario is characterized by the modern drug wave, starting in the early 1960s in the highly industrialized countries and affecting primarily urban and semiurban youth, but spreading later to more and more countries in all regions of the world. This trend has led to an enormous expansion in the misuse of cannabis, stimulants, hallucinogens, heroin, and—as the most recent threat—cocaine. Epidemiological data, as well as data on drug seizures, provide evidence of this process of a rapid worldwide spread of abuse. Within this picture a speedy increase in multiple drug abuse with a variety of rapid changes in consumption patterns is observable.

5.3. Populations at Risk

Risk factors and populations at risk have also been changing, especially during the past two decades. At first, middle- and upper-class youths, particularly students, were the main target. Increased drug use coincided with increased youth protest in some places. Those countries that were affected earlier show a definite shift in the risk to groups from deprived areas, with deficient social backgrounds and psychopathological characteristics. Earlier sex differences with a disproportionately high ratio of young males abusing drugs have almost vanished in some places, resulting in more or less equal consumption and abuse rates in males and females. The age of first drug abuse has become lower, and the rates of inhalant abusers and alcohol drinkers among schoolchildren have increased in many parts of the world.

5.4. Future Trends in Drug Abuse and Dependence

Any projection as to future trends in drug abuse must take into account several relevant factors. The most prominent are demographic trends, with special regard to age groups and other risk groups, and consumption rates in various groups, countries, and regions. Environmental events can affect risk proneness, and the mass media can influence risk awareness. Drug production, marketing, legislation, and law enforcement concerning legal and illegal drugs can affect rates of drug use and abuse.

In the United States and many other industrialized countries the birth rate has decreased considerably since 1960. In many developing countries, in contrast to this trend, a decreased infant mortality has resulted in increasing adolescent and young-adult populations. Finally, as life expectancy lengthens, there has been an increase in the elderly adult group in the developing countries, a trend that is still continuing. A similar trend can be expected in the future in juvenile drug misuse in developing countries, an increase in drug misuse by the elderly in industrialized countries, and a leveling off or decrease in juvenile and young-adult drug misuse in industrialized countries (and subsequently in other countries with reduced birth rates).

5.5. Implications for Public Health

Serious public health consequences can be predicted from the global increase in alcohol-related morbidity, the global increase in multiple-drug-use morbidity, the increase in tobacco-related morbidity in particular regions, and the increase in cocaine-related morbidity in identified population groups. An increase in the drug-related morbidity in preadolescents and adolescents has also occurred in numerous areas. The long-term prognosis of juvenile drug abuse and dependence is still a matter to be clarified. The "aging-out hypothesis" (in which adolescents were assumed to recover from drug dependence with time alone) may have to be revised in light of new evidence.

6. Morbidity and Mortality Related to Drug Abuse

Morbidity and mortality related to drug abuse must be incorporated as a consequence of a complex interaction involving a wide range of factors, including pharmacological and toxicological properties of the drug use, combination of drug use, accessibility to health care for drug abusers and their nutritional state, and route of administration. Of particular importance is the route of administration of drugs. Injecting drugs intravenously multiplies the risk owing to the possibility of contaminated needles and syringes and contaminating substances added to dilute the heroin, cocaine, and amphetamines. The excess mortality is mainly due to overdose, infections, and trauma. In alcohol abusers the probability of liver cirrhosis increases in malnourished or underfed alcoholics. There is also an increase in mortality with cocaine if inhaled or smoked rather than sniffed. With cocaine it is the difficulty of controlling the dosage rate that accounts for the additional risks.

The excess mortality risk among heroin users is very well established and reported in many countries. The main psychiatric morbidity related to amphetamine use is acute and chronic psychosis. Among the hallucinogen abusers the mortality rate is not very well studied; death occurs mainly through accident or suicide. Morbidity is mainly due to acute toxic psychosis, chronic psychosis, depressive states, and neurological symptoms. Excess mortality from use of hypnotics, sedatives, and tranquilizers is due mainly to suicide or accidental overdose. During withdrawal cerebral convulsion and even fatal status epilepticus can occur. The abuse of volatile solvents can lead to sudden death from cardiac fibrillation or to respiratory depression. Morbidity is mainly due to liver, kidney, CNS, and bone marrow damage after prolonged use. Tobacco morbidity and mortality is very well studied and documented. Large prospective studies have been conducted specifically to delineate the relationship between tobacco smoking and the development of disease.[1] These studies indicate an overall excess mortality for male cigarette smokers of 170%. A clear-cut dose–response relationship was demonstrated repeatedly, indicating a causal relationship. Excess mortality increases with the duration of smoking, the average amount of smoking, and the depth of inhalation. It decreases with the duration of abstinence from smoking. In cigar and pipe smokers the excess mortality is considerably less pronounced. As with alcohol, excess mortality is especially high in the younger and middle-aged groups. The causes of death are as would be expected from the main tobacco-related diseases: neoplasms in the respiratory and upper digestive tract, coronary heart disease, aneurysm, cerebral vascular disease, chronic obstructive lung disease, peptic ulcers, and pneumonia. The extent of tobacco-related morbidity is illustrated by hospital statistics. In Switzerland approximately 10% of hospitalized male patients over age 50 suffer from tobacco-related conditions. No specific tobacco-related psychiatric morbidity has been documented except for the psychopathological consequences of somatic conditions. In European countries it is estimated that tobacco-related excess mortality constitutes the most important fraction of avoidable mortality, in view of the high prevalence of cigarette smoking.[16] Morbidity from abuse of analgesic agents (e.g., acetaminophen) is mainly due to hematopoietic system lesions and diseases of the kidneys.

There is evidence of a worldwide trend toward multiple drug use, with a consequent impact on both mortality and morbidity. The synergistic action of drugs abused in combination has been demonstrated by increased fatalities due to respiratory depression. The severity of personality changes with corresponding social deterioration may also be exacerbated by multiple drug use. The same holds true for general health status and nutrition. The synergistic actions of alcohol and tobacco are a cause of neoplasms, respiratory inflammation, and other maladies.

7. Drug Dependence and Implications for Human Reproduction

Chromosomal damage through drug abuse has been much debated, especially with respect to lysergic acid diethylamide (LSD) and cannabis. There is some evidence of chromosome abnormalities in animal studies and in humans, but a teratogenic effect with an increased risk of fetal malformations has not been proven so far.[3,33]

Effects on pregnancy are best documented for alcohol and tobacco smoking, but have also been reported for cannabis, cocaine, and volatile solvents. Accumulated research clearly indicates that smoking during pregnancy retards fetal growth and increases the risk of spontaneous abortion, complications of pregnancy, preterm delivery, and late fetal and neonatal deaths. Maternal smoking is also associated with an increased risk of sudden infant death syndrome. An increased risk of respiratory infections in the first year of life is present if the parents smoke.[1]

Heavy alcohol consumption in pregnancy increases the risk of perinatal mortality.[15,23] A range of abnormalities has been described as the fetal alcohol syndrome.[2,14] This syndrome includes mental retardation, growth deficiency, and a variety of maldevelopments. Its incidence in central Europe is estimated to be 3 per 1000 of all newborns, and 40–50% percent of the children of alcoholic mothers are considered to be damaged.[20]

Opiate dependence, especially heroin dependence, has a nonquantified impact on stillbirth, fetal growth retardation, and neonatal morbidity. Comparable effects have been documented in association with the chronic excessive use of barbiturates, tranquilizers, amphetamines, caffeine, LSD, and cannabis.[7,10]

References

1. Ashley, MJ: Alcohol, tobacco and drugs: An audit of mortality and morbidity, in Drew LRH, Stelz P, Barclay WA (eds): *Man, Drugs and Society. Current Perspectives.* Canberra, Australian Federation of Alcoholics and Drug Dependents, 1982, pp 350–355.
2. Clarren SK, Smith DW: The fetal alcohol syndrome. *N Engl J Med* 1978; 298:1063.
3. Eberle P: Verursachgen Halluzinogene Chromosomendefekte und Missbildunger? *Nervenarzt* 1973; 44:281–284.
4. Edwards G: British policies on opiate addiction: Ten years working at the revised response, and options for the future. *Br J Psychiatry* 1979; 134:1–13.
5. Edwards G: Drinking problems: Putting the Third World on the map. *Lancet* 1979; 2:402.
6. Eve SB, Freedson HM: Use of tranquilizers and sleeping pills among older Texans. *J Psychoactive Drugs* 1981; 13:173–189.
7. Finnigan LP, Fehr KP: The effect of opiates, sedative–hypnotics, amphetamines, cannabis and other psychoactive drugs on the fetus and newborn, in Kalant OJ (ed): *Research Advances in Alcohol and Drug Problems.* New York, Plenum Press, 1980, vol. 5.
8. Ghodse AH: Morbidity and mortality, in Edwards G, Busch C (eds): *Drug Problems in Britain: A Review of Ten Years.* London, Academic Press, 1981.
9. Glantz MD, Petersen DM, Whittington FJ: Drugs and the elderly adult, in: *NIDA Research Issue no. 32.* Rockville, MD, DHHS Publication no. ADM83-1269, 1983.
10. Harvey DJ: *Marihuana '84.* Oxford, IRL Press, 1984.
11. Hughes PH, Barker NW, Crawford GA, Jaffee JH: The natural history of a heroin epidemic. *Am J Public Health* 1972; 62:995–1001.
12. Hughes PH, Canavan KP, Jarvis G, Arif A: Extent of drug abuse: An international review with implications for health planners. *World Health Stat Q* 1983; 36:3/4, 394–497.
13. Jeri FR: Coca-paste smoking in some Latin American countries: A severe and unabated form of addiction. *Bull Narcotics* 1984; 36:15–31.
14. Jones KL, Smith DW: Pattern of malformation in offspring of chronic alcoholic mothers. *Lancet* 1973; 1:1267.
15. Kaminski M, Rumeau C, Schwartz D: Alcohol consumption in pregnant women and the outcome of pregnancy. *Alcoholism: Clin Exp Res* 1978; 2:155–163.
16. Leu E, Schaub T: *Raucher und Gesundheit Eine Volkswirtschaftluche Analyse.* Basel, Institut der Sozialwissenschaften der Universität, 1985.
17. *Liver Cirrhosis Mortality and Alcohol Consumption in Selected Countries mid-1970s.* London, Office of Health Economics.
18. MacKintosh DR, Stewart GT: A mathematical model of a heroin epidemic: Implications for control policies. *J Epidem Community Health* 1979; 33:299–304.

19. Mäkelä K, Room R, Single E, et al: *Alcohol, Society and the State. A Comparative Study of Alcohol Control*. Toronto, Addiction Research Foundation, 1981.
20. Majewski F: *Untersuchungen zur Alkoholembryopathie*. Stuttgart, Thieme, 1980.
21. Müller Ch: *Altraspsychiatrie*. Stuttgart, Thieme, 1967.
22. Müller, R: *Alkoholproblems in der Schweiz, 1950–1978*. Lausanne, Switzerland, 1982.
23. Olegård R, Sabel K-G, Aronsson M, et al: Effects on the child of alcohol abuse during pregnancy. Retrospective and prospective studies. *Acta Paediatr Scand* 1979; 5 (suppl 275):112–121.
24. O'Malley PM, Bachman JG, Johnston LD: Reliability and consistency in self-reports of drug use. *Int J Addict* 1983; 18:805–824.
25. Perrine MW: Alcohol involvement in highway crashes: A review of the epidemiologic evidence. *Clin Plastic Surg* 1975; 2:11–34.
26. Smart RG, Arif A, Hughes PH, et al: *Drug Use among Nonstudent Youth*. World Health Organization Offset Publication no. 60. Geneva, WHO, 1981.
27. Smart RG, Hughes PH, Johnston LD, et al: *A Methodology for Student Drug Use Surveys*. World Health Organization Offset Publication no. 50. Geneva, WHO, 1980.
28. Sulkunen P: Drinking patterns and the level of alcohol consumption: An international overview, in Gibbons RJ, Israel Y, Kalant H, et al (eds): *Research Advances in Alcohol and Drug Problems*. New York, Wiley, 1976, vol 3.
29. Tedermann S: Alcohol, alcoholism, alcolisation. *Donees Scientifiques de Characters Physiologique Economique et Social*. Institut National d'Etudes Demographique Travaux et Documents. Cahier no. 29. Paris, Presses Universitaires de France, 1956.
30. Terry CE, Pellens M: *The Opium Problem*. Bedford Hills, NY, Bureau of Social Hygiene, 1928.
31. Walsh B, Grant M: *Public Health Implications of Alcohol Production and Trade*. World Health Organization Offset Publication no. 88. Geneva, WHO, 1985.
32. World Health Organization: *Controlling the Smoking Epidemic*. World Health Organization Technical Report Series, no. 636. Geneva, WHO, 1979.
33. Zerbin-Rudin E: Ursachen und Folgen der Drogensuchten aus genetischer Sicht, in von Volker F (ed): *Suchtgefahren in unserer Zeit* (Compendium Psychiatricum). Stuttgart, Hippokrates, 1983.

Further Reading

Johnston LD: *Review of General Population Surveys of Drug Abuse*. World Health Organization Offset Publication no. 52. Geneva, WHO, 1980.

Rootman I, Hughes PH: *Drug Abuse Reporting System*. World Health Organization Offset Publication no. 35. Geneva, WHO, 1980.

5

Etiological Factors

1. Introduction

The etiology of drug dependence has probably been of interest since the connection between drug consumption and adverse consequences was observed. There have been many explanations for psychoactive drug use, abuse, and dependence (often with some moral component). Consideration of drug dependence as a medical problem is a relatively recent phenomenon, originating in the late 1700s but gaining popularity only in the last half-century.

Hundreds of studies have examined the role of dozens of factors purported to cause drug dependence, especially alcohol dependence. The etiology of drug dependence is complex and multifactorial, depending on the interplay of many factors, including genetic, constitutional, and environmental factors.[5,14] This is the single most important finding from these studies. Ways of conceptualizing these multiple etiological factors have included the biological/psychological/sociological classification of drug dependence and the public health model. The latter model consists of the agent (the drug), the host (the individual), and the environment, along with their interactions.

Figure 1 displays a model that takes into account the diverse factors operating in the etiology of drug dependence. Note that social factors operate as both antecedents and consequences; the same is true for individual factors. The model takes into account such diverse elements as genetics, learning, and drug effects. At all levels there are feedback mechanisms which can ameliorate or exacerbate drug use, depending on the individual and the circumstances. The model represents a linking of postulates. In the model, external stimuli (such as social influences) and/or internal stimuli (such as mood states) may evoke initial or repetitive drug-taking behavior. The description of the individual takes into

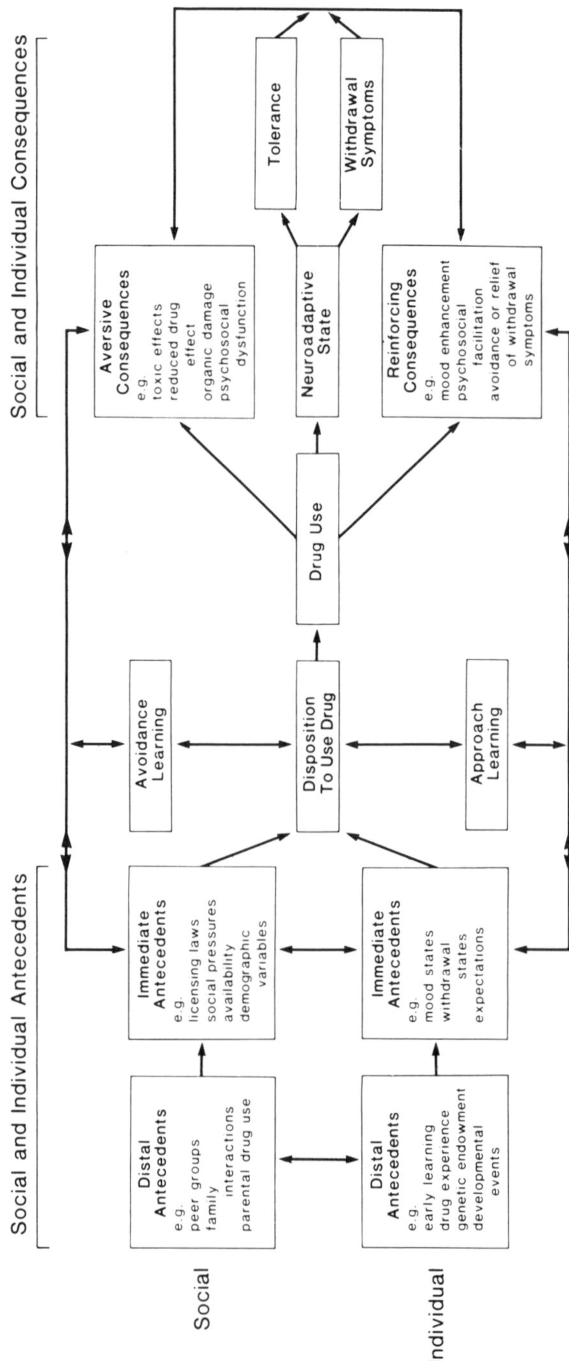

Figure 1. Factors affecting drug use and abuse. (From Ref. 6. Reprinted with permission.)

account biological and psychological attributes and previous social experiences. Drug-seeking behavior may vary in terms of specific drug(s) used, amount(s) and route(s) of administration, and the drug effects and associated behaviors. A number of internal and external responses initiate reinforcing or aversive learning processes.

Drug actions and their effects may also cause biological responses that involve tolerance and/or withdrawal symptoms specific to the particular substance. The changes associated with the neuroadaptive states may have both aversive and reinforcing properties. The withdrawal symptoms themselves may be immediately aversive, and their relief by drug-taking serves to strengthen the drug-seeking drive. Repeated withdrawal episodes and subsequent self-administration may initiate conditioning processes whereby previously neutral stimuli will first elicit withdrawal symptoms, which in turn lead to drug-seeking behavior. By a process of generalization, internal cues (e.g., anxiety) in drug-using individuals may come to elicit the same behavioral response as the drug withdrawal syndrome—drug-seeking behavior. Drug taking may become a dominant response to these internal cues, and behavior becomes a narrowed stereotyped repertoire of drug-related responses.

Permanent or temporary cessation of drug-taking behavior may be encouraged by the lack of reinforcement. This may be due to biological changes or therapeutic interventions. Aversive consequences may develop because of withdrawal symptoms, negative environmental responses, or increasing drug toxicity. Other reinforcers in the environment (besides drug effects) may become more rewarding as a result of improved social circumstances or therapeutic responses.

If drug taking is resumed after a period of cessation, the previous levels of intake and decreased flexibility may quickly develop as a result of residual biological alterations (persistent neuroadaptive changes) and previous learning.

While the traditional viewpoint has been to see dependence as located within the individual, the World Health Organization model argues for locating dependence within a system of interacting processes of which the pharmacological property of the drug is only one element.

2. Host Factors

2.1. Genetic Factors

Strong evidence indicates a genetic component to drug dependence. Such evidence comes from family, twin, adoption, and biological marker studies. These, in combination with other studies, indicate, however, that environmental factors influence the expression of the inherited predisposition to alcoholism just as they influence the expression of other inherited traits.

2.1.1. Family Studies

Many studies indicate that drug dependence runs in families, but family traits may or may not have a genetic basis. Such studies generally have found that 25% or more of the fathers and brothers of identified alcoholics are also alcohol dependent. The rate for alcohol dependence in the males from families of alcohol-dependent persons appears to be about five times the rate in the general population. This rate (for male relatives in families of alcohol-dependent persons) ranges from 25 to 50%, and the rate for female relatives in families of alcoholics ranges between 5 and 8%. Up to one-half of hospitalized alcohol-dependent persons come from homes where one or both parents have abused alcohol. In a review of 150 studies, all except one showed higher rates of alcohol dependence among relatives of alcohol-dependent persons than in the general population. It is noteworthy, however, that in many family studies a large number of alcohol-dependent subjects are found who do not have an alcohol-dependent parent or other relative, indicating clearly that in many individuals environmental factors play an important role in the etiology or pathophysiology of the disorder.[7,8,17] Opium addicts in Asia have similarly been noted to have a higher-than-expected number of relatives with opium addiction.[26]

2.1.2. Twin Studies

Twin studies have provided a valuable method for studying possible genetic diseases. Monozygous (identical) twins share the same genes, while dizygous (fraternal) twins share some of the same genes. If monozygous twins are more concordant for a trait or disease than are dizygous twins, one assumes that heredity is playing a role.

Twin studies have shown more concordance in monozygous than in dizygous twins for a variety of drinking behaviors, including the quantity and frequency of alcohol consumption and alcohol effect on brain wave function and, in one study, on alcohol dependence. Additionally, twin studies suggest genetic factors may contribute up to 50% of the variability in alcohol elimination rate and that genetic factors contribute significantly in some people to such alcohol complications as cirrhosis, psychoses, and perhaps hangovers. In summary, twin studies implicate genetic factors in the control of a variety of drinking behaviors and alcohol dependence, although they do not provide absolute evidence for a genetic component in alcohol.[10]

2.1.3. Adoption Studies

Adoption studies have contributed to our knowledge of the inheritability of alcohol dependence by examining the incidence of alcohol dependence in children of alcoholics who were adopted at an early age. There have been several large-scale, well-controlled studies in several Scandinavian countries and in North America.[2,3,7,18] From these the following tentative conclusions emerge:

- Adopted sons of alcohol-dependent fathers are three to four times more likely to be alcohol dependent than the sons of non-alcohol-dependent fathers, regardless of the drinking habits of the adoptive parents.
- Sons of alcohol-dependent fathers are no more likely to be alcohol dependent if raised by their alcoholic biological parents than if raised by non-alcoholic adoptive parents.
- There may be a mild form and a severe form of alcoholism, with a genetic basis for the severe form in males.
- Similar findings were found for women but at a much lower incidence than for men, and these are considered much more preliminary in view of the relatively small number of affected persons. Women seem more severely affected if the mother was an alcohol abuser rather than the father.
- Most such studies did not show any relationship between parental alcohol dependence and any other psychiatric condition, although some studies suggest that daughters of alcohol-dependent parents are more prone to depression if raised by their alcohol-dependent parents than if raised by non-alcohol-dependent adoptive parents. These studies suggest that both sex-linked and recessive modes of inheritance are unlikely. Dominant inheritance is suggested for some alcohol-dependent males.

2.1.4. Genetic Markers

The relationship between heredity and drug dependence has also been explored via the association between alcoholism and other characteristics known to be inherited. Such genetic markers include color blindness, blood groups, body proteins (such as the human leukocyte antigen system), finger ridge counts, and the ability to taste certain substances. The only biological marker consistently associated with alcoholism is color blindness, but it is currently believed to be associated with toxic effects of alcohol. At the present time, such studies do not provide much knowledge about the inheritance of alcoholism.[7,14]

2.2. Neurotransmitters and Enzymes

A new era in the field of drug dependence began with the discovery of specific opioid receptors in the limbic system. Subsequently, endogenous morphinelike substances, referred to as endorphins, have been identified and shown to play an important role in mediating opioid effects. The mere fact that endogenous morphinelike compounds exist suggests a possible role in the etiology of opioid dependence. In addition to their possible importance in the etiology of opioid dependence, theoretically such compounds could play a role in either the etiology or pathogenesis of other types of drug dependence. The latter possibility arises from the observation that products of alcohol metabolism can condense with dopamine and form alkaloids known as tetrahydroisoquinolines (THIQs). THIQs are also known to be intermediary products in the formation of morphine in plants. Two THIQs, salsolinol and tetrahydroisopapaverline, have so far not been identified in humans. Their potential role in the etiology of alcohol dependence remains unproven.[19,22]

Ethanol has been found to modify opioid receptor activity of neuroblastoma cells, perhaps by a nonspecific effect of cell membranes, providing an additional mechanism by which opioid receptors and/or endorphins may play a role in alcohol dependence. Ethanol is known to affect a variety of other central nervous system neurotransmitters, including norepinephrine, dopamine, acetylcholine, serotonin, γ-aminobutyric acid, and the cyclic nucleotides cAMP and cGMP. Frequently alcohol exerts a biphasic effect on neurotransmitter release or turnover, raising speculation that such compounds are directly involved in mediating central nervous system responses to alcohol, many of which are clinically biphasic. The precise roles that neurotransmitters play in the etiology of alcoholism remain unclear.

Alcohol-metabolizing enzyme systems and the products of alcohol metabolism have been implicated in the etiology of alcoholism apart from the THIQ hypothesis. There are known to be more than 20 different alcohol dehydrogenase isoenzymes and several aldehyde dehydrogenase isoenzymes. Such enzymes are under genetic control, and differences in concentrations in humans account for intra- and interindividual variations in metabolism of alcohol, as well as for some of the racial differences noted. It has been hypothesized that some individuals may have alcohol-metabolizing systems that facilitate or discourage the consumption of large amounts of alcohol. Theoretically, these metabolic systems enhance or minimize the development of alcohol dependence. An example of such a mechanism is the flush reaction to alcohol noted in some individuals consuming a small amount of alcohol. This reaction appears to result from the buildup of acetaldehyde due to the absence of a subtype of aldehyde dehydrogenase, producing symptoms of flushing of the upper torso, head, and neck; headache; perspiration; nausea; dizziness; tachycardia; and hypotension. This reaction can occur with small amounts of alcohol in susceptible persons and is similar to the reaction experienced by individuals on disulfiram maintenance therapy upon consuming alcohol. It has been postulated that this reaction may decrease both the prevalence of alcohol consumption and the amount consumed at any given time in individuals who experience this reaction, thus tending to inhibit the development of alcohol abuse or dependence.[11,23]

Benzodiazepine receptors have also been identified and are being intensively investigated for their etiological significance in benzodiazepine dependence.

Clinical studies of blocking agents have also contributed to our knowledge of drug dependence. For example, blocking agents working peripherally on the autonomic nervous system can greatly diminish the subjective and objective signs of opioid and sedative withdrawal. Drug dependence, then, need not be only a limbic–thalamic–hypothalamic phenomenon, but (depending on the drug) can be a peripheral phenomenon regulated by the autonomic nervous system.

While initial drug dependence usually occurs over months, or even years, recurrence of drug dependence may take only a few days. Laboratory research on animals has shown that, even in the naive animal, cellular tolerance to opioids takes place from the first dose. The usual delayed or gradual onset of initial drug dependence is thus related to psychological, social, or other environmental factors, rather than to drug factors alone.

In summary, several new investigations suggest a role for endogenous compounds, their receptors, and their metabolizing enzyme systems in the etiology of several types of drug dependence. Such systems may play an important role in mediating the effects of exogenous psychoactive drugs.

2.3. Psychological Factors

Hundreds of studies have examined the relationship among many psychological factors in the development, maintenance, treatment, and recovery from drug dependence. Most of these investigations have focused on alcohol and opioid dependence. Attitudes about drug use, personality developmental traits, psychopathological states, and psychodynamic formulations have been intensively studied, with many conflicting findings. In many cases it is difficult to determine whether psychopathological correlates of drug dependence are a cause or an effect of the dependence state. Additionally, it is not clear that factors that may initially influence an individual to begin using drugs are the same factors that influence continuation of drug use, further complicating our understanding of causal factors in the drug-dependent state.[4,25]

Psychoanalytic theorists and others interested in personality development have postulated defects in ego and superego functioning and have identified the presence of psychopathological states such as depression, sociopathy, and anxiety as being etiological in drug abuse and dependence. Longitudinal studies of children and adolescents have shown that rebelliousness, depressed mood, and low academic performance precede and predict drug use, although not necessarily drug abuse, since this has not been studied.[9]

Although major psychopathology sometimes precedes drug dependence, this does not occur in all cases.[21] Many people with chronic pain syndromes, anxiety, depression, grief, and other pathological states, while perhaps at increased risk for becoming drug dependent should they use psychoactive drugs, nevertheless do not frequently become drug dependent. Personality studies have failed to identify any one alcoholic or opioid-dependent personality type. Despite this heterogeneous personality distribution, certain transient or situational psychological states (such as social phobia or a major life crisis) may play a role in the etiology and pathogenesis of drug dependence.

Personality studies have described certain typical characteristics in many drug-dependent persons. These personality characteristics have included hostile dependence, suppression of emotion, a high level of anxiety in interpersonal relationships, low frustration tolerance, low self-esteem, compulsive personality characteristics, and others. It appears, however, as if many of these traits may well be acquired in the process of becoming drug dependent, and there is a remarkable similarity in the development of some of these characteristics regardless of the type of drug used. In such cases these personality characteristics often disappear with long-term abstinence, a phenomenon that has important diagnostic, treatment, and research implications.

Behavioral and learning theorists have also investigated hypotheses concerning the etiology of drug dependence. Among the most important of these have been the tension-reduction hypothesis, the field-dependence hypothesis, hypotheses on the reinforcing properties of drugs, and the career hypothesis. The career hypothesis refers to those individuals who abuse drugs while young, but mature out from drug dependence in middle age. Such studies have led to many interesting, often contradictory findings. They have also made major contributions to our understanding of the mechanism of action of many drugs and to the pathogenesis of drug dependence. Thus far, however, psychological studies have failed to provide solid evidence for a single major psychological role in the etiology of all or most forms of drug dependence.

Psychological studies to date have helped to ascertain certain psychological factors that may be important in the etiology of drug dependence (e.g., impulsiveness, nonconformity). While research has failed to define a specific addictive personality, important clues about the importance of personality characteristics in subgroups of people are currently being further examined. An example of this is the relationship between sociopathic/delinquent behavior in adolescents and subsequent development of drug abuse.

3. Agent

Pharmacological properties of drugs of abuse are considered extensively in Chapter 7. In animal experiments, most drugs of abuse reinforce or reward the animal for seeking and taking the drug. These reinforcing drugs include opioids, alcohol and other sedatives, amphetamines, and cocaine.

Environmental or social factors represent perhaps the least understood of the three major categories in the public health model of drug dependence, in part because studies of such factors tend to look at aggregate data and at levels of drug use or indicators of problem use. Dependence is only one such indicator and in fact one of the least readily measured. Further, it appears that there is much interdependence of environmental variables, thus making identification of their individual effect much more difficult.

3.1. Availability

While it is clear that drug use, abuse, or dependence could not occur in the absence of availability of a drug, this fact hides the complexity of the role of availability in the etiology of drug dependence. It seems certain that the degree of availability of drug is an important factor in initiating drug use. The most readily available drugs in a society tend to be the most widely used, a fact that may reflect societal demand as well as sanction. Drug availability is, therefore, a product of some balance between supply and demand, with these factors in turn being influenced by laws, regulations, economic factors, and other societal or environmental variables. When drug availability increases, the prevalence of use and perhaps of dependence tends to increase. When a widely available drug becomes less available, use, abuse, and dependence tend to decrease. These relationships probably operate only within limits, and history is replete with failed attempts of societies to eliminate psychoactive drug dependence by prohibition.[16,20,27]

Dependence on licit (medically prescribed and legal) drugs can be influenced by the prescribing habits of physicians, who have an obligation to be cautious in prescribing psychoactive drugs known or suspected to be associated with the development of the dependent state.

Efforts to control and reduce drug availability are often referred to as drug supply control. This is a critical factor in the overall societal approach to drug dependence, since treatment approaches are greatly undermined if easy drug availability continues.

3.2. Cost

Econometric studies of drugs and other commodities and empirical evidence indicate that the relative cost of drugs influences their overall level and pattern of consumption. The relationship between cost and consumption is not simple, however. High prices tend to minimize consumption of a commodity, and decreasing consumption is considered by some to be a valid public health approach to the prevention of drug dependence. One measure to increase prices on alcohol and nicotine by increasing taxes on these substances is being considered in several countries. Measures such as this, to decrease consumption by increasing prices, are almost invariably controversial when applied to licit substances (as alcohol and nicotine tend to be in most countries). Measures to reduce consumption of illicit drugs are less controversial. In these situations rigorous law enforcement efforts leads to increased cost of the drug.[24]

3.3. Laws and Regulations

Attempts to legislatively control the nature, extent, and patterns of psychoactive drug use have occurred throughout the world for centuries. Such laws usually arise in response to perceived problems with use of a certain substance and, therefore, vary among different societies and over time within a given society. Many countries have imposed harsh penalties, including death, for use of prohibited drugs in attempts to eliminate some forms of drug use. For example, such laws have been implemented throughout history in Asia with regard to opioid use; one South Asian country employs death as a legal stricture even today.

Although rigorous study of the effects of such policies have rarely been prospective, it is generally agreed that they rarely have been successful in eliminating use of the drug in question. In fact, antidrug laws can exacerbate preexisting drug problems. One example is certain antiopium laws which have fostered heroin use, since heroin can be transported, sold, and consumed more secretly than opium. Intensive multifaceted efforts at eliminating alcohol production and consumption have met similar fates in many countries at different times, although consumption and some problems such as alcoholic cirrhosis of the liver have been reduced in some societies. Most societies today have regulations (although these are not always codified) either prohibiting the production and sale of some drugs or controlling the manufacture, distribution, and sale of others. Such regulations attempt to minimize drug-related problems and are often simultaneously designed to produce revenue for the government, leading to potentially conflicting goals. The overall impact of such regulations on the prevalence of drug dependence is usually indirect and impossible to assess precisely. To the extent that such laws minimize overall consumption by a population or a subgroup (i.e., adolescents) they exert some impact on the prevalence of use, abuse, and dependence and hence are of etiological significance and worthy of further study. Regulations that minimize excessive consumption may also minimize the occurrence of certain adverse consequences of drug use (e.g., alcohol-related automobile accidents).

4. Environmental Factors

4.1. Culture

Cultural influences on drug consumption have been intensively studied. Four cultural attitudes towards drug use have been described, as follows:

1. Complete abstinence
2. Ritualistic ceremonial use

3. Convivial use (emphasizes social group use)
4. Utilitarian use (emphasizes the personal aspects of drug use)

The differing rates of alcohol use in different cultures are also strongly influenced by and often inseparable from religious influence. Such differing cultural rates of alcohol use are interesting, but it is difficult to prove that any one factor accounts for increased or decreased alcohol comsumption. It is hence not possible to assign etiological significance to a simple cultural or religious factor.

Cultural change, either within a society or by emigration to other cultures, is sometimes associated with increased use of psychoactive substances. Several groups with traditionally low rates of alcoholism are now experiencing escalating problems.

4.2. Family Influence

Families play an important role in influencing drug use, abuse, and dependence, aside from genetic influences. Parents and older siblings serve as important role models for drug-taking behaviors. Parental attitudes about drug taking by children also influence such behavior by offspring, although many parents feel they exert little such influence. The influence of parental behaviors and attitudes declines as children grow older. Depending on the extent of family closeness, however, elderly parents and even grandparents can sometimes exert a profound impact on drug-abusing children. Family elders may be able to motivate a younger relative to enter treatment even when the young person no longer trusts other people.

Children of drug-dependent parents are likely to have diverse problems in later life. These include not only drug dependence, but also depression and interpersonal problems.

Parental absence, either by separation, divorce, or death, is statistically correlated with higher risk of drug dependence. The overall quality of family interaction, love, and support appears to modify subsequent drug abuse in offspring, at least in its milder forms.[1,12,15]

4.3. Peers

Numerous studies have examined the influence of the peer group on drug taking, but there is no clear consensus on the role of peers in the etiology of drug dependence. People who wish to use drugs are often drawn toward peer groups with similar motivations and drug-taking attitudes, complicating our understanding of the role of peer pressure. Peer relationships are generally considered to be an important factor in the initiation of drug use, and peer influences are an important component of many treatment programs. Peer factors may be less important than other factors in maintaining drug dependence.

4.4. Secondary Reinforcers

The reinforcing properties of drugs lead to secondary reinforcers, much as Pavlov's dogs salivated at the ringing of a bell when the bell was associated with feeding. In regard to drugs, secondary reinforcers can include drug use paraphernalia, the sight or smell of the drug, drug-using companions, or the geographical setting associated with drug use. These secondary reinforcers may help to maintain drug-seeking behavior or lead to recurrences of drug dependence in a recovering person.[13] Conversely, relocation to a drug-free environment favors a better prognosis.

References

1. Andorka R, Gseh-Szombathy L: Influence of social environment and individual factors in the development of alcoholism, paper presented at the 15th International Institute on the Prevention and Treatment of Alcoholism, Budapest, Hungary, June 1969.
2. Bohman B, Sigvardsson S, Cloninger CR: Maternal inheritance of alcohol abuse. Cross-fostering analysis of adopted women. *Arch Gen Psychiatry* 1981; 38:965–969.
3. Cloninger CR, Bohman M, Sigvardsson S: Inheritance of alcohol abuse. Cross-fostering analysis of adopted men. *Arch Gen Psychiatry* 1981; 38:861–868.
4. Collins RL, Marlatt GA: Psychological collelates and explanations of alcohol use and abuse, in Tabakoff B, Sutker PB, Randall CL (eds): *Medical and Social Aspects of Alcohol Abuse.* New York, Plenum Press, 1983, pp 273–308.
5. Edwards G, Arif A, Hodgson R: Nomenclature and classification of drug- and alcohol-related problems: A WHO memorandum, *Bull WHO* 1981; 59:225–242.
6. Factors affecting drug use and abuse. *Bull WHO* 1981; 59(2):225–242.
7. Goodwin DW: *Is Alcoholism Hereditary?* New York, Oxford University Press, 1976.
8. Jellinek EM: *The Disease Concept of Alcoholism.* New Haven, CT, College and University Press, 1959.
9. Kandel DB: *Longitudinal Research on Drug Use.* New York, Wiley, 1978.
10. Kaij L: *Alcoholism in Twins: Studies on the Etiology and Sequels of Abuse of Alcohol.* Stockholm, Sweden, Almquist and Wiksell, 1960.
11. Korsten MA, Matsuzaki S, Fienman L, Lieber CS: High blood acetaldehyde levels after ethanol administration. *N Engl J Med* 1975; 292:386–389.
12. Kosviner A, Hawks D, Webb MGT: Cannabis use amongst university students: 1. Prevalence rates and differences between students who have tried cannabis and those who have never tried it. *Br J Addict* 1973; 69:35–60.
13. Kumar R, Stolerman IP: Experimental and clinical aspects of drug dependence, in Iverson LL, Iverson SD, Snyder SH (eds): *Handbook of Psychopharmacology.* New York, Plenum Press, 1977, vol 7, pp 321–367.
14. Murray RM, Gurling HMD: Alcoholism, polygenic influence on a multifactorial disorder. *Br J Hosp Med* 1982; 27(4):328–334.
15. Plant MA: *Drug-takers in an English Town.* London, Tavistock, 1975.
16. Robins LN, Helzer JE: Drug use among Vietnam veterans—Three years later. *Med World News,* October 1975; 16(23):44–49.
17. Saunders JB: Alcoholism: New evidence for a genetic contribution. *Br Med J* 1982; 284:1137–1138.
18. Schuckit MA, Goodwin DW, Winokur G: A study of alcoholism in half siblings. *Am J Psychiatry* 1972; 128:122–126.

19. Simon EJ: Opiate receptors and their implications for drug abuse, in Lettieri DJ. Sayers M, Pearson HW (eds): *Theories on Drug Abuse, Selected Contemporary Perspectives,* Monograph 30. Rockville, MD, NIDA, 1980, pp. 303–308.
20. Smart RG: An availability-proneness theory of illicit drug abuse, in Lettieri DJ, Sayers M, Pearson HW (eds): *Theories on Drug Abuse, Selected Contemporary Perspectives,* Monograph 30. Rockville, MD, NIDA, 1980.
21. Stevenson RD, Carney A: Social and psychological background of drug addicts interviewed in Dublin. *J Irish Med Assoc* 1971; 64:372–375.
22. Su CY, Lin SH, Wang YT, Li CH, Hung LH, Lin CS, Lin BC: Effects of beta endorphin on narcotic abstinence syndrome in man. *J Formosan Med Assoc* 1978; 77:133–141.
23. von Wartburg JP: Acetaldehyde, in Sandler M (ed): *Pyschopharmacology of Alcohol.* New York, Raven Press, 1980, pp 137–147.
24. Weeden R, Burchell A: Alcohol and disease: Economic aspects. *Br Med Bull* 1982; 38(1):9–11.
25. Wells B, Stacey B: Social and psychological features of young drug misusers. *Br J Addict* 1976; 71:243–251.
26. Westermeyer J: Opium smoking in Laos: A survey of 40 addicts. *Am J Psychiatry* 1974; 131:165–170.
27. Westermeyer J: Opium availability and the prevalence of addiction in Asia. *Br J Addict* 1981; 76:85–90.

Further Reading

Cohen S: Reinforcement and rapid delivery systems: understanding adverse consequences of cocaine. *NIDA Res Monogr Ser* 1985; 61:151–157.

Walsh D, Grant M: *Public Health Implications of Alcohol Production and Trade.* World Health Organization Offset Publication, no. 88. Geneva, WHO, 1985.

6

Natural Course and Psychosocial Manifestations

1. Introduction

Drug dependence may occur as an acute, chronic recurrent, or chronic progressive disorder. The course varies with the individual, the drug, and the particular environmental circumstances. Drug dependence disorders differ from many other medical disorders in that the symptoms, particularly the psychological and behavioral ones, generally appear only when the drug is currently being used (at least in the early stages). The course of the disorder is therefore greatly influenced by drug dosage, duration of use, and frequency or pattern of use. At one end of the scale, some recreational drug use may not be pathological. At the other end of the scale, advanced drug dependence produces biomedical, psychological, and social pathologies.

2. Course of Drug Dependence

2.1. Manifestations of the Course

As has been mentioned, many substances of abuse have a normal, nonpathological, or nonabusive range of use. With alcohol, this use is called social drinking. Fortunately, most individuals stay with this level of usage, but some progress into abuse and dependency. Depending on the drug, the individuals, and the society, there are differences in the proportion of those who become dependent.

Certain early, prodromal signs may suggest that drug dependence is starting. The individual may begin to think about and anticipate the next drug-using experience. Drug use becomes an end in itself. The person may begin to organize his life around drug using, planning the next occasion, and ensuring beforehand that there is enough drug available. The individual may begin to feel that no social or recreational event is pleasurable without drug use. Because of shame or guilt, the incipient drug-dependent person may begin to hide the drug use. In this early stage, many drug-dependent persons consume the drug more rapidly than before. They typically become defensive and hostile when the drug-using behavior is criticized. Later, concern about overuse typically ensues, so that the person may make efforts to control the drug usage by reducing the amount or frequency of use or by changing the drug or route of administration. Instead of social usage, individual usage may appear, especially to relieve physical or emotional symptoms.

With respect to order of progression, it is helpful to subdivide the signs, symptoms, and social markers into separate dimensions, such as biomedical, psychological, and sociocultural features. In addition to drug-taking behavior and the direct pharmacological action of the drug, there are frequently secondary biomedical, economic, family, work, legal, and interpersonal problems.

Drug users do not typically maintain constant drug dose levels, although a minority do so for various lengths of time. Others use drugs only in binges with long periods of abstinence in between. Even heavy daily drug users may decrease the amount of drug taken in certain situations, such as after appearance of some physical complication or after appearance of a social, occupational, or legal threat. These variations in drug intake may be normal cyclical variations of the disorder; they are not necessarily signs of improvement. Complete loss of control over drug use is a rare and usually late event. Most drug users can sometimes control the level of their usage, but are unable to do so consistently or predictably.

Early, middle, and late phases are elaborated further in Table I on behavioral factors, Table II on psychological factors, Table III on social factors, Table IV on biomedical factors, and Table V on treatment approaches.[22]

2.2. Factors Affecting Course

The course and progression of substance abuse and dependence are clearly influenced by the particular substance and its inherent characteristics (e.g., fast versus slow-acting, speed of absorption). The route of administration is important; there is often more rapid progression with intravenous than oral use. Likewise the availability of drugs plays an important part.[23]

Age of onset of use and excessive use appear to be important.[11] Heavy drug use beginning at age 16 would exert a different influence on the life course compared to heavy use started at age 45. Elderly drug-dependent persons are less

Table I
Phases of Drug Dependence: Behavioral Factors[a]

Characteristic	Early phase: problematic usage	Middle phase: chronic dependence, addiction	Late phase: deterioration
Drug usage	Increasing amounts and frequency of use	"Titer" or "binge" usage; attempts at abstinence	Continuous usage; uses "substitute" intoxicants
Control over usage	Begins attempts to decrease amounts or frequency of use	Begins to lose control (takes more than intended or for a longer period than intended)	Loses control most of the time
Drug-related behavior	Seeks occasions to use; chooses friends who use heavily; may begin to be secretive about usage	Increased need to use at specific times and places; develops ingenuity at obtaining, paying for, hiding, and using drug	Compulsive usage, despite many problems associated with usage and decreased enjoyment from drug or alcohol; plans daily activities around usage
Drug effects on behavior	Episodic intoxication, dysarthria, emotional lability; attempts to hide drug or alcohol effects from others	Impairment between intoxication episodes: trite and illogical expressions prevail in conversation; fatigue; decreased productivity	Poor grooming, disheveled dress; lack of interest in appearance; unconcern with opinions of others

[a]Adapted from Westermeyer,[22] with permission.

Table II
Phases of Drug Dependence: Psychological Factors[a]

Characteristic	Early phase: problematic usage	Middle phase: chronic dependence, addiction	Late phase: deterioration
Motivation	Uses to enjoy, build up confidence, relieve insomnia, anxiety, etc.; use becomes increasingly important	Uses to feel normal; use is as important as family, friends, work	Enjoys usage less, but cannot stop; use becomes the central element of person's life
Emotional concomitants	Mood swings related to usage: anger, remorse, anxiety; shamed or anxious regarding usage; feels weak, remorseful	Personality change, increasing emotional lability; ambivalent about usage; feels guilty, resentful, inadequate, inferior	Erratic, suspicious, often apathetic; defensive regarding usage; feels alone, deserted
Cognitive processes	Obsesses regarding next usage; reduced interests and ambition; focuses thoughts and conversation on chemical usage	Increasing self-pity, deteriorating self-image, self-deception regarding usage and its effects; loses sense of time	Confused, projects own problems onto others; unable to conceptualize current status objectively
Judgment, insight	Begins to exercise poor judgment; still able to extricate self from most problems; episodic insight and concern with drug or alcohol usage	Large proportion of decisions lead to problems; problem solving increasingly ineffective; avoids being insightful, though capable of insight	Extremely poor judgment in most matters; unable to solve own problems; is not insightful even during abstinent intervals

[a]Adapted from Westermeyer,[22] with permission.

Table III
Phases of Drug Dependence: Social Factors[a]

Characteristic	Early phase: problematic usage	Middle phase: chronic dependence, addiction	Late phase: deterioration
Interpersonal relationships	Changes associates, from abstainers and moderate users to heavy users	Alienates others by arguing, embarrassing, taking advantage; breaks promises, lies	Manipulates others to obtain drug or alcohol; compensatory bragging
Family	Argues with family over usage; spends less time at home; neglects family emotionally	Abuses family by lying, stealing, and/or fighting; spends most of time away from home	Alienated from family; lives away from family
Employment	"Monday morning" absenteeism; conflict with boss	Decreased job efficiency; changes jobs often or is fired; decreasing job prestige; holds jobs for shorter periods	Day labor; unemployed, on relief or social welfare
Residence	Stable residence; lives with others	Begins moving from place to place; loses roommates, family members	Lower socioeconomic neighborhood; lives alone
School[b]	Decreasing grades; complaints from teachers	Suspension from school, school dropout	Requires special educational and rehabilitation facilities
Legal effects	May have legal problems; DWI,[c] disorderly, assault	Usually has legal problems and large attorney fees; may be litigious	Defaults on contractual obligations; may be imprisoned for property offenses, manslaughter
Finances	Spends increasing funds on drug or alcohol; may take extra job to support habit; may become extravagant	Spends large amount of annual income on drug or alcohol; heavily in debt, bankruptcy	Spends most of income on drugs or alcohol; financially destitute
Social affiliations	Discontinues social activities not involving alcohol or drug usage (e.g., church, sports)	Drops formal group affiliations; begins short-lived companionship with chemically dependent persons	Becomes an involuntary client of social institutions (e.g., jail, social welfare, hospitals)

[a]Adapted from Westermeyer,[22] with permission.
[b]For drug-dependent persons of school age.
[c]DWI, driving while intoxicated.

Table IV
Phases of Drug Dependence: Biomedical Factors[a]

Characteristic	Early phase: problematic usage	Middle phase: chronic dependence, addiction	Late phase: deterioration
Pharmacology	Tolerance increases; larger doses used to relax, relieve insomnia or other symptoms	Withdrawal effects; blackout (for alcohol); morning or daytime usage to alleviate withdrawal	Decreased tolerance (early onset of intoxication or blackout); delirium tremens or withdrawal seizure
Common health problems	Injuries: vehicular or industrial, accidents, falls, burns	Infections; respiratory, urogenital, skin; injuries, accidental overdosage, suicide attempt	Parenteral users: septicemia, pulmonary edema, endocarditis; alcoholics: cirrhosis; violence; injuries, homicide, suicide; nutritional problems: vitamin, protein, mineral deficiency; acquired immune deficiency syndrome (AIDS)
Sexual effects	May initially enhance sexual function	Sexual problems; impotence, frigidity, promiscuity or extramarital liaisons, venereal disease	Difficulty obtaining sexual partner; purchase of sexual services; loss of interest in sex; prostitution to obtain funds for drug
Common symptoms	Insomnia, boredom, chronic anxiety, headache, palpitations, tachycardia, flatulence, belching, cramps, epigastric distress, irritability, puffy face or extremities	Sweating, apprehension, decreased libido, visual disturbances, myalgia, malaise, obesity, diarrhea, weight change (loss or gain), memory lapses, weak, fatigues easily, "dry heaves," depression, panic, fears	Bad taste, impotence, halitosis, cachexia, persistent abdominal pain

[a] Adapted from Westermeyer,[22] with permission.

Table V
Phases of Drug Dependence: Treatment Approaches[a]

Characteristic	Early phase: problematic usage	Middle phase: chronic dependence, addiction	Late phase: deterioration
Prognosis without treatment	Some spontaneously improve, some progress to later stages (percentages unknown)	Small percentage spontaneously improve; most progress to later stage	Virtually no spontaneous improvement; a few "plateau"; most deteriorate rapidly
Most effective treatment modalities	Self-help groups; marital, family therapy; selective use of pharmacotherapy for 1–2 years (e.g., antidepressants, disulfiram), partial hospitalization (e.g., day only, evening only, weekend only)	Initial residential treatment: hospital or detoxification unit, therapeutic community, halfway house, followed by some outpatient treatment methods, as in "early phase"	Long-term residential treatment: special long-term units, nursing home, quarter-way house, followed by "middle" or "early" treatment methods in selected cases, methadone maintenance for opioid dependence
Prognosis with optimal treatment	Good to very good: 60–80% "significantly improved" at 1 year posttreatment	Fair to good: 30–60% "significantly improved" at 1 year posttreatment	Fair to poor: 10–30% improved at 1 year; high mortality and morbidity rate in remainder
Cooperation with treatment	Willing to undertake a prolonged period of abstinence, see physician regularly, follow treatment recommendations	Does not enter treatment unless pressured by family, employer, court, friends, physician	Will not undertake abstinence voluntarily; must be coerced by society (e.g., incarceration, legal commitment into treatment)

[a]Adapted from Westermeyer,[24] with permission.

likely to have marital, employment, and legal problems associated with drug use, but more likely to have biomedical problems and social isolation as compared to younger drug-dependent persons. Women in some settings demonstrate more rapid progression than men.[27] Periods of complete or relative abstinence can moderate the course. Thus, reduced dosage or episodic abstinence can be valid treatment objectives when total lifelong abstinence is not possible or likely.

The natural history of involvement with a drug is influenced by a number of different factors. Social learning and social expectations of the culture exert a strong influence. Excessive use is favored when decisions about drug use are made by the individual rather than by other group members (e.g., family, the physician, a religious group). Earlier onset of drug dependence tends to favor heavier use and a worse outcome; younger users tend to have more antisocial and self-defeating behavior. The distressed, depressed, and maladjusted person tends to progress more rapidly. Other common factors related to stability or progression are cost of the drug and legal prohibitions. Despite wide social and cultural differences around the world, drug-dependent persons still experience a progression in the type and severity of problems which is remarkably similar from country to country for a particular drug.[1,3,5,13,18]

3. Natural Course According to Type of Drug

The natural course for several common drugs is presented here. These are the drugs which have been most thoroughly researched up to the current time.

3.1. Opioids

The course of heroin drug dependence has been shown to be more rapid in comparison to opium, as shown by a study of 51 matched pairs.[26] Heroin dependents took more doses of drug per day and spent more money on drugs, but they also sought treatment sooner than patients dependent on opium. Heroin apparently leads to a more rapid course as compared to opium.

Opium smokers in Asia as well as chronic alcoholics often stay on stable dosages for extended periods, up to a decade or two, without any rapid progression or deterioration. However, the eventual mortality among opium-dependent persons and alcoholics has been consistently higher than that among the general population. Within a decade or two of initiating heavy use, most opium-dependent persons and alcoholics make a serious attempt at abstaining from the drug. Most succeed in abstaining for a period of time even without treatment, especially if economic or legal problems are present or the drug is not available.[20,23]

A small percentage of opium-dependent persons eventually give up drugs, sometimes after two or three decades of use. This has been referred to as maturing out from drug dependence. Absence of opiate drugs in the immediate environment also greatly facilitates recovery and abstinence. There is a danger that opium-dependent patients may turn to alcohol dependence, as well as vice versa.

3.2. Alcohol

The course of alcohol dependence can be divided into four phases: the prealcoholic phase, the prodromal phase, the crucial phase, and the chronic phase.[8] The following three main symptoms can be viewed as markers:

1. The onset of amnesia while drinking (i.e., blackouts) signals the start of the prodromal phase.
2. The inability to regulate the amount or duration of drinking (i.e., loss of control) marks the start of the crucial phase; loss of control may be partial or intermittent.
3. The onset of prolonged intoxications marks the beginning of the chronic phase.

Not every alcohol-dependent person has all of these symptoms, nor do they necessarily occur in that order.

Symptom clusters have also been used to assess progression rather than individual symptoms, as follows:

1. Onset of psychological dependence (i.e., needing, planning for, and anticipating drinking).
2. Tremor, morning drinking, and amnesia (i.e., mild withdrawal).
3. Alcoholism psychosis (i.e., severe withdrawal).[12]

This general order of symptom appearance has been confirmed by observation of alcohol-abusing and -dependent persons.[15] Alcoholic drinking behaviors may be found in some nonalcoholic drinkers, but symptoms indicating marked increased tolerance, physical dependence, withdrawal reactions, and physical damage do not occur among normal drinkers. Certain behaviors appear more often in histories of alcohol-dependent drinkers than in the histories of social drinkers. These include symptoms such as tremors after drinking, frequent binge drinking, frequent blackouts, and hospitalization for effects of drinking. Certain behaviors, such as first alcoholic blackout, when present, appeared earlier in the history of nonalcoholics (average age 22.0 years) than in alcoholics (average age reported 30.8 years). Although this may seem paradoxical, such an adverse reaction in young drinkers who profit from experience may have a positive effect; the individual may learn something about controlling or reducing drinking from the experience. Those who do not experience blackout or withdrawal symptoms (i.e., hangover) until they reach higher doses or have chronic drinking habits may be at greater risk of alcohol dependence.

Various forms and courses of alcoholism have been described, as follows[9]:

1. Alpha alcoholism—a continual psychological dependence on alcohol, without loss of control or inability to abstain; this shows no tendency to progress.
2. Beta alcoholism—physical damage from alcohol, but without physical or psychological dependence.
3. Gamma alcoholism—this conforms most closely to the popular notion of alcoholism, with tolerance, physical dependence, withdrawal symptoms, and loss of control.
4. Delta alcoholism—this resembles gamma alcoholism, but instead of loss of control there is inability to abstain. There is high intake, but at a stabilized level.
5. Epsilon alcoholism—this is periodic or binge alcoholism, or dipsomania.

It is now recognized that these forms or courses of alcoholism are not at all mutually exclusive. Rather, a few or several of these categories tend to coexist over time in the alcohol-dependent person. Nonetheless, these categories may aid in understanding or describing a patient's drinking patterns.

Remissions from alcoholism can occur at all ages. Over the short term, alcoholism resembles a remitting but progressive illness. Alcoholics who experience the most severe consequences often achieve the most stable recoveries. Resumption of asymptomatic drinking (at least temporarily) is common among former alcohol dependents. Extent of previous drinking makes a substantial difference. Return to asymptomatic drinking is more possible for those who have only mild or recent alcohol-related problems, whereas chronic, severely alcohol-dependent persons tend not to have a benign course.[21] Not unexpectedly, alcoholics have high death rates in comparison with the general population.[25]

Untreated alcohol-dependent persons tend to do poorly over time.[10] However, a few do recover without formal treatment, a process sometimes called spontaneous recovery.

3.3. Cocaine

Cocaine use may occur temporarily as an occasional social or recreational habit. However, this substance creates a powerful urge to use stronger and more frequent dosages in users if use persists.

It appears that the moderate use of coca leaves by the Indians in the Andean highlands has not led to major complications,[2] but chronic heavy use of the leaves has been associated with drug-dependence problems in lowland areas of South America. The extraction of pure cocaine from coca leaves and coca paste smoking have exacerbated this situation radically.

In animal experiments where there is access to unlimited amounts of intravenous cocaine, the animals rapidly escalate drug-seeking behavior to the exclusion of eating and copulation. Monkeys in this kind of experiment have died within 5 days.[4] Although such a situation would be hard to duplicate in human beings, it is nevertheless true that cocaine users can develop severe craving and increased consumption to a point that leads to severe physical, psychological, and social problems, and even death from overdose. Cocaine is often alternated with use of other drugs such as amphetamines, opioids, and alcohol.[2]

3.4. Tobacco

Habitual tobacco smoking involves a nicotine dependence, probably reinforced by repetitive operant and Pavlovian conditioning. The one-pack-a-day smoker is self-administering approximately 70,000 boluses of nicotine a year.[17]

Tobacco dependence often begins early in adolescence, usually as a peer-influenced behavior. As with other dependence-producing drugs, psychosocial factors account for initial use while psychopharmacological factors account for continual use. If the behavior becomes intense and persists, the inhalation of smoke from burning tobacco can continue for a lifetime. Large numbers of smokers do spontaneously abstain, but 70–80% relapse within a year.[17] Programs to assist abstinence employ techniques such as immediate cessation, education, and dietary and attitudinal adjustments. These programs have good results initially, but 60–70% of clients relapse approximately 3 months posttreatment. Individual counseling, hypnosis, aversive conditioning, and nicotine chewing gum also provide encouraging initial results, with a similar high relapse after 1 year posttreatment.[14]

Tobacco dependence on cigarettes is expressed in terms of pack-years. One pack-year consists of a pack of cigarettes per day (containing 20 cigarettes) taken over a 1-year period. Ten pack-years could consist of one pack per day over 10 years, 1.5 packs per day over 6.7 years, or two packs per day over 5 years.

Physical complications associated with chronic tobacco dependence include lung cancer and heart disease. These begin to appear in a population of smokers after about 20 pack-years. Local irritative phenomena, such as sinusitis, gingivitis, laryngitis, or bronchitis, may occur much earlier.[16]

Various forms of smoking have different effects, probably in association with their greater or lesser tendency for deep inhaling into the lungs. Cigarette smoking generally leads to greater dependence than cigar or pipe smoking (although these also can be heavily abused).

3.5. Cannabis

Repeated cannabis use leads to tolerance. One of the complications of heavy cannabis use (or even lighter use in sensitive individuals) is deterioration of mental functioning. Vulnerable users may develop the amotivational syndrome, consisting of diminished ambition and drive, apathy, distractibility, impaired skills in communicating, introversion, and experiences of derealization and depersonalization. There is controversy regarding whether this syndrome is due to preexisting psychopathology, an associated personality change, or the neurotoxic effects of chronic cannabis use.[2]

3.6. Polydrug Abuse

Commonly drug-dependent persons use two or more mind-altering drugs. These may be used simultaneously (e.g., alcohol and tobacco), or they may be alternated or rotated (e.g., stimulants during the day and sedatives at bedtime). This practice has been called polydrug abuse. Use of more than one drug frequently ensues when a predominant social form of drug dependence (i.e., opioids, cannabis, alcohol) is successfully reduced in a society.

Reasons for polydrug abuse include the following:

1. Variation in availability and cost, so that the person uses drugs that are readily available and low in cost.
2. Attempts to heighten desired effects or diminish side effects, such as by using a stimulant during the day and a depressant at night.
3. Choice of a different class of drugs for different settings and times, such as using alcohol in a group and cannabis when alone.
4. Drug exploration or experimentation among individuals who try anything.[2]

Polydrug abuse can present special problems for diagnosis and treatment. For example, two drugs may be used in doses which alone would not be dependency-producing, but which together produce dependence. One drug may be used to cope with the untoward consequences of another drug, such as taking sedatives to sleep after having abused stimulants. When the patient is a polydrug abuser, treatment for only one substance can result in rebound abuse of other drugs.

4. Psychosocial Consequences of Drug Dependence

4.1. Special Aspects

A condition such as drug dependence which disables a person or has a major impact on behavior will also have repercussions on the family and other social groups. Drugs that affect behavior the most (e.g., opiates, alcohol, sedatives, amphetamine, cocaine) are most likely to affect the patient's social network, but effects on the family, friends, and co-workers can also occur in a muted fashion with other drugs as well (e.g., tobacco, cannabis, betel-areca, khat).

The immediate social context of drug use is a powerful factor in developing and sustaining psychoactive dependence. Factors favoring drug abuse include the following: drug dependence among socially significant others, tolerance of deviant drug use by significant others, other associated deviant group behavior (e.g., theft, corruption), and nonhelpfulness of immediate others. As people use drugs in a deviant fashion, they tend to associate with others who are deviant users. The latter in turn reinforce further deviant psychoactive use. As the group becomes more unlike the general population, both external pressures and internal attractions favor development of a drug subculture. Such groups have norms, values, behaviors, even jargon, dress, greetings, and symbols that reinforce their subcultural identity. This social identity may in turn reinforce further deviant drug use. Likewise, subgroups can become extremely powerful aids to recovery, as exemplified by self-help groups.

4.2. The Family

A dysfunctional family may set the stage for drug dependence, especially in adolescent offspring. Conversely, drug problems cause severe trouble for most families, even those which are otherwise structurally intact and functional.

Drugs and associated costs lead to an economic drain on family resources. Job security and earning effectiveness may be compromised. This can require that the spouse and children either support the family or accommodate to financial reverses. Behavior of a drug-dependent family member may disrupt the everyday rhythm of family life, including eating, sleeping, home maintenance, recreation, and religious observances. Marital relationships may be distorted by arguments which may escalate to physical violence, cessation of sexual relations, and cycles of mutual blame–reproach–guilt–manipulation. The nondependent spouse may be drawn into increasingly maladaptive and counterproductive behaviors—a situation aptly described as family codependence.

Children in these families have a higher incidence of reported child abuse, incest, school problems, and social delinquency. Often the children assume parenting roles (the so-called role reversal) because the marital pair have both become dysfunctional parents. These children who take care of their drug-dependent parents often feel responsible for both the drug problems and the ensuing family problems. In these situations the children may alternately manifest hostile rejection and rescuing behavior vis-à-vis their parents.

The family may deny existence of the drug-dependence problem. Several years may elapse before the family asks for help with the problem. Three family phases of drug dependence have been described, as follows:

1. Early—the family initially denies the problem, then conceals its presence from outsiders.
2. Middle—the family experiences crisis and chaos, but is confused about what to do.

3. Late—three outcomes are possible:
   a. Homeostasis—maintenance of a pathological but steady status.
   b. Restitution and rehabilitation—abstinence from drugs and recovery from drug dependence.
   c. Deterioration and destruction—a self-destructive course, with social disability and premature death for the patient and further family deterioration.

See Figure 1 for a schematic representation of restitution and rehabilitation.

Drug dependence affects family rituals, such as family celebration of holidays, having a daily meal together, and annual vacations at the same location and at the same time each year. Interference with family rituals can lead to two types of outcomes. In one type of family, the drug-dependent parent's behavior does not seriously interfere with the observance of the family ritual. The children of these families are less likely to become drug dependent later in life. In the other type of family, ritual observance by family members is adversely affected by the drug-dependent parent's behavior. The children in these latter families are more likely to become drug dependent.[28]

4.3. Types of Families in Drug Dependence[19]

No one family schema for drug dependence can be adequate for all societies, since family structure and function vary widely from one ethnic group to the next. The family systems described here are merely examples of family organization as encountered clinically among drug-dependent persons.

The functional family system is apparently stable and functional. The marital pair have reasonable sexual adjustment and maintain good parenting function; the children are reasonably well adjusted. The drug dependence is usually an individual response to life stress and individual conflict. Drug use often occurs outside the home and does not disrupt family operations.

In the enmeshed family system, members are overly involved and dependent on one another. Drug-dominated behavior interrupts normal family tasks, causes conflict, shifts family roles, and requires adjustive and adaptive responses from the family. Drug use in a parent impairs sexual desire and performance in chronic stages, further alienating the marital couple. The enmeshed family is ill equipped to cope with the added burden of dependent behavior. Excessive drug use occurs when family anxiety is high, and in turn the drug use generates more family anxiety in a vicious, self-perpetuating cycle of escalating problems.

The disintegrated family system is often a later stage of either of the two previous family systems. There is usually a history of earlier stable family life that has steadily deteriorated. By the time of entry into treatment, these family systems have collapsed. Often the parents have separated, if not divorced. There is overt hostility and alienation between the family and the patient. Relatives may

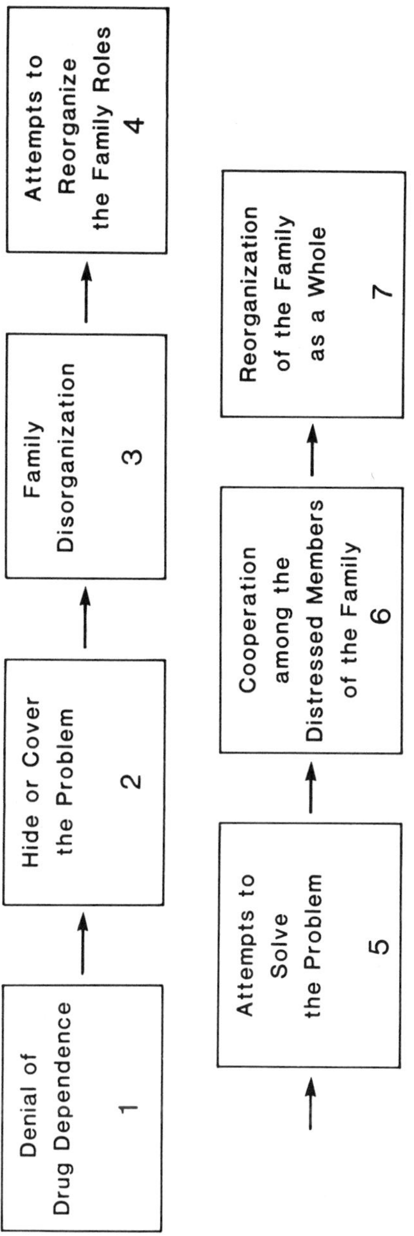

Figure 1. Adjustment to drug dependence by the family. (From Ref. 7. Reprinted with permission.)

be called in by remaining family members as allies against the patient. The patient has usually lost work, has been ejected from parent–child relationships, and has been excluded from most family activities.

The absent family system represents the end stage of family deterioration. Either all ties with family of origin have been lost, or the patient never established an independent marital/family system. Drug-dependent persons of this type have few family contacts, few friends, and no social or vocational resources. Their sparse social networks consist of other heavy drug users who offer minimal social support for recovery.

4.4. Family Health Problems

Spouses, offspring, and parents of substance abusers often present to the clinician with a variety of somatoform, psychophysiological, or allergic problems, such as palpitations, vague aches and pains, weakness or dizziness, but also migraine, tension headaches, gastritis, irritable bowel syndrome, allergic rhinitis and conjunctivitis, and eczema. At times these problems can be disabling, even life threatening when they involve disorders such as peptic ulcer, ulcerative colitis, and bronchial asthma.

Marital partners of drug-dependent individuals may seek medical care for symptoms related to dysfunctional sexuality. In female partners, dyspareunia can occur. Among male partners, impotence may result.

Typically these patients do not link their pain or dysfunction to the drug dependence in their family member. When the clinician asks about drug dependence in the family, however, the patient usually reports it readily. It is a major and overwhelming problem, which they do not know how to manage. Given the physician's support and conceptual tools regarding management, these patients can proceed on a plan to intervene in their family member's drug dependency. At least they can learn how to cope better themselves by regaining control over their lives and finding alternate means of handling the family problem.

In most cases the physician has not previously been aware of the drug dependence in the family member of the patient. It is necessary to routinely ask about drug dependence in the family when patients with somatoform or psychophysiological disorders are encountered. In cases where the clinician knows the family well, the physician may already be aware of this problem. It is then a simple matter to relate the patient's present illness to the family presence of drug dependence.

A common psychiatric disorder affecting family members of drug-dependent relatives is depression. This results from the frustration, loss, guilt, shame, and anger with the drug-dependent relative. Given the genetic and familial links between drug dependence and depression, it is not unusual that family members are at risk for depression in the presence of environmental stresses.

The most commonly affected family member is the spouse, but parents or offspring may also develop psychiatric conditions. Parents often feel responsible for the fact that their son or daughter is abusing drugs, even if the offspring is an adult. The instability within the family creates difficulty for the children, including the adolescent offspring. Whereas spouses or parents may demonstrate their emotional distress as depression, the children and adolescent offspring are more likely to manifest disturbances in conduct or academic underachievement. Children or adolescents may abandon friends and become socially withdrawn or discontinue a favorite hobby or sport.

At times the family member may relate the psychiatric disturbance directly to the fact that another family member is dependent on drugs. At other times he may not make that link himself and thus may neglect to tell the clinician about it. Thus, it is important that the physician inquire in such cases whether there is a drug-dependent family member.

Clinicians may first encounter the family member as a victim of violence at the hands of a drug-dependent relative. The violence is at times inadvertent. For example, the family member may be victimized when the drug-dependent person has caused a vehicular accident or started a fire. At other times the violence may be purposeful, such as an assault. The family member may make a suicide attempt, possibly as a means of calling attention to the family distress. Victims of family violence may range from newborns to the elderly. Dependent or disabled family members may suffer from neglect, with inadequate food or clothing, when a drug-dependent person refuses or is unable to provide for them.

It is not unusual for the spouse or offspring of a drug-dependent patient to begin themselves abusing drugs. In most situations this consists of a wife who begins to use drugs along with her husband, sometimes after opposing the use unsuccessfully over a period of time. Adolescent offspring may also begin to abuse drugs. When preteenage children or even younger children in elementary school begin abusing drugs, the clinician should investigate whether one or both parents are drug dependent.

5. Recovery

5.1. Chronology of Recovery

The time frame of recovery varies from patient to patient. Most biomedical recovery occurs by 1 year after becoming drug free, depending on the duration of drug exposure and on relapses. Physiological recovery continues over several weeks to several months. Complete adaptation to sobriety varies with intensity of educational and treatment effort and patient motivation, but probably is not complete for 2 years in most cases. Grief work, psychological maturation, and social reintegration may take up to 5 years.

Figure 2 demonstrates the relapse rate after treatment for heroin, cigarette smoking, and alcohol dependence. This graph combines several studies done prior to 1970. At that time the interventions were time-limited, with little continuing care (sometimes referred to as aftercare). With more modern approaches and early case finding, the treatment outcome has improved. However, this classical graph does demonstrate clearly the trend for most relapse to occur in the first 3 months. After 6 months, the rate of recurrence decreases. The recurrence rate after spontaneous abstention among rural opium smokers in Asia is remarkably similar.

The person recovering from drug dependence must make a series of physical, behavioral, psychological, social, and sometimes even spiritual or ideological changes. These vary in intensity depending on the drug type and the severity of drug dependence. Nonetheless, the changes occur in a fairly predictable sequence at various stages in recovery. It is helpful for clinicians, patients, and their families to appreciate these phases and their temporary nature.

5.2. Psychological Concomitants of Recovery

When a dependent person ceases using drugs, a consistent series of physical and psychological events follows. The central nervous system begins healing, but low-grade withdrawal symptoms and signs may continue for several months. When the dependent person is safely abstinent, people in the social network may dare to become distraught and express their own needs and feelings. However, the

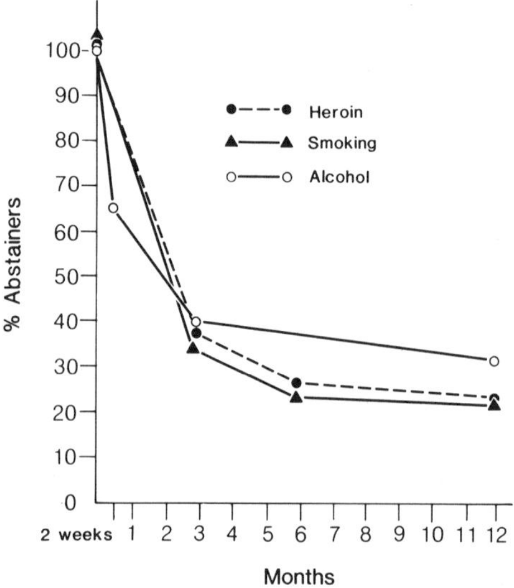

Figure 2. Relapse rate over time for heroin, smoking, and alcohol. (From Ref. 6. Reprinted with permission.)

recovering person may still be in trouble at work or before the law for things done while using drugs. These changes and challenges produce intense, stormy feelings. Now the recovering person can no longer use the drug to suppress these feelings. Emotional reactions buried under drugs for years may surge forth. Feelings and memories not previously dealt with may well up. At this stage the recovering person needs help accepting and living through these strong feelings.

Even those who have not yet damaged their health, family, or career still have many losses. At the least, they have lost time from their lives, missed opportunities, and ignored life's rewarding experiences. They may have lost social status. And, in recovery, they further lose drugs, which they may have perceived as their only reliable and soothing companion. Self-esteem has usually been undermined from loss of control over drugs and from guilt or shame over transgressions while intoxicated. Relationships, financial or career standing, and health may be destroyed or undermined. These losses must be acknowledged, borne, and put in perspective during recovery.

5.3. Social Concomitants of Recovery

It is natural for drug-dependent persons to protect themselves from their helplessness by denial and by regressive feelings of omnipotence and grandiosity. Or they may react to guilt by blaming others. These defense patterns, erected to protect or compensate for drug use, may become habitual, with an existence of their own. Upon stopping drugs, the recovering person must replace these childish defense patterns with mature patterns. This maturation process can be fostered in group settings, especially in self-help groups. It may take years and is not always completely accomplished.

Recovery varies not only from drug to drug, but from culture to culture. When a drug is illegal or deviant in a given culture, users have different psychological characteristics from those using legal drugs. For example, European and American women took legal opiate remedies in the nineteenth century. They appear to have had more in common vis-à-vis their recovery needs with alcohol-dependent women and prescription drug abusers in the twentieth century than with twentieth-century urban opiate abusers. This is so because the legality of the drug influences the type of problems sometimes more than the pharmacological properties of the drug being abused.

5.4. Clinical and Demographic Considerations

Different populations of drug abusers have special recovery needs: patients with serious psychiatric or physical illnesses, elderly people, ethnic minority groups, women, and adolescents. For example, adolescents using a range of hallucinogens, cannabis, tobacco, alcohol, cocaine, phencyclidine, and sedatives need treatment approaches that reflect sophistication about their developmental needs as adolescents in addition to their drug use. Adolescents' denial of difficulty with drugs is usually related to their expectations that nothing bad can ever happen to them. A common proverb states, "Young people believe they will live forever." As a normal part of adolescence, there is a greater willingness to accept risks. Conversely, denial of drug dependence among geriatric populations is often supported by a doctor or pharmacist, who provides the drug to the elderly person.

5.5. Recovery According to Different Drugs of Abuse

Differences occur in recovery patterns for different drugs of abuse. The differences result from the varying pharmacological effects of the drugs, as well as from characteristics of drug use in a particular social or legal context. In particular, early recovery depends strongly on the type of drug since abstinence syndromes and medical complications vary widely among drugs. For example, sedatives and opioids can produce severe withdrawal, while neither cocaine nor psychedelic drugs typically cause a severe abstinence syndrome.

Treatment of abuse of alcohol, other sedatives, and opioid drugs must take into account two characteristics: the addictive property of the drug, and the cumulative production of mild to moderate central nervous system dysfunction (from the drug or associated biomedical conditions) which persists after cessation of use. Patients usually look and feel ill during excessive drug use and show considerable healing the first 3–12 months after becoming drug free, with decreased desire to take drugs and improved subjective well-being and mood regulation.

Stimulants and hallucinogens may produce disorganization of psychological function to the point of confusion or even psychosis. Recovery is marked by a period of depression and lethargy. Some individuals require psychiatric hospitalization and treatment during this phase of recovery. Much of their psychopathology usually improves within a few weeks of being drug free, although this may require several months to a year in chronic users. Patients are usually relieved to hear that some of their depression and mental dysfunction is part of healing, an expected effect of the drug leaving the brain. Once aware that these symptoms can be expected to improve in most cases, recovering patients can usually tolerate them during the early months of abstinence.

References

1. Berger LJ, Westermeyer J: World traveler addicts in Asia: II. Comparison with "Stay at Home" addicts. *Am J Drug Alcohol Abuse* 1977; 4:495–503; abstract in *Yale Psychiatr Q*, Spring 1979.
2. Cohen S: *The Substance Abuse Problems*. New York, Haworth Press, 1981.
3. Dudley DL, Roszell DK, Mules JE, Hague WH: Heroin vs alcohol addiction—Quantifiable psychosocial similarities and differences. *J Psychosom Res* 1974; 18:327–335.

4. Grinspoon L, Bakalar J: Cocaine, in Dupont R, Goldstein A, O'Donnell J (eds): *Handbook on Drug Abuse*. Rockville, MD, NIDA, 1979, chap 22.
5. Halikas JA, Rimmer JD: Predictors of multiple drug abuse. *Arch Gen Psychiatry* 1974; 31:414–418.
6. Hunt WA, Barnett LW, Branch LG: Relapse rates in addiction programs. *J Clin Psychol* 1971; 27:455–456.
7. Jackson JK: The adjustment of the family to the crisis of alcholism. *Q J Stud Alcohol* 1954; 15:562–586.
8. Jellinek EM: Phases of alcohol addiction. *Q J Stud Alcohol* 1952; 13:675–684.
9. Jellinek EM: *The Disease Concept of Alcoholism*. New Haven, CT, College and University Press, 1959, pp 36–41.
10. Kendall RE, Staton MC: The fate of untreated alcoholics. *Q J Stud Alcohol* 1966; 27:30–41.
11. Kissin B: The pharmacodynamics and natural history of alcoholism, in Kissin B, Begleiter H (eds): *The Biology of Alcoholism*. Vol 3: *Clinical Pathology*. New York, Plenum Press, 1974, chap 1.
12. Orford J, Hawker A: Note on the ordering of onset of symptoms in alcohol dependence. *Psychol Med* 1974; 4:281–288.
13. Park P: Developmental ordering of experience in alcoholism. *Q J Stud Alcohol* 1973; 34:473–488.
14. Peckacek TF: Modification of smoking behavior, in Krasnagor NA (ed): *The Behavioral Aspects of Smoking*. NIDA Research Monograph 26. Washington, DC, U.S. Government Printing Office, 1979.
15. Pokorny A, Kanas T, Overall J: Order of appearance of alcoholic symptoms. *Alcoholism: Clin Exp Res* 1981, 5:216–220.
16. Russell MAH: Smoking problems: An overview, in Sarvik ME, Cullen JW, Gritz E (eds): *Research on Smoking Behavior*. NIDA Research Monograph 17. Washington, DC, U.S. Government Printing Office, 1977.
17. Schiffman SM: The tobacco withdrawal syndrome, in Krasnagor NA (ed): *Cigarette Smoking as a Dependence Process*. NIDA Research Monograph 23. Washington, DC, U.S. Government Printing Office, 1979.
18. Schuckit MA, Russell JW: Clinical importance of age at first drink in a group of young men. *Am J Psychiatry* 1983; 140:1221–1223.
19. Steinglass P: Experimenting with family treatment approaches to alcoholism, 1950–1975: A review. *Family Process* 1976; 15:97–123.
20. Vaillant GE: The natural history of narcotic drug addiction. *Semin Psychiatry* 1970; 2(4):486–498.
21. Vaillant GE, Milofsky E: Natural history of male alcoholism. IV. Paths to recovery. *Arch Gen Psychiatry* 1982; 39:127–135.
22. Westermeyer J: *A Clinical Guide to Alcohol and Drug Problems*. New York, Praeger, 1986.
23. Westermeyer J: *Poppies, Pipes and People, Opium and Its Use in Laos*. Berkeley, CA, University of California Press, 1983.
24. Westermeyer J: *Primer on Chemical Dependency: A Clinical Guide to Drug and Alcohol Problems*. Baltimore, Williams & Wilkins, 1976.
25. Westermeyer J, Peake E: A ten-year follow-up of alcoholic Native Americans in Minnesota. *Am J Psychiatry* 1983; 140:189–194.
26. Westermeyer J, Peng G: Opium and heroin addicts in Laos. II. A study of matched pairs. *J Nerv Ment Dis* 1977; 184:351–354.
27. Wilsnack SC: Alcohol abuse and alcoholism in women, in Pattison EM, Kaufman E (eds): *Encyclopedic Handbook of Alcoholism*. New York, Gardner Press, 1982, chap 57.
28. Wolin SJ, Bennett LA: Family rituals. *Family Process* 1984; 23:401–420.

III

Pharmacological Factors

7

Pharmacology of Dependence-Producing Drugs

1. Introduction

This chapter presents information on psychoactive drugs that are liable to abuse, including such substances as alcohol, tobacco, betel-areca, industrial solvents, and khat. Even milder psychoactive substances (e.g., caffeine, betel-areca) are covered since patients often present in the clinical setting with combined use of psychoactive substances. Patients may substitute certain of these substances for other substances. Increasingly in recent years, new drugs are available in communities where formerly only a few traditional drugs were prevalent. Highly potent "designer drugs" (see Chapter 10) are now being synthesized by sophisticated chemists who produce illicit or dangerous substances for their own profit. The clinician must therefore be familiar with a spectrum of drug types. Pharmacological principles as they relate to drugs of abuse are stressed.

2. Metabolism and the Drugs of Abuse

2.1. Absorption

Unless drugs are taken intravenously, they must cross the surface of the pulmonary alveoli, nasal or oral mucosa, or some portion of the intestine. Some alcohol absorption takes place in the stomach.[30] Drugs may also enter the fetal circulation via cell membranes in the placenta.

The route of administration markedly affects the onset and the degree of drug effect. For example, cocaine in the chewed coca leaf is slowly absorbed via the buccal mucosa. It is absorbed rapidly, however, when the purified cocaine powder is inhaled nasally, injected, or when cocaine freebase is combusted and smoked.

Absorption of drugs through biological membranes generally is characterized by the following:

1. Drugs in high concentration diffuse into areas of low concentration.
2. Compounds higher in lipid solubility tend to cross membranes more readily.
3. Movement of charged particles of weak acids or bases depends on the pH of the environment, so that gastric acid or the alkaline intestine influences the rate of absorption.

2.2. Drug Distribution

Drugs that are soluble in body water and cross membranes readily may be distributed into nearly all body water. This occurs with ethyl alcohol. Charged compounds do not readily cross cellular membranes.

The cellular barrier of the blood vessel endothelium generally has gaps or maculae, which make it relatively easy for drugs to exit. Some areas of the body, such as the central nervous system (CNS), may resist penetration by some drugs. After psychoactive drugs are ingested, they must reach the blood stream and be so distributed that they reach the effector site in the brain and provoke the effect. The area of highest concentration of a drug may not be the site of action. For example, tetrahydrocannabinol is widely distributed to sites outside of the CNS; it is then metabolized in these sites.[48]

Some drugs are simply distributed as solutes in blood, but other drugs are associated with blood constituents. The most important example is the binding of drug to plasma protein, usually albumin. Such binding may significantly affect the distribution of the drug to other sites in the body. The binding, by decreasing the amount of free drug in the plasma, may retard the movement of free drug and decrease the amount available for transfer across the capillary endothelium to sites of action, metabolism, and excretion. Hence, both the effect and the elimination of the drug may be altered. Since the binding is reversible and in equilibrium, free drug will be replenished by bound drug dissociated from the drug–protein complex. Binding may constitute a reservoir for drugs. For example, methadone has a prolonged effect, in part because it is highly bound to plasma protein. Drugs may be distributed to body stores and later released slowly. This may occur with chronic cannabis use, as the cannabis is stored in body fat.

There is a physical basis for the blood–brain barrier. Capillaries in the brain do not permit entrance or exit of drugs as readily as do capillaries elsewhere. More important, the brain capillaries do not permit direct access to the interstitium. Interposed between the capillary endothelium and the brain's extracellular space is another membrane in close apposition to the capillary wall. This barrier is made up of lengthy processes of astrocytes, which form a sheath around the capillaries. It is a barrier only to water-soluble molecules which are not actively transported. Lipid-soluble substances diffuse across this double barrier efficiently. Heroin, sodium thiopental, and cocaine all cross very rapidly. Since the brain receives nearly one-fifth of the cardiac output, lipid-soluble drugs are rapidly distributed to the brain.

The volume of drug distribution is a theoretical volume that describes the distribution of drug in body water. For example, if a drug is injected into the blood stream and it never penetrates the capillary endothelium, it remains in the intravascular space. Such a drug would be mixed and diluted in approximately 3 liters of plasma water. Its volume of distribution then would approximate 3 liters. However, if a compound's lipid solubility enables it to traverse both the capillary endothelium and the membranes of cells, then it is equally distributed in both intra- and extravascular water. Such a drug will have a volume of distribution equal to total body water, which is about 40 liters. Ethyl alcohol is an example of one such drug.

2.3. Termination of Drug Actions

Single doses of drugs have a relatively brief effect on most organisms. Termination is of three types: redistribution, metabolism, and excretion, the latter two processes generally being most important.

2.3.1. Drug Metabolism (Biotransformation)

Drug metabolism refers to chemical modification of drugs which usually diminishes their activity and promotes their excretion. Since most drugs are lipid soluble and enter tissues readily, they are not easily eliminated from the body without modification. Highly lipid-soluble drugs, which pass through the glomerulus, easily diffuse or are actively transported back into the renal tubular cells and reenter the circulatory system. In general, biotransformation yields compounds (called metabolites) that are more water soluble and more easily excreted in urine, sweat, and bile. Drug metabolites almost always have a diminished volume of distribution and do not readily penetrate cellular membranes.

Not all metabolites are inactive. Occasionally the process of chemical change yields an active compound (perhaps even more active than the original compound), which may then be further metabolized. For example, about 10% of codeine is transformed to morphine. Codeine may exert little or no effect by itself prior to the transformation. Morphine is then conjugated to glucuronic acid and excreted in the urine as morphine glucuronide. Heroin is also biotransformed to morphine and ultimately excreted as the glucuronide. Urine screening for heroin usually depends on morphine excretion as an indicator. These factors are important for criminal justice programs which use urine screening methods to detect opioid use or abuse, since sufficient quantities of codeine can mimic morphine or heroin abuse on certain sensitive urine screen methods.

The enzymes that metabolize drugs in humans are generally nonspecific. Alcohol dehydrogenase is one of the enzymes responsible for metabolizing ethanol, but it also metabolizes methanol, isopropyl alcohol, and diethylene glycol. The mixed-function oxidase or cytochrome P-450 enzymes associated with the endoplasmic reticulum in the liver (the microsomes) and other organs (e.g., lungs) are nonspecific and may alter substances of widely differing structure as long as they are lipid soluble and can attain entrance to hepatic and other cells.

Another common means of metabolism is conjugation, in which the drug is attached to a glucuronide or sulfate radical, as in the metabolism of morphine and heroin. Other psychoactive drugs, including phenobarbital, amphetamine, and meperidine (pethidine), are oxidized by microsomal enzymes. Ethanol is oxidized by the nonmicrosomal enzymes alcohol dehydrogenase and aldehyde oxidase. Some compounds are subject to both synthetic and conjugative biotransformation. The synthetic reaction often provides a center for conjugation. For example, chlorpromazine and diazepam are oxidized by P-450 and may then be conjugated.

Studies of enzyme-catalyzed biochemical reactions have generated concepts that are useful in understanding rates of biotransformation and elimination of drugs. Basically, two rates of enzymic reactions occur: first order and zero order. In first-order reactions, the concentration of drug is far below the level that would saturate the enzyme. The reaction velocity is proportional to the concentration of the drug. With more drug there will be more metabolite. A first-order rate will yield a constant proportion of metabolite to amount of remaining drug. For example, if 100 units of drug interact with an enzyme, a first-order rate would produce 50 units of metabolite per unit of time; 1000 units of drug, 500 units of metabolite; and so forth. Most psychoactive drugs so react. For a zero-order rate, the concentration of drug saturates the enzyme so that the evolution of metabolite is characterized by a fixed amount per unit time. For example, if 100 units of drug interact with an enzyme system, a zero-order rate might produce 50 units of metabolite per minute; 1000 units of drug still results in 50 units of metabolite; and so forth. Ethyl alcohol is an important example of a drug whose metabolism is zero order at ordinary concentrations. Some drugs have first-order kinetics at low concentration and zero-order at higher concentrations. (Phenytoin is one example.)

Drug-metabolizing enzymes may be inhibited or induced. Enzyme inhibition can occur through many mechanisms. One well-understood process, competitive inhibition, occurs when another substance serves as a substrate for the enzyme. The chemical structure of an inhibitor may be in some ways similar to that of the usual substrate. Such inhibition may be overcome by increasing the concentration of the original substrate. One example of inhibition in psychopharmacology is the inhibition of acetaldehyde dehydrogenase (oxidase) by disulfiram.[25] This inhibition provokes severe symptoms in ethanol drinkers who cannot metabolize the acetaldehyde generated by the initial step in the metabolism of ethanol. Noncompetitive inhibition occurs when an agent unrelated in structure to the substrate is capable of binding in a distorting fashion to the enzyme to prevent normal interaction between the substrate drug and enzyme. Such inhibition may not be overcome by an increased concentration of substrate. Frequently, metabolism of one drug is induced by previous use of another drug. For example, in heavy tobacco smokers, chlorpromazine is metabolized at an abnormally rapid rate.[47] Alcohol-dependent persons also metabolize barbiturates at a rapid rate.

Drug-metabolizing enzymes, particularly those associated with the rough and smooth endoplasmic reticulum of the cell, undergo alterations in drug-transforming ability by pretreatment with a variety of drugs and chemicals, including phenobarbital.[13] Compounds may, by induction, hasten their own metabolism or the metabolism of other compounds, such as meprobamate and glutethimide.

2.3.2. Drug Excretion

Drugs or their metabolites may be excreted in body fluids, the most important of which is urine. Drugs may also appear in sweat, bile, breast milk, or expired air. Compounds or metabolites that are water soluble generally remain in the urine and are excreted, while those that are lipid soluble may be passively reabsorbed back into the blood stream. Without metabolic oxidation, a lipid-soluble drug like phenobarbital would require approximately 100 years for final removal from the body. A compound that ionizes as a weak base or acid in solution may exist in two forms, depending on the pH of the medium. The ionized form will be more water soluble and is unlikely to be passively reabsorbed into tubular cells and the blood stream. Relatively uncharged (e.g., unionized) compounds are higher in lipid solubility and more likely to be reabsorbed. Since systemic administration of acid or base is reflected by a change in urine pH, we can modify the degree of ionization of some compounds in the urine. Alkalinizing the urine can enhance the excretion of some weak acids, such as phenobarbital. Acidifying the urine can enhance the excretion of basic compounds, such as amphetamine, methadone, nicotine, and phencyclidine (PCP).

The liver excretes many drugs, often in conjugated form, via the bile into the duodenum. Some compounds are not excreted in the feces but are reabsorbed through the intestine into the blood stream, to be finally excreted into the urine (or resecreted by the liver into the gut). Glutethimide and PCP are subject to extensive enterohepatic recycling of this sort.

2.4. Quantitative Characterization of Drug Action

Drug effects usually rely on binding to a cellular component which alters the function of the cell in some way. The biological or reactive entities that bind the drug are referred to as receptors. This binding is usually unstable, and a dynamic equilibrium exists between free drug and drug bound to receptor. Quantitative drug effects are based on a semilogarithmic or S-shaped dose–response curve, in which there is an initial slow appearance of drug effect with increased dose, then a rapid increase, followed by a gradual leveling off of drug effect which does not increase even with higher doses. Figure 1 is a typical dose–reponse curve in which two drugs are compared in their ability to elicit an effect.

In Figure 1, drug A evokes a response at a lower dose and is more potent than drug B. If a group of drugs is compared via dose–response curves, the most potent drug will lie closest to the ordinate. In Figure 1, drugs A and B vary in potency but their efficacy is the same. The plateaus at the peak of the effect are clearly the same (100%), so the drugs have the same efficacy. Drug users often confuse the issue of potency with efficacy. For example, fentanyl, an opioid effective in doses of 0.05–0.1 mg, has been popular for its potency in some drug-using communities.[41] Its potency is impressive, but that does not mean that the drug is more effective in relieving pain, inducing euphoria, depressing respiration, or provoking constipation than other opioids. It merely means that it can achieve the same effect at lower doses.

Figure 2 contains a dose–response curve for codeine, indicating that it is a less powerful drug. Despite increased dosage, it never approaches the efficacy of other opioids. Codeine has its major effect through its coversion to morphine, a conversion so slow that the drug never reaches opiate efficacy.

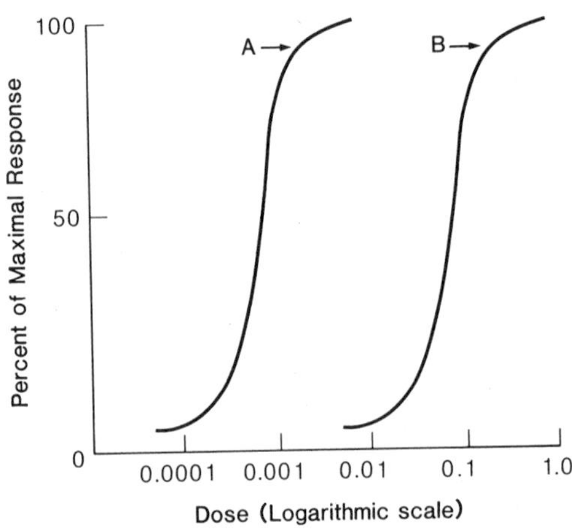

Figure 1. Typical dose–response curves.

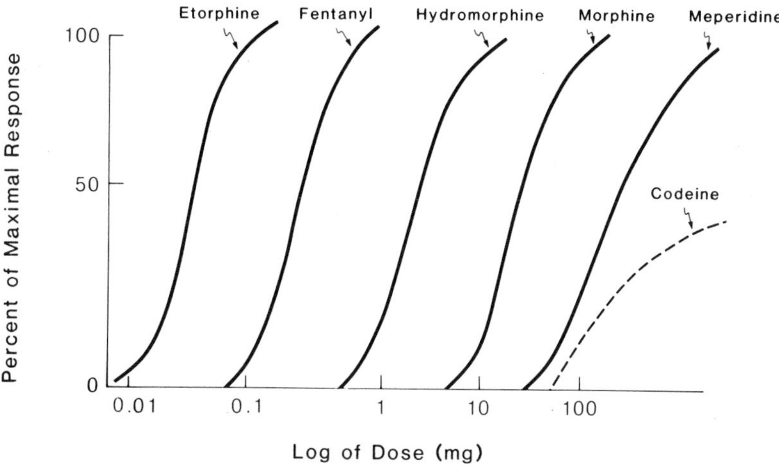

Figure 2. Dose–response curves of opioid drugs. (From Ref. 53. Copyright 1986 by Praeger Publishers, a division of Greenwood Press. Reprinted with permission.)

Compounds called antagonists bind to receptors and provoke no effect or less effect than other drugs in the same class. These drugs may, however, alter the action of effective drugs by competition for the same receptor(s). In this situation, depicted in Figure 3, drug B shifts the dose–response curve away from the ordinate and acts as a competitive inhibitor or antagonist. Drug B's effects are surmountable by increasing the concentration of drug A. Drug B may have no or little effect itself. Some drugs may act as agonists (effectors or stimulators) at the receptor, but in the presence of other drugs they act as antagonists. Pentazocine is a mixed opiate agonist–antagonist, while naloxone and naltrexone are pure antagonists with no agonist effect. In Figure 3, A could be morphine and B could be naloxone or naltrexone.

Quantification as it focuses on drug distribution, metabolism, and elimination is referred to as pharmacokinetics. Figure 4 portrays the typical disappearance of a drug from the plasma after three different methods of administration. Oral ingestion is slowest, since most drugs must progress to the small intestine before entering the blood stream. Intravenous injection requires only the time for blood to course through the veins, to the right side of the heart, to the pulmonary bed, to the left side of the heart, through the arteries, and thence to the tissue capillaries, where the drug exerts its effect—a process that is complete in about a quarter of a minute (depending on the individual's circulation time). Nasal inhalation takes about the same amount of time (perhaps a second or two faster than antecubital injection). Pulmonary inhalation or "smoking" has onset of effect that is several seconds faster than injecting, since the drug enters the blood stream directly at the pulmonary bed (thereby bypassing the system vein, the right side of the heart, and the pulmonary arteries). Injection not into the

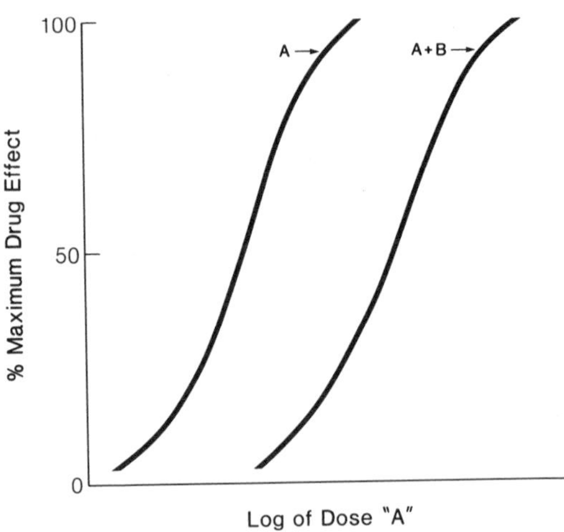

Figure 3. Competitive inhibition of agonist (A) and antagonist (B).

blood stream produces blood levels similar to oral ingestion, but more rapidly under some conditions (e.g., certain drugs, muscle injection) and sometimes more slowly under other conditions (e.g., certain drugs, poor vascular perfusion, subcutaneous injection).

For most drugs, processes of interaction with tissue are first order. With first-order kinetics, the process proceeds in such a fashion that a constant proportion of drug present is handled per unit time. In Figure 5, the plasma concentration of drug present is plotted logarithmically against time, which is plotted arithmetically. Since the disappearance from plasma is exponential, this semilog

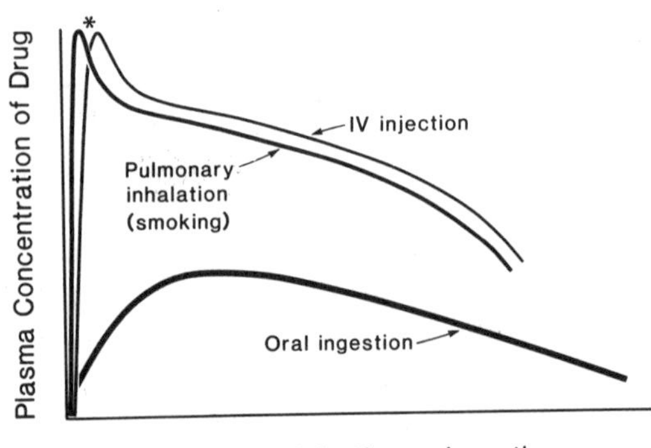

Figure 4. Changing serum concentration of a drug following injection, smoking, and ingestion. *, The time difference has been exaggerated for graphic purposes.

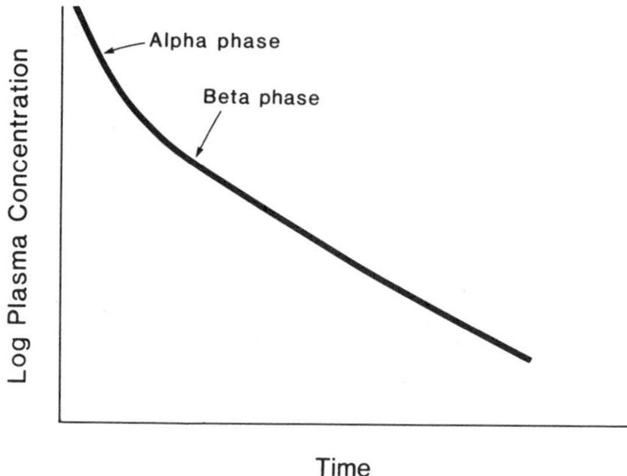

Figure 5. Disappearance of drug from plasma.

plot yields a straight line. The alpha or initial phase usually relates to distribution following injection, while the beta or later phase reflects metabolism and excretion. Most drugs follow this pattern of first-order kinetics. Occasionally a drug will not follow this pattern, as with the disappearance of alcohol from the plasma, which, for practical purposes, follows zero-order kinetics.

Half-life refers to a drug's persistence in the blood or plasma. This reflects the time it takes for a drug to decrease in concentration by 50%. Alcohol does not have a half-life because its decline in the serum (and its duration of effect) is related to the initial dose. (This is occasionally called dosage-dependent kinetics.) The plasma half-life may have clinical use. Meperidine (e.g., pethidine) has a short half-life and must be given every 2–3 hr as a clinical analgesic. Morphine's half-life is longer and its analgesic duration of action is generally longer. The half-life of methadone given at a low dose for the first time is brief (i.e., a few hours), but much longer (20–30 hr) in a heavily tolerant individual taking repeated high doses since the enzyme capacity is exceeded and the kinetics become zero order.[22]

If a drug is given at intervals that approximate or are less than the half-life, the drug will begin to accumulate in the body. At each dose, some of the previous dose will remain and a stepwise increase in concentration will occur. If the dosage interval is markedly prolonged, then no accumulation occurs because the previous dose will be excreted before the next dose is administered. A drug constantly administered is subject to constant excretion. The point of balance at which the rate of drug administration approximates the rate of excretion is referred to as the steady state.

An important concept of the steady-state concentration is illustrated in Figure 6. The dosage markedly affects the steady-state concentration but the time to reach the plateau is independent of dosage. High doses yield a high steady-state

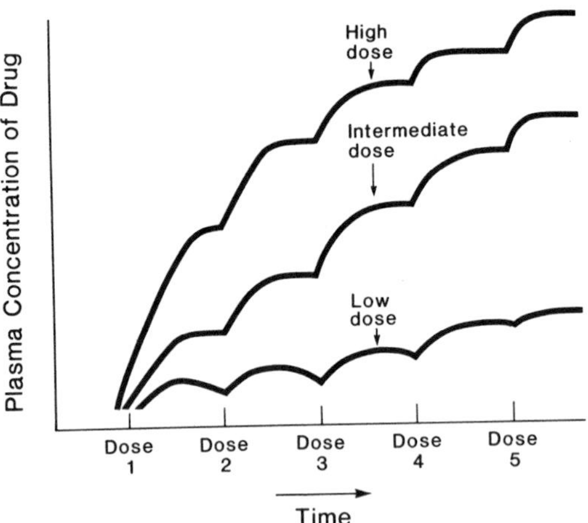

Figure 6. Cumulative plasma levels and increasing dose.

concentration; low doses yield a low steady-state concentration. A confusing point to many is the fact that the time to reach steady state is not a factor of dose but a factor of the half-life of the drug. The plateau concentration will be reached after four to five half-lives of the drug. For example, patients taking a single daily dose of methadone will reach a steady-state concentration in 4–5 days (i.e., $4–5 \times t_{1/2}$), since the half-life at maintenance doses is about 24 hr. The patient taking 100 mg will have a higher steady-state concentration than the patient taking 25 mg but the time before equilibration will remain the same. To achieve a rapid approximation of the steady-state concentration, clinicians may give a loading dose or a higher initial dose with lower subsequent doses.

2.5. Special Pharmacological Issues Related to Drugs of Dependence

Current language is often inadequate to explain the pharmacological effects of psychoactive drugs. For example, drug abusers report feeling "high" or "good" or "relaxed" as reasons for drug use. These subjective states are virtually impossible to operationalize objectively for research purposes. New terms, such as "primary reinforcing properties" (for early use) or "secondary reinforcing properties" (for chronic use), are proving useful in studying the abuse potential of drugs and the drug-seeking behavior of users.[32]

Another critical issue to our understanding is psychotoxicity, or the drug's ability to alter brain function sufficiently so that the user is intoxicated. Certain drugs, such as opioids, alcohol, sedatives, and potent stimulants (cocaine, amphetamine), can seriously impede judgment or psychomotor function. Other drugs, such as tobacco, caffeine, khat, or betel-areca, seldom do so, at least in an obvious disabling way.

2.5.1. Tolerance

Many psychoactive drugs lose their effect on repeated use. Consequently, an individual who wishes to achieve an effect may need a larger dose. This phenomenon is referred to as tolerance. Tolerance comes about by essentially two mechanisms, which often act together: dispositional tolerance and pharmacodynamic tolerance. Repeated exposure to a drug that provokes improved rate of elimination, nearly always due to an improved metabolic capacity through hepatic enzyme induction, is a reflection of dispositional tolerance. Tolerance to drugs, particularly to opioids, sedative–hypnotics (including benzodiazepines), cocaine, and ethanol, is mediated by a diminishing cellular response to the agent—so-called cellular or pharmacodynamic tolerance.

The opioid drugs do not exhibit cross-tolerance to ethanol and sedative–hypnotics. Tolerance to all effects of opioids does not occur equally. For example, analgesic and sedative effects to the opioids decrease most markedly. Thus, chronic opioid-dependent persons may still experience the constipating effects of the drug, but no analgesic effects.

Tolerance to ethanol and sedatives can also be considerable, but it never reaches the degree often described for opioids. This has two important consequences. First, users of these drugs can usually achieve a state of intoxication. Second, they are not nearly so tolerant to the respiratory suppressant effect of their nonopioid agents. Thus, death secondary to respiratory depression is not unusual in a habitual sedative user. An individual who has achieved intoxication by overcoming a high degree of tolerance to the drug's cortical effects may need only a small additional dose to cause respiratory arrest.

Tolerance to cocaine, amphetamine, and psychedelic drugs occurs readily. Users may develop profound tolerance to both the cardiovascular and euphoric effects but remain at high risk for the development of psychosis, especially after chronic, high-dose usage.[16]

Cross-tolerance exists among opioids. Cross-tolerance in the broader class of alcohol–sedative drugs is pronounced. An individual tolerant to alcohol will also be tolerant to barbiturates, meprobamate, benzodiazepines, methaqualone, ethchlorvynol, glutethimide, and the gaseous anesthetics. There is little or no cross-tolerance between the opioids and the alcohol–sedative drugs.

2.5.2. Dependence and Withdrawal

Physical dependence signifies an altered physiological state, produced by repetitive use of a drug. Its presence is manifested by the emergence of a withdrawal or abstinence syndrome upon cessation of drug use. The continued administration of the drug prevents emergence of the abstinence syndrome. This may be a compelling reason why individuals continue chronic use of some agents. The most severe and stereotyped withdrawal syndromes are associated with the depressant drugs: opioids, ethanol, and the sedative–hypnotics (including benzodiazepines). Milder withdrawal occurs with tobacco and stimulants (including cocaine).

Withdrawal from opioids begins at various intervals after cessation of drug use, depending on the particular opioid being consumed. Severity of the syndrome and its duration vary depending on the particular opiate drug, the dose, and duration of use. Withdrawal in a dependent individual may be easily precipitated by administration of an opiate antagonist, such as naloxone. Withdrawal is easily treated with opioid drugs, although other treatments ranging from a supportive milieu to benzodiazepines have been effective in young healthy individuals with mild withdrawal. The nonopioid clonidine has also been used to relieve withdrawal symptoms.[18]

Withdrawal from alcohol or the hypnotic–sedatives can be severe, even life-threatening. Sedative drugs that persist for a long time in the body (some barbiturates and benzodiazepines) have a delayed onset of the abstinence syndrome, as long as several days or even weeks. Drug-free withdrawal of mild withdrawal conditions is certainly possible.[54] Long-acting benzodiazepines are probably most commonly used today for alcohol or sedative–hypnotic withdrawal treatment, though phenobarbital is also effective.[42] Phenothiazines lower the seizure threshhold and should not be used for withdrawal treatment from these drugs.

Adverse symptoms may follow the cessation of chronic psychostimulant use, but these are probably due in large part to stress of insomnia, dehydration, fatigue, disturbances in metabolism due to their anorexigenic effects, and psychological factors.[40] A mild physical dependence syndrome to mild stimulants such as caffeine probably develops in chronic, high-dose users.[19] Tobacco smoking induces a mild dependence syndrome apparently due to pharmacological and psychological factors.

The term *addiction* often takes on social meaning. It is sometimes used to describe the thoughtless expenditure of resources for obtaining and using a psychoactive drug. Conversely, the use of opioids for 48 hr in surgical patients will often be followed by a mild withdrawal syndrome, yet such patients rarely become drug dependent. Pharmacological factors alone cannot explain why some individuals adhere to psychoactive drug use as a cardinal, rather than an incidental part of life.

Clinical manifestations of dependence and withdrawal depend on such mechanisms as cellular tolerance, neurotransmitter–receptor effects, and central as well as peripheral nervous system effects. These are discussed in Chapter 5, "Etiological Factors," in Section 2.2, on neurotransmitters and enzymes.

3. Opioids

3.1. Sources of Opioids and Their Antagonists

Opiates obtained from the poppy include the phenanthrene alkaloids of opium: morphine, codeine, and thebaine. Crude opium is a resin extracted by incising the ripe capsules of the poppy and allowing the juice to air dry.

Some important opiates are semisynthetic. They are produced by chemical manipulation of thebaine or morphine. Important representatives include heroin, hydromorphone, and oxycodone.

A number of entirely synthetic opioids do not structurally resemble morphine. These include methadone, meperidine, fentanyl, and propoxyphene. The general term *opioid* includes the natural opiates as well as the synthetic opiatelike compounds.

Certain synthesized agents have morphinelike effects (i.e., are agonists) at the same time that they antagonize the characteristic morphine effects (usually at higher doses). These are labeled mixed agonist–antagonists. Pentazocine is a mixed agonist–antagonist which has some analgesic (i.e., agonist) properties at moderate doses and antagonist properties at higher doses. Addicted persons may take antihistamines along with drugs like pentazocine in order to reduce the antagonistic effects. The most important pure antagonist is naloxone, a drug that has no agonist properties.

3.2. Administration, Absorption, Distribution, Metabolism, Excretion

All opioids are less potent when taken by mouth than by other routes, not only because some are poorly absorbed but because they are readily metabolized in the liver.[33] Most opioids are subject to significant first-pass effects through the liver and have an oral/parenteral potency rate much less than 1.0. Opioid-dependent persons usually prefer the sudden effect (or rush) from intravenous injection, smoking, or nasal insufflation, but some are content to take oral opioids. Opioids also readily cross the placenta from mother to fetus.

The opioids are widely distributed in the body. Heroin (diacetylmorphine) enters the CNS more rapidly than morphine because of its high lipid solubility. Heroin is quickly deacetylated to morphine in the brain.

Many important opioids (morphine, meperidine. methadone) are significantly bound to plasma protein, an important clinical factor. Methadone's greater than 80% binding is in part responsible for its relatively lengthy stay in the body.

Most opioids are metabolized in the liver. Heroin is deacetylated to morphine. This morphine ultimately appears in the urine, usually conjugated to glucuronide. Other hepatic reactions that increase water solubility of opiates include oxidation, hydroxylation, and *N*-dealkylation. Some agents, which are more effective orally, may undergo less first-pass degradation in the liver; these include codeine, oxycodone, and methadone.

3.3. Effects

The CNS effects of opioids include suppression of the cough reflex and respiratory depression. Large doses of meperidine may provoke excitation and occasionally convulsions. The analgesic effect is secondary to an interference with pain perception. The respiratory effects also result from a general depressant effect in the CNS secondary to binding at opioid receptors in medullary centers. The mechanism of death in overdose is usually respiratory depression and anoxia. After an early elicitation of nausea and vomiting, opioids may subsequently suppress vomiting. Virtually all opioids cause miosis which is not antagonized by atropine. Opioids generally diminish enteric secretions (biliary and pancreatic). Their constipating effect probably occurs by interfering with propulsive rhythmical contraction, although they may increase muscle tone in the gastrointestinal (GI) and biliary tract. Opioids produce peripheral vasodilatation, probably through a central action, which may cause hypotension. Rapid injection of morphine and heroin may cause histamine release which contributes to vasodilatation and causes itching, flushing, and sweating. Opioids stimulate the release of antidiuretic hormone but inhibit the release of adrenocorticotropin and gonadotropins and have direct effects on testicular cells, which may contribute to diminished sexual interest and activity in the chronic opioid user.[32]

Intravenous heroin use is occasionally associated with pulmonary edema. The mechanism of production of this syndrome is poorly understood. The pulmonary edema does not respond to naloxone injection, while typical opioid overdose (manifested by coma or respiratory depression) does rapidly respond to intravenous naloxone injection.

3.4. Tolerance, Dependence, Abstinence Syndrome

The WHO Expert Committee on Drug Dependence has described opioid dependence as a state arising from repeated administration of this type of drug on a periodic or continuous basis. The characteristics of drug dependence include (1) an overpowering desire or need to continue taking the drugs, which are obtained by any means, the need being satisfied by the drug taken immediately or by another drug with similar types of properties, (2) a tendency to increase the dose owing to development of tolerance, (3) a psychic dependence on the effect of the drug related to subjective and independent appreciation of these effects, and (4) physical dependence on the effect of the drugs requiring its presence for maintenance of homeostasis. This results in a characteristic abstinence syndrome when the drug is withdrawn.

Intermittent use of small quantities produces little evidence of toleran Perhaps as many as 50% of recreational opioid users in some settings do not advance beyond such intermittent use. A degree of tolerance develops to analgesic doses in 48–72 hr. Evidence of acute dependence even after a single analgesic dose has also recently been demonstrated for opiate-naive subjects. Tolerant morphine and heroin users have received 1.0-g doses or more, intravenously, without serious effect. Tolerance can be marked to certain effects while to certain other effects (e.g., constipation, miosis) there is little or no tolerance.

With chronic opioid dependence, the individual develops a second reason for continued drug administration: the prevention of drug withdrawal. When the dependent person stops taking the drugs, withdrawal ensues in 4–24 hr following the last dose, depending on the drug (e.g., shorter for morphine and heroin, longer for opium and methadone). The symptoms grow worse and peak in 24–72 hr. The acute symptoms will generally end within 4 or 5 days (up to 7–10 days for opium or methadone).

4. Alcohol (Ethanol, Ethyl Alcohol)

4.1. Forms of Alcohol

There are numerous forms of alcohol, including ethanol and methanol, for example. Ethanol is the chief beverage alcohol in common use. Ethanol used for beverage purposes is generally made by the fermentation of various carbohydrate sources with yeast. A concentration of 12–14% alcohol is usually enough to affect the yeast and stop the natural fermentation process. Most wine has 10–12% alcohol. In fortified wine, pure alcohol is added to the wine to increase the ethanol to about 20%. Beer, which contains 4–6% alcohol, incorporates the carbon dioxide from the fermentation; so does sparkling wine. Most distilled spirits contain 20–50% alcohol.

4.2. Administration, Absorption, Distribution, Metabolism, Excretion

Alcohol can traverse many biological membranes, including the rectal, gastric, and small-intestinal mucosa. The absorption proceeds without enzymatic action or degradation and is relatively complete. Gastric absorption occurs, but most absorption occurs in the small intestine. Increasing its concentration up to a certain maximum progressively speeds the rate of absorption, although high alcohol concentrations reduce absorption. Concurrently ingested food decreases the rate of alcohol absorption. The delay in absorption occasioned by food relates in large part to the food's retardation of gastric emptying. Since the intestine is the most important site of alcohol absorption, any delay in gastric emptying (e.g., anticholinergic drugs, food, certain intestinal diseases, a high concentration of alcohol) will retard absorption.

Alcohol is distributed throughout all tissues essentially in body water. Its apparent volume of distribution approximates 40 liters. Since women generally have a lower proportion of body water and a higher proportion of body fat than men, the distribution volume is usually smaller for a woman than for a man of equal weight. Equilibrium between alcohol concentration in the blood and other body tissue may vary. Brain concentration rapidly approaches that of the blood. The placenta is also readily permeable to alcohol.

The degree of intoxication and its potential impact are generally estimated by measuring the blood alcohol level (BAL). An indirect estimate of the BAL can be obtained by measuring the concentration of ethanol in expired air, since the latter bears a constant relationship to blood alcohol concentration and is usually approximately 1/2000 of the BAL. However, care must be taken when testing expiration for alcohol content. The breathalyzer cannot discriminate between alcohol from the lungs and residual alcohol in the oral cavity. This is especially true if a breath test is carried out within 0.5–1 hr after a person drinks alcoholic beverages. The amount of alcohol present in the blood is generally reported as the number of grams of alcohol present in 100 ml; e.g., 200 mg per 100 ml = 0.2 g/100 ml or (simply) 0.2%. Legislation in many countries states that any concentration greater than 0.08–0.12% in a motor vehicle operator can be used as firm evidence of driving while intoxicated. See Table I for the BAL as

Table I
Approximate Blood Alcohol Percentage[a]

Number of drinks[b]	Body weight (lb)							
	100	120	140	160	180	200	220	240
1	0.04	0.03	0.03	0.02	0.02	0.02	0.02	0.02
2	0.06	0.06	0.05	0.05	0.04	0.04	0.03	0.03
3	0.11	0.09	0.08	0.07	0.06	0.06	0.05	0.05
4	0.15	0.12	0.11	0.09	0.08	0.08	0.07	0.06
5	0.19	0.16	0.13	0.12	0.11	0.09	0.09	0.08
6	0.23	0.19	0.16	0.14	0.13	0.11	0.10	0.09
7	0.26	0.22	0.19	0.16	0.15	0.13	0.12	0.11
8	0.30	0.25	0.21	0.19	0.17	0.15	0.14	0.13
9	0.34	0.28	0.24	0.21	0.19	0.17	0.15	0.14
10	0.38	0.31	0.27	0.23	0.21	0.19	0.17	0.16

[a]Subtract 0.01% for each 40 min.
[b]One 120-ml glass of wine (10% alcohol) = one 360-ml bottle of beer (3.5% alcohol) = one 360-ml shot glass of distilled alcohol (40% alcohol or 80 proof).

a function of alcohol dose and body weight. This table should be applied with caution to those with relatively high amounts of body fat, since the latter will have a higher BAL at a given dose of alcohol as compared to lean persons.

Most ethanol is completely oxidized, ultimately to CO_2 and H_2O. A small portion, usually less than 5%, is excreted unchanged in the urine and in expired air. These excretory processes generally follow first-order kinetics (see Section 2.3). The oxidation processes occur primarily in the liver, where most of the alcohol dehydrogenase exists. Alcohol dehydrogenase can oxidize other alcohols, including the small amount of alcohols formed in the large intestine by bacteria. Ethanol is first oxidized to acetaldehyde, which is further oxidized to acetate and carbon dioxide. This process readily handles low volumes of alcohol.

The rate of alcohol metabolism is not increased by higher alcohol concentration. This means that detoxification is constant, regardless of consumption. It is not particularly rapid: the average rate of metabolism is 30 ml of 86-proof (43%) whiskey per hour for a 70-kg man.

Alcohol can also be metabolized to acetaldehyde by another enzymatic system, the microsomal mixed-function oxidase system. This system normally metabolizes insignificant amounts of alcohol but may become important when large volumes of alcohol are consumed. Even with voluminous consumption, the amount metabolized by this alternate microsomal ethanol-oxidizing system (MEOS) may not exceed 25% of consumed alcohol. The biological importance of the MEOS system and its activation is uncertain, but its discovery has sparked much speculation. The MEOS may be induced by heavy drinking because it is part of the cytochrome P-450 (mixed-function oxidase) system. This has been offered as an explanation for some metabolic tolerance of alcohol. The existence of a second system producing acetaldehyde has caused attention to focus on the toxicity of acetaldehyde, itself, in the heavy consumer.

The presence of an inducible system may explain some clinical observations. Alcohol-dependent people, when exposed to anesthetic agents while sober, are tolerant to their effects. Yet when intoxicated with alcohol, these individuals are exceedingly sensitive to coadministered sedatives and anesthetics. In the first instance, the drinker is resistant because the induced microsomal system may rapidly metabolize the other drugs. However, if intoxicated, the drinker may be exposed to a high concentration of the other drug because of competition between alcohol and sedative for shared microsomal metabolic sites.

Acetaldehyde is oxidized by the enzyme acetaldehyde dehydrogenase. This enzyme is inhibited by the drug disulfiram. The resultant accumulation of acetaldehyde, if one drinks alcohol while taking disulfiram, provokes a syndrome of flushing, headache, nausea and vomiting, sweating, hypotension, and dizziness. The syndrome occurs rapidly after ingestion of alcohol. The disulfiram is slowly eliminated from the body and individuals may not be able to drink for several days, even after stopping the drug. A number of other compounds, including the inky-cap mushroom (*Coprinus atramentarius*), some cephalosporins, metronidazole, and the sulfonylureas, provoke the acetaldehyde syndrome in sensitive people. Disulfiram also inhibits dopamine β-hydroxylase enzyme needed for synthesis of norepinephrine and epinephrine and numerous other enzymes that use copper as a cofactor, since disulfiram chelates this metal.

4.3. Effects

Alcohol's effect in the CNS (or other organs) can probably be attributed to binding to more than one receptor. It may also act like many other anesthetic agents by altering membrane structure and function. It has further been postulated that alcohol somehow alters opioid receptor function. Condensation of dopamine or catecholamine products and acetaldehyde may result in the production of unusual endogenous compounds: opiatelike alkaloids called tetrahydroisoquinolones. These may bind to opioid receptors and in some systems have been shown to exert physiological or pharmacological effects.[15] While still a possible mechanism whereby alcohol dependence is produced, it is an unsettled issue.

Alcohol markedly modifies cellular and organ function. It alters nerve cell penetration by sodium and potassium ions, and it affects monoamine metabolism rates. Alcohol increases the flow of saliva and the flow of gastric hydrochloric acid, inhibits transport and metabolism of carbohydrate, and causes fat to accumulate in the liver. It is a potent vasodilator, affecting vasopressin (ADH) levels and urine flow, altering temperature regulation, and possibly altering mechanical performance of the heart.

Alcohol is, like many hydrocarbons, a neurophysiological depressant of the entire CNS. All brain functions appear to be affected. It affects such widely diverse areas as social behavior, cognition, motor performance, sexuality, and respiration. Alcohol interferes with motor function and judgment simultaneously. By degrees, the centers that normally exercise the restraints responsible for social behavioral inhibition are released and conduct is changed, often to a more aggressive attitude. Alcohol has often been described as a disinhibitor, and although no mechanism is known for the description, it remains useful. Alcohol seems regularly to provoke euphoria (or to relieve dysphoria). With increasing doses psychomotor activity is slowed and impaired. Continued drinking leads to depression and ultimately to somnolence, coma, and even death.

The CNS effects correlate to some degree with BAL. At 0.03% (30 mg/100 ml), there is little effect in the nontolerant person; at 0.05%, responses and reactions will slow and skilled integrative behavior may deteriorate; at 0.10–0.15%, most drinkers are noticeably intoxicated and demonstrate ataxia and slurred speech. The occurrence of a BAL higher than 0.20% is thought to be strong supportive evidence of alcoholism. A BAL of 0.30% is virtually pathognomonic of alcoholism. A BAL of 0.40% is associated with coma and 0.50% with death. Experience with alcohol also influences its effects. For example, similar performance effects have been found at 0.03% for abstainers, 0.07% for moderate drinkers, and 0.10% for heavy drinkers.[36]

Chronic ingestion may lead to CNS organic impairment even if nutrition is otherwise judged adequate. Unlike most other psychoactive substances of abuse, alcohol can produce considerable tissue damage outside the CNS. Erosive gastritis may provoke even fatal hemorrhage. Alcoholics may undergo esophageal–gastric tears due to severe vomiting. There is an increased incidence of peptic ulcer in alcoholics. Alcoholism can cause acute pancreatitis; repeated episodes of pancreatitis may lead to pancreatic insufficiency with decreased pancreatic enzymatic secretion. Repeated pancreatitis with inflammation and scarring may even be a causative factor in diabetes mellitus. Alcohol increases the concentration of fat deposited in the liver by increasing fat synthesis and by causing mobilization of fat from peripheral stores. The increased lipid synthesis is, in part, a response to excess hydrogen ion resulting from alcohol oxidation. The initial accumulation of fat may be reversible, but eventually the changes become irreversible and the chronic dysfunctional scarring of cirrhosis ensues. In addition to these changes, an acute inflammatory reaction, alcoholic hepatitis, may occur. Alcoholic cardiomyopathy (beer drinker's heart) is related to excessive consumption.[46]

Alcohol has, as even social drinkers well know, a diuretic effect. This relates to an inhibition of secretion of antidiuretic hormone and a decreased renal tubular reabsorption of water. Alcohol stimulates the release of adrenocortical hormones by increasing the secretion of ACTH. Additionally, the drug increases the concentration of circulating epinephrine; sympathomimetic effects (e.g., hyperglycemia, pupillary dilatation, and hypertension) are seen early in intoxication. Large doses of alcohol can also produce severe hypoglycemia.

Damage to the fetus can be caused by a drinking mother.[17] Fetal alcohol syndrome (FAS) includes diminished birth weight and size, small head circumference, a variety of facial abnormalities (including microophthamalia and micrognathia), mild to moderate mental retardation, and sometimes skeletal, cardiac, pulmonary, or renal abnormalities. Fetal alcohol effect includes a range of growth deficiencies and birth defects related to maternal alcohol intake, but does not include all of the elements needed for a diagnosis of FAS. There is no defined threshold dose, so some experts recommend that pregnant women not drink at all.

4.4. Tolerance, Dependence, Abstinence Syndrome

Individuals who repeatedly drink large amounts of alcohol become tolerant to many of its effects. This tolerance in humans is not clearly based on changes in drug disposition or metabolism, but is caused by adaptational changes of CNS cells (cellular or pharmacodynamic tolerance). Those tolerant to alcohol may on occasion have incredibly high blood alcohol concentrations; a few have survived concentrations of 700 mg/100 ml. Even so, the tolerance is incomplete and individuals can always achieve some degree of intoxication and impairment. The physical dependence accompanying tolerance is profound, and withdrawal produces a series of adverse events that may lead to death. Individuals tolerant to alcohol are cross-tolerant to many other CNS depressants (e.g., barbiturates, nonbarbiturate hypnotics, and benzodiazepines).

A continuum of symptoms and signs accompanies alcohol withdrawal, usually beginning 6–8 hr after cessation of intake. Occasionally, the onset of withdrawal may not occur until 3 or more days after withdrawal (if the drinker also uses long-acting sedatives) or can actually start during a period of high alcohol intake (perhaps due to incomplete absorption from illness). The mild withdrawal syndrome includes tremor, weakness, diaphoresis, hyperreflexia, and gastrointestinal symptoms. Autonomic lability occurs in mild withdrawal and is evidenced by a pulse rate of 100–120/min, a temperature of 37.2–37.8°C (99–100°F), and elevated blood pressure. The severe withdrawal syndrome, or delirium tremens, begins after 48 hr and often includes anxiety, increasing confusion, poor sleep, and marked sweating. Marked delirium, with gross disorientation and cognitive disruption, is often associated with extreme restlessness and a pulse rate greater than 120/min, a temperature over 37.8°C (100°F), and hypertension.

Initially, fleeting hallucinations and nocturnal illusions that arouse fear and restlessness may occur. Visual hallucinations involving threat of assault and presence of dangerous animals are frequent and often incite terror. The patient is overly responsive to all sensory stimuli, particularly to objects seen in dim light. Vestibular disturbances may cause the patient to believe that the floor is moving, walls are falling, or the room is rotating. Some patients may suffer generalized grand mal seizures, usually not more than two in short succession (alcoholic epilepsy or rum fits). As the delirium progresses, a persistent coarse tremor of the hand at rest develops; this tremor sometimes extends to the head and trunk. Marked ataxia is present. Symptoms vary among patients but are frequently the same with each recurrence for a particular patient.

Temperature may be elevated during the withdrawal of any sedative agent, but elevated temperature in alcohol withdrawal is a poor prognostic sign. The mortality of untreated delirium tremens may be as high as 15%. However, the course is usually self-limiting, terminating in a long sleep. The acute period persists from 2 to 10 days, but can be more prolonged in severe withdrawal syndromes. Delirium tremens should begin to clear within a day or two. If there is no evidence of marked improvement within this interval, other causes may be contributing.

Drugs frequently used to treat alcohol withdrawal are similar to alcohol in pharmacological effect. Paraldehyde, commonly used in the past, is now used infrequently due to difficulties in storage (a short shelf life) and problems with intramuscular injection (painful, possibility of sterile abscess and nerve damage).

Short-acting barbiturates (pentobarbital and secobarbital) are also seldom used today, but phenobarbital, with its longer persistence, is quite useful. Some older clinicians still prefer to prescribe chloral hydrate for withdrawal. Benzodiazepines, such as chlordiazepoxide and diazepam, have become the most common drugs for withdrawal therapy due to their greater margin of safety. Phenothiazines are not recommended; they may not control severe delirium tremens and they lower the seizure threshold. The routine administration of phenytoin is not necessary. Magnesium sulfate is indicated if the patient has had a recent seizure or has a history of previous seizures.

5. Sedatives (Including Benzodiazepines)

5.1. Forms of the Drugs

This category includes sedatives, hypnotics, and anxiolytics. The lack of similarity between the structure of barbiturate, benzodiazepines, glutethimide, ethchlorvynol, methaqualone, and related drugs has made it difficult to propose a common receptor or mechanism. The benzodiazepines may bind to a receptor protein in the cerebellum and cerebral cortex.[44] This material which will stereospecifically bind benzodiazepine has an association with the putative inhibitory neurotransmitter γ-aminobutyric acid and its receptor, but the two sites are not identical.[14] All representatives show cross-tolerance to each other and to ethyl alcohol as well.

The broad class called barbiturates refers to any derivative of malonylurea. The first was introduced in 1903. These drugs vary in their onset and duration of action. Short-acting barbiturates are more highly valued by drug abusers. Longer-acting barbiturates (such as phenobarbital) produce a smoother, less stormy withdrawal.

Glutethimide has all the disadvantages of barbiturates and a distinct one of its own: a lengthy duration of effect which contributes to its association with fatal overdose. Ethchlorvynol is shorter acting than glutethimide and is the only therapeutic sedative besides ethanol that is also an alcohol. Methaqualone, a quinazolone, produces less cardiovascular and respiratory depression and is a favorite of sedative abusers. Chloral hydrate can induce tolerance and dependence similar to those of the barbiturates. Two carbamates, meprobamate and tybamate, resemble the barbiturates in terms of sedation, tolerance, dependence, and overdose liability, and they show cross-tolerance to the barbiturates.

The benzodiazepines, introduced into clinical medicine in the early 1960s, are utilized as antianxiety, sedative–hypnotic, anticonvulsant, and muscle-relaxant drugs. Their margin of safety is wide, although their use can lead to dose escalation, tolerance, dependence, and withdrawal.

5.2. Administration, Absorption, Distribution, Metabolism, Excretion

Barbiturates include long-acting and short-acting types. Two shorter-acting barbiturates, secobarbital and pentobarbital, are well absorbed from the upper GI tract, with most absorption occurring in the small intestine. A larger volume of water consumed with the drugs enhances absorption because of better dispersion and solubility. The intravenously administered anesthetic thiobarbiturates are highly lipid soluble and undergo a rapid uptake into the CNS. Secobarbital and pentobarbital are also lipid soluble, but to a lesser extent. They are also widely distributed into the CNS and other tissues including the placenta. The more lipid-soluble compounds are widely distributed, rapid in onset, and completely reabsorbed from tubular urine after glomerular filtration. Phenobarbital, which is not often abused, but is a useful drug in the treatment of withdrawal, is less lipid soluble, less degraded by hepatic metabolism, and secreted in the urine. The half-life of both secobarbital and pentobarbital in humans varies widely and may exceed 40 hr.

Methaqualone is also well absorbed from the GI tract; the hydrochloride salt is more rapidly absorbed than the base. One hundred percent of an oral dose will be absorbed in 2 hr; the onset of action is rapid (10–20 min).

Glutethimide is erratically absorbed from the GI tract, and wide variations in both serum concentration and the time of peak concentrations are seen, often with usual doses. The glucuronide metabolites pass into the enterohepatic circulation where some are hydrolyzed and reabsorbed; this explanation is offered as one contribution to persistent coma after overdosage. Effects of glutethimide appear soon after ingestion and peak plasma concentrations occur 1–2 hr after ingestion.

Meprobamate is well absorbed from the small intestine. Maximum plasma concentrations are reached 1–3 hr after ingestion. The half-life is often reported as 6–18 hr but greater variation has led to the suggestion that some dose-dependent kinetics may occur.

Ethchlorvynol has a rapid onset of effect and a fairly brief duration. It acts within 15 min, with a peak blood concentration seen in 1–1½ hr. Its wide distribution and lengthy half-life (16–25 hr) may account for the delayed withdrawal syndrome, which can occur days or weeks after the drug is discontinued.

Benzodiazepines have become widely used. Most are used for anxiolytic purposes. Flurazepam is prescribed mainly as a hypnotic, and clonazepam is recommended only as an anticonvulsant. The benzodiazepines are readily absorbed from the GI tract. These agents are highly lipid soluble, widely distributed, and highly bound to plasma proteins. Oxazepam and lorazepam are metabolized in the liver to inactive glucuronides and have a relatively brief half-life compared to diazepam.

5.3. Effects

The chief effect of these agents is to inhibit or impair the transmission of nervous impulse. Most will initially increase total sleep time and decrease the time to onset of sleep in insomniac patients. These salutary effects are short lived—usually a few days. Nearly all hypnotics (and many other psychoactive drugs) diminish rapid eye movement (REM) sleep and time spent dreaming. REM suppression is followed by REM rebound in which the dream state may take up 50% of the night (normal is 25%).[24] This may cause vivid dreams and nightmares.

Sedative drugs, with the possible exception of benzodiazepines, have the ability to depress CNS function so profoundly as to cause respiratory depression and death. At high doses some may depress cardiovascular function as well. These agents are prime candidates for suicide attempts. There is no specific antidote or antagonist; treatment of overdose consists of supporting respiration, maintaining hydration and urine output, facilitating the disposition of the drug, and dialysis.

5.4. Tolerance, Dependence, Abstinence Syndrome

This type of sedative drug when taken on a continuous basis, generally in amounts exceeding therapeutic dose levels, can lead to dependence (i.e., tolerance, a tendency to increase the dose, psychic dependence, possible physical dependence, and abstinence symptoms when the drug is withdrawn).

Chronic use of sedatives is associated with a diminished effect. Individuals may become mildly tolerant to even a single dose of these drugs. They eventually are not sedated at blood concentrations higher than the original sedating blood concentrations. A loss of sedative properties occurs more completely than loss of neurotoxic effects. The chronic user, in order to achieve a desired effect, may need larger doses to achieve the desired effect and thereby become ataxic, dysarthric, and retarded in movement and thought. Such a user is still at a risk of overdose, respiratory depression, and death because tolerance to effects on brain stem functions develops much more slowly than cortical function impairment.

Withdrawal from the short-acting sedatives (e.g., sodium amytal, lorazepam) is more likely to produce convulsions, as compared to the longer-acting sedatives. This may or may not be followed by delirium tremens, with hallucinosis. On the other hand, the long-acting sedatives (e.g., phenobarbital, diazepam) may produce hallucinosis with or without confusion. Since patients withdrawing from the long-acting sedatives may not convulse, appear toxic, or show confusion, clinicians may confuse this syndrome with other conditions (e.g., schizophreniform psychosis, affective psychosis).

6. Amphetamines

6.1. Administration, Absorption, Distribution, Metabolism, Excretion

Amphetamine and methamphetamine stimulate the CNS. They mimic the effects of the catecholamines (e.g., norepinephrine). They are effective when given orally. After oral administration, the effects generally appear within 30 min. These drugs tend to act for prolonged periods.

Several hepatic pathways are available for amphetamine degradation, including *p*-hydroxylation and N-demethylation. Significant amounts of unchanged amphetamine ordinarily appear in the urine. Excretion of amphetamine is considerably enhanced in acid urine.

6.2. Effects

Many effects of amphetamine relate to its peripheral, indirect stimulation of alpha and beta receptors by facilitating release of norepinephrine from sympathetic nerves, but other pronounced effects in the CNS have less certain mediation. Amphetamine increases systolic and diastolic blood pressure and generally increases pulse pressure. Although beta activity exists, the heart rate in humans is often reflexively slowed. With large doses, however, tachycardias and tachyarrythmias may occur. Cardiac output is not enhanced by usual doses.

Smooth muscle responds as it does to sympathomimetic compounds. Bronchial muscles are relaxed. The bladder is stimulated, and pain and difficulty in urination may occur. Amphetamine usually slows the movement of intestinal contents and may cause constipation. By slowing gastric emptying, amphetamine slows delivery of some other drugs to the absorptive intestinal surface and thus interferes with absorption.

Amphetamine increases metabolic rate and oxygen consumption and occasionally body temperature, although this may depend on ambient temperature and level of motor activity. There is a regular increase in plasma free-fatty-acid concentration.

Amphetamine markedly stimulates the CNS in humans. The *d* isomer is several times more potent in the CNS than the *l* isomer. A single dose in the 5- to 10-mg range of *d*-amphetamine produces increased wakefulness, alertness, and a decreased sense of fatigue. Mood is elevated, accompanied by increased initiative and confidence, even elation. There is a general increase in psychomotor activity. Performance of repetitive, simple tasks improves, and physical performance in other spheres may improve as well.[52] A decrease in total sleep is accompanied by a decrease in REM sleep to very low levels, and withdrawal after repeated use provokes a sleep-disturbing rebound in REM sleep.

6.3. Tolerance, Dependence, Abstinence Syndrome

A WHO Expert Committee on drug dependence[55] has defined drug dependence of amphetamine types as a state arising from repeated administration of amphetamines or an agent with amphetaminelike effects on a periodic or continuous basis. Its characteristics include (1) a desire or need to continue taking the drugs, (2) development of tolerance by consumption of increasing amounts to obtain the desired euphoric effect, (3) psychic dependence on the effect of the drug related to the subjective and individual appreciation of the drug effect, and (4) no characteristic abstinence syndrome when the drug is discontinued.

Tolerance to the anorexiant effect of amphetamine may readily occur. Marked tolerance, often accompanied by dosage increase, occurs to the mood-elevating and euphoriant effects sought by the recreational amphetamine user. In chronic users, daily doses in excess of 1500 mg of amphetamine have been reported.

Tolerance to amphetamine may be partially mediated by displacement of norepinephrine at the sympathetic neuronal storage sites by an amphetamine metabolite, 4-hydroxynorephedrine. Animal studies indicate that this mechanism does not explain the central tolerance. The development of tolerance is not consistent, and some effects (for example, its efficacy as a treatment for narcolepsy) may not be subject to the development of tolerance.

Withdrawal effects are highly variable from person to person. Some patients show severe transitory depression or paranoia, while others do not. Postintoxication psychiatric conditions do occur, and these may be erroneously identified as a stimulant withdrawal syndrome.

Central toxic effects include nervousness, agitation, tremor, insomnia, fever, confusion, and, in some patients, delirium and panic states. Paranoid ideation is not uncommon, and amphetamine abuse should be considered in the differential diagnosis of schizophrenia, paranoid type. Stimulation of the cardiovascular system may provoke headache, tachycardia, palpitations, and even cardiac arrhythmias. Both hypertension and hypotension have been reported. Excessive sweating may occur. Abdominal cramps, nausea and vomiting, and diarrhea have been reported.

There are a few documented cases of death from overdoses of amphetamine, usually associated with hyperthermia, and life may end in hyperpyrexia, cardiovascular shock, and convulsions. Fatalities have occurred among bicycle riders or other athletes who have taken amphetamine in large doses on a hot summer day. On the other hand, users may die from cerebrovascular hemorrhage.

The toxic dose varies widely, but excessive symptoms are rare in doses of less than 15–30 mg of amphetamine. Nontolerant users have survived doses of 400–500 mg, but death has resulted from as little as 120 mg intravenously.

Psychosis may accompany amphetamine administration.[16] Previously psychotic individuals may become psychotic with very small doses.

Related stimulants, methylphenidate and phenmetrazine, have also been abused. Their profile of use and abuse resembles that of amphetamine.

7. Cocaine

7.1. Forms of the Drug

Cocaine, the active alkaloid of coca leaf, was extracted first from the leaves in 1860. Soon thereafter its local anesthetic properties were noted. It was widely sold legally as an ingredient in wine, tonics, and soft drinks until the early part of the twentieth century. For centuries Andean mountaineers have chewed coca leaves, especially in association with hard physical labor at high altitudes.

An intermediate form between coca leaves and purified cocaine is coca paste. The leaves are extracted utilizing kerosene and sulfuric acid solvents. The resultant paste or semisolid may contain 80% cocaine sulfate. The paste can be further processed to cocaine base or hydrochloride, or it can be smoked by sprinkling it on tobacco or other smoking materials. Recently, the smoking of alkaloidal or basic cocaine has become popular in some areas. Concurrent use of fire and ether (necessary for preparation) has led to serious burn injuries. The difference in physiological effect between chewing a coca leaf and smoking alkaloidal cocaine is great. Processed cocaine is crystalline cocaine hypochloride. When distributed illicitly, it is usually diluted with sugars (e.g., mannitol, lactose) or local anesthetics (e.g., procaine, lidocaine).[10]

7.2. Administration, Absorption, Distribution, Metabolism, Excretion

The most common administration is by nasal insufflation (sniffing or snorting) of the hydrochloride salt. Some absorption of material through the buccal mucosa probably occurs. Orally ingested esters are often completely hydrolyzed in gastric juice, but this is apparently not true of cocaine. Cocaine is absorbed from the GI tract following chewing of leaves, swallowing of the leaf quid, or administration of the drug in gelatin capsules.[49] The alkaline compound is probably ionized and poorly absorbed in the stomach, and most absorption occurs in the upper small intestine. Cocaine may also be injected intravenously (i.v.). The hydrochloride salt is soluble in water. A mixture of cocaine and heroin has been popular from time to time in various places.

Pulmonary absorption and central effect of cocaine are rapid, occurring within a few seconds. Smokers of coca paste or freebase experience intense euphoria almost immediately on smoking, followed quickly by a descending dysphoria which provokes more use until all available drug is consumed.

Since cocaine is a potent vasoconstrictor it may diminish its own rate of absorption from the nasal or GI mucosa. Its half-life in plasma is approximately 1 hr.

Cocaine is hydrolyzed in plasma. This hydrolysis is prevented by cholinesterase inhibitors such as physostigmine. The drug is poorly hydrolyzed in the plasma of individuals with atypical serum cholinesterase.[49] Small amounts of cocaine may be excreted unchanged in the urine.

7.3. Effects

Cocaine is an effective stimulant of the CNS. This stimulation may be related to the drug's ability to potentiate the actions of catecholamines, especially dopamine. Cocaine interferes with the reuptake of catecholamines into nerve terminals, thus prolonging their effects. There is some evidence that other local anesthetics cause euphoria and even CNS stimulation on nasal inhalation.[50]

Cocaine's effect on the CNS is manifested by euphoria, alertness, and psychomotor excitement. With larger doses, marked agitation and even convulsions have been noted. An acute psychosis may occur in association with either brief or chronic use.

Psychosis from chronic use, indistinguishable from that described for amphetamine, may occur, especially in high-dose users and freebase smokers.

The adrenergic stimulation of peripheral organs by catecholamines may lead to tachycardia, vasoconstriction, hypertension, and mydriasis. Large intravenous doses may provoke tachyarrythimias.

The euphoric effect of cocaine disappears rapidly, even while significant drug remains in the plasma. Some tolerance to convulsant and cardiovascular effects has also been reported, but there is also evidence of an increased response of the CNS to repeated doses.[27] Development of tolerance and mild withdrawal syndrome (with anhedonia, anergy, fatigue, depression), both indicating a form of physical dependence, occurs in heavy chronic users.

7.4. Tolerance, Dependence, Abstinence Syndrome

The WHO Expert Committee on Addiction-Producing Drugs[55] has recognized and identified the characteristic of cocaine dependence as the most reinforcing drug known for many users.[35] Animals and humans become compulsive users, especially when the rapid delivery systems, such as intravenous use, freebase or coca paste smoking, are employed. The reward is immediate and the return to baseline mood levels or below occurs rapidly. Both the intensive euphoria and its disappearance can drive vulnerable persons back to more cocaine.

It is clear that cocaine is a powerful reinforcer which can lead to life-attenuating behavior. Although certain people, because of personality structure or life situations, might become more easily overinvolved, anyone with access to cocaine risks becoming a compulsive user.[11] Under conditions of access to large amounts of cocaine the human response remarkably resembles that of the laboratory animal. Cocaine-dependent humans prefer cocaine intoxication to all other activities. They continue using the drug until they or the cocaine is exhausted. They exhibit behavior markedly different from their precocaine life-style. Cocaine-driven humans relegate all other drugs and pleasures to a minor role in their lives. The drive for cocaine compels them to engage in acts previously unacceptable to their former standard of conduct. If the cocaine-seeking behavior is extinguished, either cocaine or environmental cues associated with prior use will cause physiological and behavioral changes resembling cocaine use and will tend to result in a relapse.[7,45] After a prolonged series of stimulations and dysphoric reactions to cocaine, sudden cessation can lead to a stimulant withdrawal syndrome characterized primarily by a substantial depression. In an effort to relieve the depression, self-treatment with cocaine may be resumed with little impact on the depressive process, but with a relapse back to compulsive cocaine use.[45] These positive and negative concomitants—i.e., (1) the intense euphoria, (2) the effort to avoid dysphoria, (3) self-treatment of a distressing postcocaine depression, and (4) the painful or dysphoric residual phase—predispose the patient to relapse. The fact that only a sizable minority of users become compulsive users means that the majority can convert new consumers by proclaiming that it is safe.[2]

8. Cannabis

8.1. Forms of the Drug

Cannabis preparations come from the plant *Cannabis sativa L.*, which is an annual plant occurring in male and female forms. There are substantial differences in the amount of psychoactive materials contained in different varieties of *Cannabis sativa L.* The amount is also influenced by a variation in the climatic conditions, weather, soil, time of harvest, and condition and length of storage. The plant produces resinous substances which contain the major part of the psychoactive and intoxicating ingredients. The substances occur primarily in the flowering tops and upper leaves and are sometimes separated from the rest of the plant for use as hashish. The stalk and seeds contain a negligible amount of psychoactive ingredients.

Various cannabis preparations include beverages, soups, cakes, and other foods. Cut and dried flowering tops and leaves are smoked. Most of the psychoactive effect is probably due to delta-9-tetrahydrocannabinol (THC), although other psychoactive materials may exist in the plant. The potency of various preparations varies enormously. Preparations made from laborious scraping of resin from the plant's leaves (hashish) may contain much higher concentrations of THC. Purified delta-9-THC is exceedingly difficult to prepare, and hence expensive.

8.2. Administration, Absorption, Distribution, Metabolism, Excretion

THC is well absorbed from the pulmonary mucosa, although much psychoactive material is lost in smoking. Using a 1% THC cigarette made up of 500 mg of material, an experienced smoker would only obtain one-half of the available THC, or 2.5 mg. Effects occur rapidly after inhalation, and plasma concentrations reach a maximum after 10–30 min. The effects from a single cigarette decrease after 3 hr. Hashish preparations can be smoked or ingested orally. Onset of action after oral ingestion is 30 min to 1 hr, and time of effect is 5–7 hr. Even though GI absorption is complete, the potency is diminished because GI metabolism or hepatic first-pass effects are profound.

Delta-9-THC has at least one active hepatic metabolite, an 11-hydroxy derivative. Other metabolites, including 8,11-dihydroxy-THC, appear in the urine and feces. Enterohepatic recirculation may occur. Little unmetabolized compound appears in the urine.

There is rapid distribution of delta-9-THC to lipoid tissues and a slower subsequent elimination phase, with a half-life that may last days.

8.3. Effects

Cannabis or THC produces changes in mood, time sense, memory, and other aspects of brain function. The reinforcing effect is relaxation and well-being. Short-term memory is impaired so consistently that conversation is disjointed because planned expressions are not carried out. This is one reason why laughter erupts often. Coordination, balance, and stance are regularly affected, but relatively simple motor tasks are unimpaired until higher doses are used.

Other confirmed effects include dry mouth and throat, increased hunger, and an altered time sense. Minutes may seem like hours. Effects in the human electroencephalogram occur temporarily. Most investigators believe that higher doses (particularly of delta-9-THC) may produce severe thought disruption with hallucinations and delirium.

Cardiovascular effects consistently include tachycardia and reddening of the conjunctiva. Systolic blood pressure is often slightly elevated, probably secondary to the increase in heart rate. The dose-related tachycardia is opposed by beta blockade, but this intervention does not alter the subjective and behavioral effects. Pupillary size is unaltered, but intraocular pressure is lowered.

Conflicting data have been reported on human levels of sex hormones and sperm form and motility. Testosterone concentrations are diminished in regular cannabis smokers.[29]

Pulmonary consequences have been studied, but one methodological problem in humans is that almost all smokers of marijuana are also smokers of tobacco cigarettes. The mode of marijuana inhalation and the larger volume of smoke might lead to a greater adverse pulmonary effect of marijuana smoke. The tar produced by marijuana hydrolysis is carcinogenic. Hoarseness, bronchitis, and chronic cough are reported by chronic users.

Pharmacodynamic tolerance to some cannabinoid effects has been demonstrated in animals. Similarly, studies in humans have demonstrated some adaptational decrease in changes in heart rate, skin temperature, intraocular pressure, and other drug effects. Physical dependence occurs in humans.

For further study of the effect of cannabis the reader can refer to the joint study conducted by the Addiction Research Foundation, Toronto, Canada, and WHO on the adverse and behavioral consequences of cannabis use.[37]

9. Tobacco/Nicotine

9.1. Forms of the Drug

Tobacco products may be chewed, taken by nasal insufflation as snuff, or combusted and inhaled using pipes, cigars, or cigarettes. Nicotine is the chief psychoactive agent sought by users of tobacco.* Its use has spread during the last few centuries, and it is used in every country today.

Nicotine was isolated from the leaves of the tobacco plant in 1828. The compound was named for Jean Nicot, who promoted European importation and cultivation because of his commitment to the compound's medical values. Nicotine is one of a very few natural alkaloids that is liquid. Its pKa is 8.5 and it is readily soluble in water. It has no current medicinal use, although it is being evaluated for certain conditions. In addition to its recreational use, it is occasionally used as a pesticide, since it is quite poisonous in pure form.

Cigarette tar is made up of polycyclic aromatic hydrocarbons which are carcinogens. Among the list of hazardous compounds are carbon monoxide, polonium 210, hydrocyanic acid, acetonitrides, DDT, and literally thousands of others, including natural products, pyrolysis products, and residual chemicals sprayed on the leaf.

*When people ingest natural products such as coca leaf, opium, beer, and tobacco cigarettes they may ingest dozens or hundreds of chemicals. The pattern for study of such products has been the isolation and identification of a chief chemical or principal psychoactive product. Other products may be important in alleviating, diluting, or provoking the effect of the product.

9.2. Administration, Absorption, Distribution, Metabolism, Excretion

Nicotine is readily absorbed from the respiratory tract and buccal mucosa. It can also be significantly absorbed through the skin. Nicotine as a relatively basic compound is poorly absorbed from the stomach, where it is largely ionized, but it is better absorbed from the small intestine. The latter issue is of importance in nicotine poisoning, which occurs with accidental ingestion of insecticide or tobacco. The latter occurs usually when a child eats a tobacco cigarette. The fatal dose of nicotine for an adult is approximately 60 mg. A cigarette may contain as much as 20 mg of nicotine, of which less than 1% may be delivered in the smoke. The dose of a single eaten cigarette may be severe or even fatal to a small child. Still, oral absorption is slow, and GI atony (which may occur) slows it further. Induction of vomiting may eliminate the poison.

The nicotine in cigarette smoke arrives suspended on minute particulate matter and is quickly absorbed from the lung. The rapidity of nicotine delivery in smoke is even faster than that of i.v. injection (about 7 sec versus 14 sec). The drug reaches the CNS seconds after inhalation. Smokers who do not inhale (confined largely to those who smoke pipes and cigars) absorb some nicotine from the buccal mucosa. Cigarette smokers who inhale have higher blood levels of nicotine than noninhaling cigar or pipe smokers. The compound is widely distributed. It appears in breast milk and crosses the placenta. Peak concentrations of nicotine occurring in the plasma average 25–50 ng/ml.

Nearly 90% of ingested nicotine is altered metabolically in the liver. This prominent first-pass effect may account for the poor efficacy of oral nicotine or nicotine chewing gum for reducing the number of cigarettes smoked in experimental and treatment trials. A significant fraction of inhaled nicotine is metabolized by the lung, and some portion of the drug is metabolized in the kidney. The metabolic system generates cotinine and nicotine-1-*N* oxide. All metabolites and a small portion of unmetabolized drug are excreted in the urine. The rate of urinary excretion is dependent, in part, on the urinary pH. If the urine is alkaline, significant portions of the nicotine are passively reabsorbed in the renal tubule. The half-life is about 1–2 hr.[56]

9.3. Effects

Recent work suggests the existence of specific CNS receptors for nicotine. Acetylcholine receptors at ganglionic sites, and to some extent at striated muscle sites, are described as nicotinic because nicotine mimics the effects of acetylcholine there. Importantly, the drug has initial stimulant properties and later depressant properties due to conduction blockade. To emphasize, small doses of nicotine stimulate the autonomic nervous system and skeletal muscle by stimulating cholinergic receptors at autonomic ganglia and neuromuscular synaptic sites. Larger doses inhibit or even paralyze these functions. Users may learn to vary the time and dose to obtain either of these biphasic effects.

Nicotine effects are complex and dependent on physiological interactions and duality of effects. As an example, the drug can cause tachycardia by exciting sympathetic cardiac nerves while inhibiting parasympathetic pathways. It can cause bradycardia by stimulating the parasympathetic cholinergics or inhibiting the sympathetic impulses to the heart.

The drug stimulates the CNS. Large doses generate muscle tremors possibly directly secondary to its CNS action. Very large doses by oral ingestion may produce convulsions. Respiration may be stimulated and vomiting may follow central stimulation of the chemoreceptor trigger zone. An alerting pattern is seen in the electroencephalogram (EEG) and behavioral arousal is seen. Nicotine improves cognition and memory,[4] decreases aggression,[9] and decreases body weight.[51]

Peripheral effects are also important. There is generally an inhibition of gastric contractions, slowing of gastrointestinal emptying, acceleration of heart rate, and other effects secondary to release of norepinephrine. Some degree of peripheral vasoconstriction and a drop in extremity skin temperature are common. There may be initial stimulation of salivary and bronchial secretion.

Evidence that nicotine is the active substance in tobacco smoke has been gathered in a number of direct and indirect experiments. The bolus of nicotine that reaches the brain within seconds of inhaling a cigarette constitutes the pharmacological reinforcer. Smokers correlate nicotine content with proper strength and satisfaction. Low or nonnicotinic cigarettes fare poorly in the marketplace. Smokers given the centrally active ganglionic (nicotinic) blocker mecamylamine increase their consumption of cigarettes, while smokers given nicotine intravenously decrease their cigarette consumption much more than controls given saline intravenously.

Heavy smokers adjust their plasma nicotine concentrations by consuming a cigarette every 20–40 min. Smokers will increase cigarette consumption when given low-nicotine cigarettes or will increase the depth of inhalation and duration of each puff when limited to shorter cigarettes. They essentially titrate their nicotine levels.[23] Some smoking reinforcers and stimuli that encourage smoking behavior (e.g., meeting friends, relaxing after a meal) have nothing to do with the pharmacological effects of nicotine. However, the arousal and alerting effects of the drug are essential to the development and maintenance of tobacco dependence.

The tendency of smokers to increase their inhalation efficiency calls into question the likelihood that low-nicotine-content cigarettes are useful. Some smokers actually increase consumption of other deleterious chemicals to titrate the nicotine level.

9.4. Tolerance, Dependence, Abstinence Syndrome

Dizziness, nausea, and vomiting occur only in the nontolerant individual. Increased tolerance to the depressant effects of the drug can be caused by a few doses. There is some evidence that even in heavy smokers the degree of effect diminishes. The most dramatic cardiovascular response occurs with the first cigarette of the day.[22] Tolerance to nicotine may occur anew each day rather than over longer periods.

Dependence, manifest by subclinical abstinence syndrome, occurs with tobacco/nicotine. The onset and duration of withdrawal symptoms are poorly characterized, although abstinence produces significant discomfort, bradycardia, EEG slowing, and blood pressure changes. Craving for tobacco may be associated with restlessness, headache, impairment of concentration, and other symptoms. Smokers excrete nicotine faster than nonsmokers.[6]

10. Caffeine

10.1. Forms of the Drug

Caffeine, along with the closely related alkaloids theophylline and theobromine, occurs in a variety of plants whose geographical distribution ensures widespread use. Tea, cola beverages, and coffee are important sources of caffeine. Caffeine in tablet form is incorporated in analgesic preparations, stimulants, anorexiants, and coryza remedies.

10.2. Administration, Absorption, Distribution, Metabolism, Excretion

Caffeine is well absorbed after oral consumption in solution. It appears quickly in the plasma, although highest concentrations are not seen for 30–45 min. It is distributed into all body compartments and crosses the placenta. Caffeine is minimally bound to plasma proteins, has high lipid solubility, and appears in fairly high concentrations in the cerebrospinal fluid. See Table II for sources of caffeine and typical dose levels.

Only 10% of administered caffeine appears unchanged in the urine. It is chiefly metabolized in the liver and has a plasma half-life of 3½ hr in humans. The important metabolities in urine are 1-methyluric acid and 1-methylxanthine.

10.3. Effects

Pharmacological effects of caffeine and the other methylxanthines[20] include the following:

1. Translocation of intracellular calcium with a resultant alteration of excitation, contraction, or secretion properties.
2. Increased accumulation of cyclical nucleotides, particularly cyclic AMP, secondary to inhibition of phosphodiesterase.
3. Blockade of some receptors, mainly adenosine.
4. Activation of adenosine receptors in the CNS.

The drug diminishes drowsiness and fatigue. Under certain circumstances it enhances mental acuity and the performance of some tasks. Larger doses may be associated with excitement, anxiety, and insomnia.

Caffeine produces tachycardia and an increased force of cardiac contraction. Systemically, vessels are dilated. The drug increases gastric secretion and acidity. Caffeine may relax some smooth muscle (bronchi) and slightly augment skeletal muscle contraction. It also has direct diuretic properties.

10.4. Tolerance, Dependence, Abstinence Syndrome

Mild tolerance may develop even in daily users who consume small quantities. Tolerance and dependence exist in high-dose users (>600 mg caffeine per day). Components of the abstinence syndome include headache, irritability, restlessness, lethargy, and excessive yawning. High-dose coffee drinkers who acquire their habit at work are particularly prone to develop symptoms on nonworking days. They soon learn that some consumption of coffee (or other caffeine source) is necessary on weekends.[19]

11. Volatile Solvents–Inhalants

Numerous psychoactive substances have been inhaled as gases or the vapor of volatile liquids. Use of volatile substances occurs primarily among young

Table II
Caffeine Content in Beverages

Beverage	Volume per serving (ml)	Caffeine per serving (mg)
Ground coffee	150	80–180
Instant coffee	150	40–100
Tea	150	30–80
Hot chocolate	150	50–70
Most cola drinks	350	35–55
Decaffeinated coffee	150	3
Ovaltine	150	0

people, although some workers exposed to the agents also abuse them. These compounds are widely available commercially and in the home as solvents and glues. They provoke a brief euphoria or a giddy intoxication similar to acute alcohol intoxication. The principal effect is CNS depression, with a disinhibition euphoria. Many popular commercial preparations are mixtures of volatile substances, and specific drug effects are difficult to pinpoint.

Volatile chemicals that are abused include: *n*-heptane, *n*-hexane, benzene, naphthalene, styrene, toluene, xylene, freons, methyl chloride, nitrous oxide, tetrachloroethylene, trichloroethylene, amyl nitrite, butyl nitrite, ethanol, isopropanol, methanol, ethyl acetate, amyl acetate, butyl acetate, acetone, methyl ethyl ketone, and methyl butyl ketone. These are included in adhesives, paint thinner, gasoline, kerosene degreasers and industrial solvents, rubber cement, shoe polish, aerosol sprays, foam dispensers, antiangina drugs, room deodorants, antifreeze, and windshield-washing fluids.

11.1. Aromatic Hydrocarbons

The aromatic hydrocarbons are a series of cyclical compounds all related to benzene. Coal and petroleum are the chief sources of the compounds. Despite benzene's myelotoxic potential,[43] it is still widely used in hydrocarbon mixtures.

Inhaled benzene is rapidly absorbed and widely distributed. The brain quickly accumulates the lipophilic substance. As much as 50% of inhaled benzene is exhaled. Adipose tissues may retain the material longer, and obese individuals may actually metabolize more drug than thin individuals who exhale large amounts. The remaining material is metabolized in the liver to phenolic derivatives which are excreted conjugated with sulfates and glucuronides. Many other metabolites may be found.

The acute hydrocarbon solvent effects are all relatively similar. Users experience euphoria, giddiness, dizziness, vertigo, and headache. There is some evidence that elevated concentrations may produce acute cardiac effects and even fatal arrhythmias. Benzene has been known to damage blood-forming elements in the body. Severe myelotoxicity occurs with benzene alone; simple alkyl substitution of the ring will remove this potential. Most myelotoxicity has occurred in relationship to industrial chronic exposure. However, blood dyscrasias have been reported in solvent abusers and these are likely to relate to benzene's content.

Toluene (methyl benzene) shares many chemical and solubility characteristics with benzene. In the past toluene preparations were often contaminated with benzene. Reports of toxicity have been those of mixed-solvent exposure.

Toluene depresses the CNS and may produce fatigue. In abusers, liver and kidney injury have been reported. Most reports of chronic damage to abusers are neurological, including cerebellar dysfunction, encephalopathy, and polyneuropathy.[31]

Xylene (dimethyl benzene) is a volatile flammable liquid, insoluble in water but easily miscible with other organic liquids. Upon absorption it is metabolized to benzoic acid and readily excreted.

Other potentially important aromatic hydrocarbon inhalants include naphthalene and styrene.

11.2. Aliphatic Hydrocarbons

The aliphatic hydrocarbons (paraffins) include straight and branched-chain hydrocarbons with various degrees of saturated single and unsaturated double bonds. The intermediate-length compounds *n*-hexane and *n*-heptane are the most important agents from a toxicological standpoint. The aliphatic compounds are water insoluble but miscible with other organic agents.

n-Hexane is readily absorbed on inhalation and concentrated in lipoid tissue. It is readily metabolized by the enzymes to metabolites that may be neurotoxic. Peripheral neuropathy may ensue, and there is speculation that spinal cord damage may occur in humans as it does in animals.[39]

11.3. Halogenated Solvents and Propellants

Many important halogenated hydrocarbons have been or are still used as anesthetic agents. A number of fluorinated hydrocarbons (freons) have been utilized as propellants. Some of the first abused aerosol propellants contained these fluorocarbons. Serious toxicities were occasionally reported, but the specificity of the fluorocarbons to human toxicity is uncertain. Certainly they can produce hydrocarbon CNS depression. The fluorinated propellants have been largely banned because of evidence that they were adversely affecting the ozone layer in the ionosphere.

11.4. Trichlorinated Solvents

Methyl chloroform, trichlorethylene, and chloroform were all once used as general inhalational anesthetics. Their use for this purpose has ceased, but all are used as commercial solvents and degreasers. They have been subject to inhalation abuse.

Trichloroethylene has been most subject to abuse of these agents. Hepatic necrosis and nephropathy have been reported.

11.5. Inhalational Anesthetic Drugs

Ether and nitrous oxide have been used as recreational intoxicants for over a century. Although many such gases have the potential to be misused, nitrous oxide is the one most commonly abused. Some increase in use by health professionals and students has been noted.[38] Most reports have not been associated with prominent toxicity. The usual sources are industrial or hospital tanks or whipped-cream cans or cartridges.

11.6. Aliphatic Nitrites

Amyl nitrite was used for years as a treatment for angina pectoris. The inhaled nitrite produces significant systemic vasodilatation, which causes peripheral pooling and a diminution of myocardial oxygen consumption. The drug is widely available over the counter in crushable glass ampules.

Nitrites are readily absorbed on inhalation. Both organic nitrates (C-O-NO_2) and nitrites (C-O-NO) are systemic vasodilators. Speculation now is that the vascular effect of nitrates or nitrites or other nitrogen-containing compounds is mediated through nitroxide, which can be formed from either agent.

Pharmacists in many urban locations report the purchase of large amounts of amyl nitrite ampules. The generalized vasodilatation produced by inhaling the drug causes hypotension, dizziness, flushing, and tachycardia. Some view this effect as enhancing sexual pleasure; delaying ejaculation or to be used at the time of orgasm. These drugs have been implicated as possibly contributing to the spread of the acquired immune deficiency syndrome (AIDS) in two ways: (1) by lessening inhibition to engage in casual sexual relationships, and (2) by suppressing or damaging the immune system, such that it becomes more vulnerable to the AIDS virus.

12. Phencyclidine

Formerly used as a general anesthetic in veterinary medicine, PCP is readily and inexpensively synthesized in simple laboratories.

12.1. Administration, Absorption, Distribution, Metabolism, Excretion

Fairly specific binding of PCP to a CNS cellular preparation has been reported.[57] This has raised the discussion of a PCP receptor. There is recent evidence that PCP may bind to one of the subspecies of opioid receptors.

Phencyclidine is apparently well absorbed from the GI tract. The onset of action after injection, smoking, or nasal insufflation occurs within a few minutes but may be delayed for 30–45 min after oral ingestion. Plasma concentrations vary widely and values between 40 and 200 μg/ml have been reported. The half-life of the parent compound in serum is relatively short but effects are prolonged.

Hepatic metabolism produces hydroxylated metabolites (some of which are conjugated with glucuronide). Certain of these metabolites are probably psychoactive. Insignificant portions of the drug are excreted unchanged. Phencyclidine dissociates in solution as a weak base; it is ionized below pH 5. Acidifying urine with ammonium chloride or ascorbic acid markedly enhances urinary excretion. Systemic acidification may decrease concentration in the cerebrospinal fluid and shorten drug effect. Interestingly, the compound (like other weak bases) passes in high concentration into gastric fluid. Such material might well be subject to reabsorption. Continuous gastric suctioning prevents this reabsorption and has been reported to be of value in the treatment of overdose.[3]

12.2. Effects

Neurological effects include ataxia, dysarthria, tremors, muscular hypertonicity, and hyperreflexia. The patient may complain of paresthesias. Analgesia with indifference to painful stimuli may be present, although reflexes remain intact. Posturing or severe dystonic reaction may occur. Myoclonic jerks and seizures may progress to status epilepticus. At higher dose levels, depression of reflexes may take place. Pupils are most often constricted, although light reaction is retained. Ptosis occurs, as well as horizontal, vertical, and even rotatory nystagmus.

Systolic and diastolic blood pressure levels are often elevated. These effects may be mediated through the α-adrenergic receptors and are reversible, using the α-blockading agent phentolamine. Phencyclidine potentiates adrenergic effects by inhibiting the neuronal reuptake of catecholamines. Such effects may operate centrally and could be important in the drug's psychostimulant action.

Phencyclidine acts as a myocardial depressant, inhibiting the force of contraction and slowing conduction in isolated cardiac tissue. Tachycardia may ensue, along with arrhythmias. Phencyclidine has anticholinergic effects in certain preparations, but these are short-lived and significantly less than those of atropine.

With lower doses, euphoria usually ensues. Frequent bursts of anxiety, lability of mood, and hostile expressions may follow or accompany the intoxication. Hallucinations can occur, although perceptual errors are more frequent. These often involve bizarre distortions of the body image; some users may panic when these occur. The impaired clarity of thought and perception, accompanied by anxiety, may produce psychotic states. Indeed, the drug might be classed as a deliriant. Many investigators have been struck by the drug's consistent ability, even in low doses, to derange interpretation of sensory input. The literature often compares the drug's effects to states of sensory deprivation. Horizontal or vertical nystagmus, muscular rigidity, and hypertension in a patient who is agitated, psychotic, or comatose and whose respiration is not depressed are typical for PCP intoxication. Animal studies indicate the efficacy of α-blocking agents. Animal experiments have also indicated tolerance to the drug.

13. D-Lysergic Acid and Related Compounds

Lysergic acid diethylamide (LSD) was a compound made in a series of syntheses in the late 1930s. The drug is exceedingly potent and may exert its effects in dosages as small as 25 μg. It is synthesized illicitly from ergot alkaloid precursors and may be supplied on pieces of blotter paper or gelatin tabs or dropped onto medications or even sugar cubes. Its use has probably diminished since the late 1960s, but it remains available in many places.

Several classes of drugs besides this one may produce perceptual and cognitive changes described as illusions, delusions, hallucinations, or psychoses. This particular grouping induces a psychedelic syndrome described as having a "capacity reliably to induce or compel states of altered perception, thought and feeling that are not (or cannot be) experienced otherwise except in dreams or at times of religious exaltation."[22] Most of the drugs included here are indolealkylamines or phenethylamine (methoxylated amphetaminelike compounds).

After oral administration LSD is rapidly absorbed and distributed throughout the body. Relatively high concentrations are found in the lung, liver, and kidney, and only a small proportion of administered drug enters the brain. Lysergic acid diethylamide is oxidized by hepatic microsomes, and a large proportion of the drug appears in the feces. The half-life is about 3 hr after an i.v. dosage,[1] but this is in contrast to the fact that 50–100 μg of LSD can induce effects that last for 12 hr.

The described syndrome has been principally studied relative to LSD. Other hallucinogens (with the exception of the atropinelike substances and PCP) produce remarkably similar phenomena. Most individuals who take LSD briefly do not require medical attention. Experienced and confident users dwell on the mood effects that are, to some, enjoyable.

There are somatic, perceptual, and affective components of the syndrome. The effects appear within 30–40 min of the consumption of extremely small doses of LSD (50 μg may be sufficient) or larger doses of other related compounds. The basic clinical syndrome includes somatic symptoms of dizziness, weakness, tremor, nausea, drowsiness, and occasionally paresthesias; perceptual symptoms of altered shapes and colors, difficulty in focusing on selected stimuli; finally, psychic symptoms including alterations in mood, disorientation of time sense, depersonalization, and, rarely, hallucinations.

Physiological effects are few. Some increased muscular tension, hyperreflexia, incoordination, and ataxia have been reported. Somatic symptoms and perceptual symptoms precede psychic changes. The psychic effects of a single dose may last 8–12 hr.

Other drugs in the category of psychedelic drugs include methoxylated amphetamine compounds, anticholinergic substances, and the harmine alkaloids.[21] The agents have multiple actions at multiple sites in the CNS.

A high degree of tolerance to the effects of LSD develops after a few doses, but responsiveness returns quickly after a brief drug-free interval. There is considerable cross-tolerance between LSD, mescaline, and psilocybin. Withdrawal phenomena are not seen.

13.1. Indolylalkylamines

Psilocybin and the related psilocin are indolylalkylamines found in certain mushrooms of the psilocybe species. Psilocybin is a phosphate ester of a 4-hydroxy dimethyltryptamine and is more potent than the 5-hydroxy dimethyltryptamines described below. Psilocybin has about 1% of the potency of LSD. It does not appear as a synthetic compound, but may occasionally be present in authentic mushrooms marketed for psychoactive uses.

Bufotenine is a plant alkaloid 5-hydroxy dimethyltriptamine. It was, however, first isolated from the skin of toads (*Bufo* species). It is weakly active by mouth and is 0.1% as potent as LSD. This example of psychedelic exotica seldom appears on the street. A snuff used by the Caribbean natives called cohoba is prepared from the seeds of various American plants (anadenanthera, mimosa, virola). Other snuffs used by American indigenes include niopo (Colombia) and yopo (Orinoco basin). These products all contain bufotenine and related indole alkaloids. Some versions of the plant products are prepared as infusions to be used as enemas. Harmine is a depicted indolylalkylamine. There are a variety of plant harmala alkaloids and they have some psychedelic activity. They make up the psychoactive principles in *Banisteriopsis caapi,* vinelike creeping plants used by South American natives near the Amazon in a variety of religious and social recreational events. Caapi is a snuff preparation of the dried *Banisteriopsis* and yage is prepared in Colombia by macerating the stem with another plant containing dimethyltryptamine and thus preparing a mixture for drinking.

13.2. Phenylalkylamine Derivatives

From this group came the bewildering three-letter abbreviations used to describe various psychedelic exotica (DOM, DMA, MDM, TMA, STP, DOB).

Mescaline (3,4,5-trimethoxyphenylethylamine) was identified as a psychoactive constituent of the Mexican cactus *Lophophora williamsi.* It is approximately 1/1000 as potent as LSD. Although widely discussed and frequently sold as more organic and safer than LSD, it seldom appears for sale. Purported mescaline samples may contain LSD or PCP.

The dried top of the cactus is called the peyotl or peyote. It is indigenous to Mexico and the Southwestern United States. The peyote button is a small, smooth, flattened sphere, sometimes called the mescal button. The plant is consumed legally as part of the rituals of the Native American Church of North American Indians. The button is chewed or eaten and swallowed.

14. Atropinelike Substances

Drugs that have anticholinergic effects often stimulate the CNS. Anticholinergic drugs such as atropine, scopolamine, and hyoscine may cause extreme excitation. Plants with such properties (deadly nightshade, datarum stramonium, morning-glory seeds, Jimson weed) may be ingested. Clinical problems include tachycardia, hyperthermia, confusion, hallucinations, and delusions. Treatment, if necessary, has consisted of the use of physostigmine to restore central cholinergic function.

15. Betel-Areca

Betel-areca chewing, as it is called, is well established from South Asia to Southeast Asia, the Malay Archipelago, and parts of Oceania. There is evidence indicating impaired judgment of the driver–users in motor vehicle accidents. Children can become intoxicated while chewing, and a reversible psychosis can occur in adults; both responses are rare. Users point to its breath freshener properties, its work-promoting effects in humid tropical climates, its promotion of social relationships, and presumed teeth-protecting qualities. About 200 million people chew daily at the present time.

There is a basic nucleus of three essential ingredients in betel-areca chewing, which are almost invariably admixed where the practice is customary. They are areca nut (*Areca catechu*), the slaked lime (calcium hydroxide) procured from burnt seashells, coral, or mountain lime, and the betel fruit or vine (*Piper betle*). In different countries various condiments have been added (e.g., cloves, camphor, nutmeg, and aloes). The areca nut, which tastes like nutmeg, is hot and acrid with marked astringent qualities. The purpose of the betel pepper is primarily as an aromatic. The quid, made up of the three basic items, is applied to the buccal mucous membrane, kept in place by the tongue as it is sucked. This has a local irritative effect. A CNS stimulant effect is due to arecaidine, arecoline, guvacine, *iso*-guvacine, guvacoline, and choline. The most psychoactive are arecoline and arecaidine; the former is hydrolyzed to the latter by the calcium hydroxide. The chewing produces a bright-red color which stains the teeth and gums.

The inexperienced betel-areca chewer notes nausea, vertigo, dizziness, and cold perspiration and complains of a sore tongue. With habituation these side effects disappear. There is little clouding of consciousness and an increased capacity for activity. Parasympathomimetic effects include contracted pupils; excessive sweat, tears, and saliva; and looseness of stools.

With regular use, dependence is soon established. If a supply is unavailable, the established chewer suffers headache, restlessness, and poor concentration. Oral cancers have been reportedly due to chronic use.[8,34]

16. Khat (Chat, Qat)

The *Catha edulis* plant is used for stimulant effects in some parts of East Africa and the Red Sea area. Recently a compound referred to as cathinone has been isolated as a psychostimulant ingredient with amphetaminelike effects. This drug may be metabolized to phenethanolamines such as phenylpropanolaline or norephedrine. Its fresh leaves are chewed for their effects, often in a social setting.

Its use has important economic effects in several countries. In exporting countries, khat plantations have replaced sorghum and other essential crops. Some suporting countries lose a large proportion of their gross income to khat expenditures. As much as 25–75% of some families' income is spent to purchase khat.

Heavy khat use can lead to insomnia. Some users then drink alcohol or take sedatives in order to sleep. Withdrawal symptoms such as fatigue, tremors, and nightmares suggest the presence of a mild dependence syndrome. Occasional gastrointestinal and urinary symptoms indicate a local irritant effect.[5,26]

17. Combined Drug Effects

A number of different types of interactions have been identified between drugs. One parsimonious description is as follows:

> Two drugs may be similar or opposite in their pharmacological effects in which case the coadministration of another drug with ethanol would cause either an increase or decrease in the ethanolic effect. The effect of the other drug would then be considered either "synergistic" (additive) or "antagonistic." However, the "additive" effect may be the sum of each of the drugs administered separately or it may be greater, i.e. "supra additive."[28]

Almost all drugs have certain additive or supraadditive effects when combined.[12] The supraadditive effect, also referred to as the potentiating effect, may result in drug fatalities at a low dosage of both drugs. For example, a blood alcohol level of 0.10 combined with a barbiturate level of 0.05 has been fatal. Diazepam has an additive effect with alcohol: diazepam blood levels have been found to be higher when alcohol is consumed.[12] Combined alcohol and marijuana, even at low dose levels of both drugs, have a dangerous effect on a driving task, which is greater than that created by either drug separately.[12]

References

1. Aghajanian GK, Bing OHL: Persistence of lysergic acid diethylamide in the plasma of human subjects. *Clin Pharmacol Ther* 1964; 5:611–614.
2. Arif A: *Adverse Health Consequences of Cocaine Misuse*. Geneva, WHO, 1987.
3. Arnow R, Done A: Phencyclidine overdose: An emergency concept of management. *J Am Coll Emergency Physicians* 1978; 7:56–59.
4. Ashton H, Stepney R: *Smoking: Psychology and Pharmacology*. New York, Tavistock, 1982.
5. Baasher T, Sadoun R: The epidemiology of khat. Madagascar, International Conference on Khat, 1983.
6. Beckett HA, Gorrod JW, Jenner P: The effect of smoking on nicotine metabolism *in vivo* in man. *J Pharm Pharmacol* 1971; 23(suppl):625–675.
7. Bridger WH, Schiff SR, Cooper SS, Paredes W, Barr GA: Classical conditioning of cocaine's stimulatory effects. *Psychopharmacol Bull* 1982; 18(4):210–214.
8. Burton-Bradley BG: Arecaidinism: Betel chewing in transcultural perspective. *Can J Psychiatry* 1979; 24:481–488.
9. Cherek DR: Effects of smoking different doses of nicotine on human agressive behavior. *Psychopharmacology* 1981; 17:339–345.
10. Cohen S: Coca paste and freebase: New fashions in cocaine use. *Drug Abuse Alcoholism Newsletter* 1980; 9:1–3.
11. Cohen S: *Cocaine Today*. Rockville, MD, American Council on Drug Abuse, 1981.
12. Cohen S: Combined alcohol, drug abuse and human behavior, in Solomon J, Keeley KA (eds): *Perspectives in Alcohol and Drug Abuse*. Boston, John Wright, 1982, pp 89–116.
13. Conney AH: Drug metabolism and therapeutics. *N Engl J Med* 1969; 280:653–660.
14. Costa E, Guidotti A, Mao C: Evidence of involvement of GABA in the action of benzodiazepines. Studies on the rat cerebellum. Mechanism of action of benzodiazepines. *Adv Biochem Psychopharmacol* 1975; 14:113–130.
15. Davis VE, Walsh MJ: Alcohol amines and alkaloids: A possible basis for alcohol addiction. *Science* 1970; 167:1005–1007.
16. Ellinwood E: Amphetamine psychosis. 1. Description of the individuals and process. *J Nerv Ment Dis* 1967; 144:273–283.
17. Finnegan LP: The effects of narcotics and alcohol on pregnancy and the newborn, in Millman RB, Cushman P Jr, Lowinson JH (eds): Research developments and drug and alcohol use. *Ann NY Acad Sci* 1981; 362:136–157.
18. Gold MS, Redmond DE Jr, Kleber HD: Clonidine in opiate withdrawal. *Lancet* 1978; 1:929–930.
19. Goldstein A, Kaizer S: Psychotropic effects of caffeine in man. 3. A questionnaire survey of coffee drinking and its effects in a group of housewives. *Clin Pharmacol Ther* 1969; 10:477–488.
20. Greden JF: Caffeinism and caffeine withdrawal, in Lowinson JH, Ruiz P (eds): *Substance Abuse: Clinical Problems and Perspectives*. Baltimore, Williams & Wilkins, 1981.
21. Grinspoon L, Bakalar JB: *Psychedelic Drugs Revisited*. New York, Basic Books, 1980.
22. Jaffee JH: Drug addiction and drug abuse, in Gilman AG, Goodman LS, Gilman A (eds): *The Pharmacological Basis of Therapeutics*, ed 6. New York, Macmillan, 1980.
23. Jaffee JH, Kanzler M: Smoking as a psychiatric disorder, in Pickens RW, Heston LL (eds):

Psychiatric Factors in Drug Abuse. New York, London, Toronto, Sydney, San Francisco, Grune & Stratton, 1979.
24. Kales A, Bixler EO, Tan TL, Sharf MB, Kales JD: Chronic hypnotic-drug use: Ineffectiveness, drug-withdrawal, insomnia, and dependence. *JAMA* 1974; 227:513–517.
25. Kelly MG: Pentazocine: A strong analgesic with low abuse potential. *Br J Addict* 1977; 72:250–252.
26. Kennedy JG, Teague J, Rokaw W, Cooney E: A medical evaluation of the use of qat in North Yemen. *Social Sci Med* 1983; 17:783–793.
27. Kilbey MM, Ellinwood EH Jr: Reverse tolerance to stimulant-induced abnormal behavior. *Life Sci* 1977; 20:1063–1076.
28. Kissen B: Interactions of ethyl alcohol and other drugs, in Kissen B, Begleiter H (eds): *The Biology of Alcoholism, Clinical Pathology.* New York, Plenum Press, 1974, vol 3, pp 109–162.
29. Kolodny RC, Masters WH, Kolodner RM, Toro G: Depression of plasma testosterone levels after chronic intensive marihuana use. *N Engl J Med* 1974; 290:872–874.
30. Levine RR, Pelikan EW: Mechanisms of drug absorption and excretion. *Annu Rev Pharmacol* 1964; 4:69.
31. Lewis JD, Moritz D, Mellis LP: Long-term toluene abuse. *Am J Psychiatry* 1981; 138:368–370.
32. Mello NK: Alcoholism and the behavioral pharmacology of alcohol: 1967–1977, in Lipton MA, DeMascio A, Killam KF (eds): *Psychopharmacology: A Generation of Progress.* New York, Raven Press, 1978.
33. Misra AL: Metabolism of opiates, in Alder ML, Manara L, Saminin R (eds): *Factors Affecting the Action of Narcotics.* New York, Raven Press, 1978.
34. Patel TB: Cancer problem—Its epidemiology and prevention with special reference to Gujarat State. *Gujarat Med J* 1979; 25:5–9.
35. Post RM: Psychomotor stimulants as activators of normal and pathological behaviour, in Male SJ (ed): *American Behaviour in Excess.* New York, Free Press, 1981.
36. Ray O: *Drugs, Society and Human Behavior,* ed 3. St. Louis, Mosby, 1983.
37. Report of an ARF/WHO Scientific Meeting on Adverse Health and Behavioural Consequences of Cannabis Use. Toronto, Ontario, Canada, Addiction Research Foundation, 1981.
38. Rosenberg H, Orkin FK, Springstead J: Abuse of nitrous oxide. *Anesthesia Analygesia: Curr Res* 1979; 58:104–106.
39. Schaumburg HH, Spencer PS: Degeneration and central and peripheral nervous systems produced by pure *N*-hexane: An experimental study. *Brain* 1976; 99:183–192.
40. Seevers MH: Drug dependence vis-à-vis drug abuse, in Zaeafonetis CJ (ed): *International Conference on Drug Abuse* (Proceedings), Ann Arbor, MI. Philadelphia, Lea & Febiger, 1970, pp 9–16.
41. Shephard N Jr: Statistics suggest U.S. faces new drug abuse problem. *New York Times,* Sept 10, 1981, p 19.
42. Smith DE, Wesson DR: A phenobarbital technique for withdrawal of barbiturate abuse. *Arch Gen Psychiatry* 1971; 24:56–60.
43. Snider R, Docsis J: Current concepts of chronic benzene toxicity. *Crit Rev Toxicol* 1975; 3:265–288.
44. Squires RF, Braestrup C: Benzodiazepine receptors in rat brain. *Nature* 1977; 266:732–734.
45. Stewart J: Conditional and unconditional drug effects and relapse. *Prog Neuropsychopharmacol Biopsychiatry* 1982; 7(4–6):591–597.
46. Stimmel B: Alcohol-related cardiomyopathies, in Stimmel B (ed): *Cardiovascular Effects of Mood-Altering Drugs.* New York, Raven Press, 1979.
47. Swett C: Drowsiness due to chlorpromazine in relation to cigarette smoking. *Arch Gen Psychiatry* 1974; 31:211–213.
48. Truitt EB: Biological disposition of tetrahydrocannabinols. *Pharmacol Rev* 1971; 23:273–278.
49. Van Dyke C: Cocaine, in Lowinson JH, Ruiz P (eds): *Substance Abuse: Clinical Problems and Perspectives.* Baltimore, Williams & Wilkins, 1981.

50. Van Dyke C, Jatlow P, Barash PG, Ungerer J, Byck R: Cocaine and lidocaine have similar psychological effects after intra nasal application. *Life Sci* 1979; 24:271–274.
51. Wack JT, Roden J: Smoking and its effects on body weight and the system of caloric regulation. *Am J Clin Nutr* 1982; 35:366–380.
52. Weiss B, Laties BG: Enhancement of human performance by caffeine and amphetamine. *Pharmacol Rev* 1962; 14:1–36.
53. Westermeyer J: *A Clinical Guide to Alcohol and Drug Problems*. New York, Praeger, 1986, p 34.
54. Whitfield CL, Thompson G, Spencer V, Lamb A, Pfeifer M, Browning-Ferrando M: Detoxification of 1024 alcoholic patients without psychoactive drugs. *JAMA* 1978; 239:1409–1410.
55. WHO Expert Committee on Addiction Producing Drugs. Thirteenth Report. *Technical Report Series,* no. 273. Geneva, WHO, 1964.
56. WHO Expert Committee on Smoking Control Strategies in Developing Countries. 22–27 No. Geneva, WHO, 1982.
57. Zukin SR, Zukin RS: Identification and characterization of (3H)phencyclidine binding to specific brain receptor sites, in Domino EF (ed): *PCP (Phencyclidine): Historical and Current Perspectives*. Ann Arbor, MI, NPP Books, 1981.

Further Reading

Carlton PL: *A Primer on Behavioral Pharmacology: Concepts and Principles in the Behavioral Analysis of Drug Action*. New York, Freeman, 1983.

Iverson LL: Neurotransmitters and CNS disease. *Lancet* 1982; 2:914–918.

IV

Diagnosis and Management

8

Clinical Diagnosis and Assessment

1. Introduction

The purpose of assessment is to ascertain the severity of the problem, as well as the patient's biological, psychological, and social resources. Identification of both problems and resources is needed in order to determine need for and type of treatment.

Diagnosis is not an end itself. Mere labeling of drug dependence can do more harm than good. Instead, diagnosis should enable the physician and patient to achieve the following:

1. Become aware of the problem and its prognosis.
2. Choose treatment alternatives likely to be successful.
3. Facilitate communication among family members and professionals.

2. Background Factors

Patients with drug dependence present to clinical settings much as do other patients, but with certain additional and special characteristics. They often feel (and are) stigmatized because of being drug dependent and thus may fear the physician's response to them. At times they want help for their medical complications from drug dependence, but are ambivalent about giving up their dependence on drugs. They may seek medical help at the insistence of others, rather than on their own. These background factors must be known and understood in undertaking thorough clinical assessment.

2.1. Interaction between the Physician, Patient, and Community

Complete assessment requires collaboration from the patient as well as other significant persons (e.g., family, employer, or teacher). Information will be available to the extent that the informant feels safe, is taken seriously, understands the purpose of the assessment, and trusts the clinician. Emphasis, sequence, wording, and the information provided by the clinician all influence this collaboration to a considerable extent.

The clinician must be prepared to deal with divergent information, needs, opinions, and definitions of the problem. Patient or family may use the physician not only as a health resource, but as a partisan, a control agent, a pressure valve, or a means of avoiding responsibility. In such circumstances the physician's role and prestige can be either an asset or a liability, depending on how they are used. Awareness of these potential dilemmas is a major step in dealing with them.

Some patients initially test the clinician by presenting a part of the problem, or a different problem, before coming to the real issue. Their ambivalence about being helped, shame about being weak or a failure, and guilt feelings or fear of giving up drugs can interfere with the interview process. Feeling accepted and understood by the clinician is an important factor in establishing physician–patient rapport.

Helpful approaches on the part of the physician include the following:

- Empathy with and acceptance of the patient as a person do not imply acceptance of drug habits.
- Readiness to listen and understand before coming to premature conclusions.
- Being clear and firm regarding one's own role, functions, abilities, powers, limits, and boundaries.
- Avoiding ambiguous messages.
- Awareness of one's own feelings toward the patient (e.g., distrust, sympathy, repulsion, interest, identification, fear).
- Appreciating the patient's ethical concerns while avoiding moral judgments.
- Inquiry should be guided by the intent to help the patient in coping with the situation, and not simply by the intent to find the patient guilty of drug dependence.

There are special circumstances in which the physician serves two masters: the patient and a social institution (e.g., army, school, prison, corporation). It is helpful at the outset to make clear the doctor's role and potential authority. If this is done from the beginning, unrealistic fears and expectations can be avoided.

Even outside of social institutions, the physician may still be caught between the patient and other persons, such as the family. Differences should not be covered up, nor should the physician prematurely take sides. Acting as a mediator is an especially useful physician role in such circumstances. This consists of clarifying divergent viewpoints of the various parties, interpreting the diverse needs of the parties, determining alternatives for managing the current problem, and negotiating for common, shared objectives. The physician may then support and perhaps assist with the agreed-upon plan and goals.

2.2. Reason for Consultation

A prime issue to be clarified during the assessment is the reason for seeking consultation. This motivation may originate from the patient, the family, or others. A biomedical problem may be the rationale for consultation, whereas a marital or legal problem is the main concern.

A frequent experience among physicians is that the patient seeks treatment for a drug-related problem such as an abscess, headaches, or depression. While the patient genuinely wants help with the drug-related problem, help with the drug dependence itself may not be desired. This creates a professional and an ethical dilemma for the physician. Treating the secondary problem while ignoring the drug dependence is like treating typhoid fever symptomatically with aspirin while ignoring the etiology. It may actually be easier to simply treat the symptomatic manifestation and ignore the basic problem. Holistic patient care demands that we do more than merely treat symptoms, however. The patient's concern regarding drug-related problems acts as therapeutic leverage in motivating the patient to address the drug-dependence problem.

3. History Taking

Success in acquiring information about the presence, severity, duration, and effects of drug dependence requires more clinical skill than is customarily needed for the usual medical history. Patients with drug-related problems rarely present with these as the chief complaint. Rather these patients are often evasive and attempt to conceal their drug dependence. Indeed they may actually believe that their medical problems are not related to drug dependence. And while that may be true for the presenting problem, it is rare that the presence of drug dependence has no clinical relevance for the management of any medical problem, even one unrelated to drug dependence.

The medical model for history taking (i.e., chief complaint, present illness, past history, review of systems, family history, and psychosocial history) employed by physicians offers a familiar and inclusive structure for diagnosing drug dependence. Certain parts of the inquiry must receive special attention.

3.1. Content and Process of History Taking

Questions concerning type of drug, consumption, pattern, and frequency of use may lead to factual data about a suspected drug problem. However, observation of nonverbal communications must accompany acquisition of information. Resistance, anxiety, or discomfort in answering certain questions comprises valuable information.

Process pertains to the emotional and relational component of the patient–physician interaction. Content refers to the cognitive factors and information. Both components are necessary to secure an adequate database. Awareness of this process may yield information of greater clinical significance than that secured by sole attention to content.

Acquisition of both process and content information can be encouraged if physicians attempt to answer questions put to themselves, as well as to the patient. What is the problem? What does the patient say is his problem? What communication style does the patient use to convey the complaint: symbolic, cryptic, defensive? Is there a seeming disparity between what the patient says is wrong and the physician's intuitive feeling that the chief complaint covers some other underlying problem? People dependent on drugs may become accomplished in duplicity and in their facility to manipulate the physician into providing psychoactive drugs. Why at this particular time does this patient make the decision to seek help?

There is usually an element of coercion, either from an external source or from an internal one. External pressure may come from the family, employer, or police. For example, the wife may say to her husband, "I have had enough. Either you get some help with your drug problem or I am leaving." An employer may issue an ultimatum to his employee to seek out and follow a treatment program or lose his job. The patient may have been apprehended committing a crime while under the influence of alcohol. As an alternative to serving time in jail, the judge may offer the option of finding professional help. The drug-dependent patient experiences emotional disturbance—guilt, shame, remorse, fear, hopelessness, anxiety, panic—which may prompt medical consultation. Or physical problems may prompt a move to seek help. Whether the coercion is external and/or internal, this represents a crucial time for the perceptive physician to initiate an intervention of the drug dependence.

The patient's mode of response to questions about use of drugs—i.e., the manner in which the patient denies, projects, evades, or rationalizes—is more important generally than the information that the patient readily volunteers. For example, the physician may ask, "Do you take drugs?" The patient may reply, "Yes, I use a lot of drugs, but it's no problem." In which case, the physician will want to know, "Why does the patient answer thus?" Or the patient may respond, "Sure, but I can quit anytime I want."

Physicians contribute to the interview process, also. Their attitudes are vital to the encounter with the drug-dependent patient. Moralistic and judgmental attitudes are quickly perceived by the patient. These can bring an early termination to the physician–patient relationship.

3.2. Chief Complaint

The person who presents the chief complaint to the physician may provide an important cue. This person may be the spouse, parent, friend, or the drug-dependent person. Parents may bring their adolescent offspring to the doctor with the complaint, "Doctor, I believe my son is taking drugs and I want you to talk to him about it." Or the person's spouse may say, "My wife takes too many sedatives and I am worried about her." Another situation may be that the mother of a young child brings the child to the doctor as a facade for her real concern. Near the end of the consultation she may say, "By the way, I want to tell you about my husband's drinking."

3.3. Present Illness, Review of Systems, Family History, and Social History

The history of the *present illness* should encompass questions about the onset, duration, severity, and vicissitudes of the drug dependence, as well as what measures have been tried for relief (e.g., cutting down on amounts, trying abstinence, consulting doctors, changing drugs, and other measures).

The *review of systems* consists of a review of symptoms referable to the various body systems (e.g., cardiovascular, neuromuscular, gastrointestinal). It is deserving of meticulous and thorough inquiry for the reason that most often early drug-dependence problems are found in this area of the patient's health. Neurological, cardiovascular, gastrointestinal, autonomic, appetite, sleep, and psychiatric disturbance should be investigated. Frequently present are feelings of shame or remorse, anxiety, and fear about impaired control over the use of the drug and hopelessness because of a growing drug dependency. The drug-dependent person usually does not volunteer these symptoms, but will reveal them if asked. A review of systems with particular reference to drug dependence requires that the physician has an understanding of the potential effect of the opioids, sedative/hypnotics, alcohol, cocaine, stimulants, hallucinogens, and volatiles. Symptoms of intoxication, dependence, tolerance, and withdrawal for each classification of drugs should be asked about (e.g.. constipation with opioids).

Past history should inquire of medical and surgical problems. Inquiry of significant life events may also aid in understanding the genesis of the drug problems. Some people may have come to rely on drugs to help them manage stress or major life changes.

The *family history* can elicit significant information about genetic vulnerability to alcoholism, psychosis, affective and personality disorders, and neurosis. Adequate parenting may not have occurred owing to the loss of a parent in childhood, by separation from death or divorce, or by emotional deprivation by a parent who is abusing drugs or suffering from mental illness. Information about the parents' attitudes toward and use of all drugs (prescription, proprietary, legal, and illicit) is important. Drugs may have been forbidden, used in ritualistic manner or for religious observations, taken for festive occasions, consumed with meals, or used without any guidelines or controls. Patterns of drug use that occurred during early formative years often have had considerable influence and shaped the patient's present use of these agents.

Social history is also important, since drug-related social problems often appear early, before biomedical problems. Difficulties in relationships with family members, particularly the patient and the parents, spouse, and children, should be reviewed. Occupational and financial problems can be associated with declining productivity, on-the-job accidents, absenteeism, and conflicts with supervisory personnel and fellow workers. The housewife–mother may neglect child care and domestic duties. Adolescents may manifest problems at home, at school, or in the community. In the elderly patient drug dependence may be difficult to differentiate from or may accentuate dementia. Inquiry about leisure time activities can also provide diagnostic clues. Drug dependence may accompany the patient's recreational pursuits, or it may even be the main focus of leisure time pursuits. Change in religious practice often results from drug dependence; the patient may reduce or abandon customary religious practice. First indications of drug dependence can occur when the patient is apprehended by the criminal justice system. Examples include the following: operating a motor vehicle while intoxicated; being a public nuisance and charged with disorderly conduct; violent behavior, such as battering spouse or children, or fighting with friends; being apprehended for possession or distribution of illicit drugs.

3.4. Drug Use History

A drug use history consists of questions such as "Do you smoke?" "What drugs do you use?" "Do you drink? How much?" If these questions are asked in a hurried fashion, the patient feels that the doctor does not consider them important. Some patients are content not to be questioned further about these matters, and they respond in a similar hurried fashion.

Drug use questions should be inclusive and relate to all drugs that can be used—prescription drugs, those which can be purchased legally without a doctor's prescription, and illicit drugs. Not only the kind of drugs used, but the amount and patterns of use are important.

It is well to precede actual questioning by an introductory statement such as "Now, I would like to know about your use of drugs. By drugs I mean any substance you use which a doctor may have prescribed, or that you purchase at the store or pharmacy, or from someone else.'' Later clarifying questions might include ''How much tea, coffee, or caffeine-containing drinks do you use? How much do you smoke? What do you smoke? What medications do you take? Do you take medications for sleep, or to relieve feelings of being anxious or depressed? How much alcoholic beverages do you drink? Do you use marijuana, cocaine, narcotics, hallucinogenics, amphetamines? Have you ever snuffed drugs? Or injected drugs?''

This questioning should be done incrementally in a detailed, careful manner. Physicians must convey the impression to patients that they believe that the answers to the questions are important and relevant to the clinical assessment.

Additionally, questions should be posed about the patient's own feelings and concerns regarding this use, as well as about the feelings of the spouse, family, and others toward the patient's drug use. Useful examples include ''Have you ever felt you should cut down on your use of alcohol?'' ''Have you ever thought that your use of drugs has been out of your control?'' Questions directed at the symptoms of dependence, episodic or intermittent withdrawal, memory impairment, and tolerance must be asked. Behavioral consequences of drug dependence should be assessed by questions that relate to the patient's self-esteem, productivity, and relationship to people.

4. Physical Examination

Drug dependence can affect any organ or system of the body. Each substance of abuse has its particular pathological effect on certain target organs or systems, as follows:

- Opioids—gastrointestinal system, autonomic nervous system.
- Alcohol—central nervous system; liver, pancreas, and stomach; cardiovascular system (i.e., hypertension, dysrhythmias).
- Sedatives—central nervous system.
- Stimulants—central nervous system, cardiovascular system.
- Hallucinogens—central nervous system.

Modes of administration also produce biomedical problems as follows:

- Ingestion—oral and pharyngeal inflammation and tumors, peptic ulcer.
- Snuffing—sinusitis, nasal septum perforation.
- Chewing—gingivitis, leukoplakia, oral tumors.
- Smoking—bronchitis, emphysema, tumors of respiratory tract.
- Parenteral injection—septicemia, abscess, bacterical endocarditis, hepatitis.

Other nonspecific health problems result from lifestyle or social problems due to acute or chronic drug dependence. These include

- Nutrition—hypoproteinemia, muscle wasting, peripheral neuritis, various vitamin deficiencies.
- Infectious disease—dermatitis, pediculoses, hepatitis, venereal disease.
- Trauma—fights, accidents, victimization.
- Psychiatric disorders—depression, panic, organic mental disorders.

Factors that affect the physical findings include the patient's gender, age, ethnic, or cultural background. For example, women are more vulnerable to alcoholic liver damage than men; elderly persons' metabolism of drugs of all kinds is slower than that of younger persons; some Asian people react to alcohol as though they were taking low doses of disulfiram. Other factors that may affect drug metabolism, and consequently alter the physical findings, are the kind, amount, rate of consumption, and patterns of use of the substance. For example, binge use, sporadic controlled use, intermittent loss of control, or chronic use can lead to different problems, as follows:

- A high dose of opioids in a naive or occasional user may result in coma or even death while not affecting a long-term addict.
- A heavy bout of drinking over several days may cause reversible fatty infiltration of the liver whereas cirrhosis may be irreversible.
- Chronic heavy amphetamine use may cause a paranoid psychotic state whereas acute doses in nonvulnerable subjects may not produce mental illness.

In general, it can be stated that drugs which depress the central nervous system, including the opioids, produce a hypometabolic state during intoxication and a temporary hypermetabolic rebound reaction during withdrawal. The opposite reaction occurs with the psychostimulants; i.e., a hypermetabolic state during intoxication is followed by a hypometabolic condition during withdrawal.

The physician can learn a great deal in the first few minutes of contact with the patient. Clues obtained in this early contact may indicate that special attention to some organ or system should be undertaken. For example, an ataxic gait may indicate intoxication with alcohol, sedative, or opioid drugs. Or cerebellar degeneration may suggest chronic alcohol use. Or icteric sclerae could indicate alcoholic hepatitis or infectious hepatitis due to use of contaminated needles.

Aspects of the physical examination often neglected, yet important for assessing drug dependence, include the following: the vital signs, autonomic nervous system, mental status, and neurological examinations. Frequent abnormalities of vital signs are as follows:

- *Temperature*
  Fever with the infectious complications of intravenous and other sources of contamination of drugs abused, and with sedative–alcohol withdrawal (including delirium tremens).
- *Pulse*
  Irregularities with heavy use of caffeine, tobacco, alcohol, and amphetamines.
  Bradycardia with opioid overdose.
- *Blood pressure*
  Hypertension from chronic alcohol use or alcohol withdrawal.
  Hypotension may occur with overdosage of many drugs, but is especially characteristic of opioid overdose.
  Phencyclidine (PCP) intoxication may cause hypertension or hypotension.

While general impressions can be formed from initial patient contact, the performance of a formal mental status examination yields much more specific data about the patient's affect, memory, cognition, and speech. It can indicate the following:

- *General behavior*
  Poor personal hygiene: chronic drug dependence.
- *Interpersonal relationship to examiner*
  Evasive, suspicious, avoiding relationship, manipulative, seductive, directs the interview, seeking nontherapeutic ends from the relationship: chronic drug dependence.
- *Mood*
  Sad, euphoric, irritable, anxious, rapid shift in mood.
- *Thought processes*
  1. Logical: does the patient make sense?
  2. Connected: can you follow the patient's train of thought?
  3. Appropriate: are the patient's concerns relevant to the doctor–patient relationship?
  4. Delusions: fixed, unlikely beliefs.
  5. Hallucinations: perceptions without apparent stimuli.
- *Orientation*
  1. Time: year, month, date, day, season, time of day.
  2. Place: country, province or region, community, building, or clinic.
  3. Person: name of self and examiner.
  4. Current situation and its purpose.
- *Memory*
  1. Remote: childhood, birthplace.

2. Recent: events of recent days and weeks.
3. Immediate: can recall memory tasks during the interview (such as numbers or objects).

Physical examination should include the following organs and systems, taking note of the following suggestive signs:

- *Head*
  Recent and/or old trauma, including a subdural hematoma or depressed skull fracture; pediculosis infestation.
- *Eye*
  1. *Pupils:* constricted with opioid intoxication; dilated with opioid withdrawal, dilated and nonreactive with alcohol or sedative overdose.
  2. *Conjunctiva:* congestion with cannabis and alcohol, pallor with anemia due to hematopoeitic suppression from several drugs or malnutrition.
  3. *Lacrimation:* associated with opioid withdrawal.
  4. *Sclerae:* icteric with liver disease.
  5. *Oculomotor:* ophthalmoplegia with Wernicke's syndrome (thiamine deficiency); PCP causes both horizontal and vertical nystagmus.
  6. *Toxic amblyopia:* tobacco, alcohol, methanol in wood alcohol or illicit distilled alcohol.
- *Nose*
  Rhinorrhea; septal ulceration and perforation from snorting drugs; rhinophyma and acne rosacea with heavy alcohol use.
- *Ears*
  Gouty tophi: due to alcohol-related increased serum uric acid.
- *Mouth*
  1. Fetor oris—odor of alcohol; poor oral hygiene; odor of tobacco and cannabis.
  2. Lips—malignant or premalignant lesion of lips and tongue due to combined use of alcohol and tobacco, cyanosis in heavy smokers.
  3. Perioral rash: solvent use.
  4. Teeth: dental caries and periodontal infection; almost any drug, but especially chewed drugs.
  5. Tongue: tremors—during withdrawal from depressants.
  6. Uvular edema—heavy hashish use.
  7. Pharynx: inflammation or tumor with alcohol or tobacco or betel.
- *Neck*
  Nodding during opioid intoxication. Muscle rigidity and spasm may occur with PCP intoxication.
- *Chest*
  Inspection and palpation.

1. Spider angiomata: liver damage.
2. Gynecomastia in the male: liver damage and testosterone deficiency.
3. Fracture of ribs: due to trauma while intoxicated.

Percussion and auscultation

Lungs: signs of bronchitis or emphysema with heavy smoking of opium, tobacco, marijuana, or hashish. Lung abscess from aspiration during acute intoxication. Acute pulmonary edema may occur with opioids. Lysergic acid diethylamide, cannabis, opium, and other drugs may precipitate asthmatic attacks in predisposed individuals. Cor pulmonale in chronic smokers.

- *Heart*

1. Cardiomegaly: alcoholic cardiomyopathy: acute cardiac dilatation from inhalant intoxication.
2. Cardiac murmurs: bacteremia in parenteral injection, causing valvulitis and endocarditis.
3. Dysrhythmias: alcohol, solvents, tobacco, caffeine, stimulants.

- *Abdomen*

Inspection

1. Distension due to ascites from chronic alcohol or inhalant dependence.
2. Dilated superficial veins due to portal vein obstruction.
3. Surgical scars from peptic ulcer, liver biopsy, parecentesis.
4. Hematemesis from esophogeal varices due to hepatic cirrhosis.

Palpation

1. Hepatomegaly with and without tenderness.
2. Tenderness of right upper quadrant—hepatitis; periumbilical or epigastric—alcoholic pancreatitis.
3. Ascites: fluid wave.

Auscultation

1. Decreased peristaltic sounds: opioids, stimulants.
2. Increased peristaltic sounds: alcoholic malabsorption syndrome; opioid withdrawal.

Percussion

1. Shifting dullness due to ascitic fluid.
2. Hepatomegaly.

- *Genitourinary*

Some of these findings may be indirect effects of the life-style of the drug-dependent person.

Male

1. Penile lesions (e.g., chancre, herpes progenitalis).
2. Urethral discharge (gonorrhea, trichomonal).
3. Testicular atrophy, loss or decrease in pubic hair among males—alcohol or opiate dependence.
4. Pediculosis pubis.

Female

1. Chancre, herpes (external genitalia, vagina, cervix).
2. Urethral and vaginal discharge (gonococcal, trichomonal, monilial, nonspecific).
3. Cervicitis—changing sexual partners.
4. Amenorrhea—alcohol or opiate effect on ovaries.

- *Musculoskeletal*
  1. Muscle wasting.
  2. Muscle spasm and rigidity with PCP intoxication.
  3. Fractures due to trauma, accidents.
  4. Osteomyelitis and septic arthritides from parenteral injection.
  5. Muscle tenderness (especially of calf muscles) with alcoholic neuropathy.
  6. Muscle pain, tenderness, swelling, and weakness due to acute rhabdomyolysis from intravenous administration.
- *Neurological*
  1. Tremors: liver flap with hepatic encephalopathy; withdrawal from alcohol or sedative drugs.
  2. Gait: alcoholic cerebellar degeneration.
- *Dermatological*
  1. Stains may be seen on the fingers of those who smoke heavily, whether cannabis, opium, or tobacco.
  2. Intravenous injection may be apparent by finding tracks (pigmented linear marks along the course of superficial veins). Thrombophlebitis may result. Those who inject opiates in the fatty tissue of the thigh or upper arm (so-called skin poppers) may show abscesses or depressed areas from previous abscesses in these areas.
  3. Pruritus, chronic papular seborrheic dermatitis.
  4. Cheilosis from vitamin deficiency, stress.
  5. Perspiration from opioid or alcohol–sedative withdrawal.
  6. Piloerection (gooseflesh) from opioid withdrawal.
  7. Pyoderma from poor hygiene or from white-blood-cell suppression with alcoholism.
- *Lymphatic system*

  Enlarged lymph glands associated with acquired immune deficiency syndrome.

Early Signs and Symptoms

Physicians should be alert to the early diagnosis of drug dependence, so that intervention and treatment may occur before irreversible physical, psychological, or social damage. Frequent headaches, recurrent gastrointestinal complaints, recent absences from school or work based on vague physical complaints, or sudden unexplained mood changes are possible early symptoms of drug dependence. More advanced symptoms may ensue with the continued use of drugs even after having problems while using drugs. Increased frequency of use despite blackouts, antisocial, or belligerent behavior while under the influence of chemicals, or confrontations by spouse or friends about usage, are frequently symptoms of loss of control over drug use. In order to validate the diagnosis in some suspected cases, the physician may ask the patient if a family member could be present during a subsequent visit.

Frequent injuries or cigarette burns due to drowsiness may be other symptoms of drug intoxication. Unexplained mood changes and history of physical display of anger may be other indications of a chemical use problem. Cutaneous signs of drug dependence should be learned, as should the signs and symptoms of stimulant intoxication and withdrawal, and opioid intoxication and withdrawal.

In adolescence, an unexplained drop in grades, chronic tardiness, increased absenteeism, deterioration in personal hygiene, or a decrease in physical recreation activities are all possible symptoms of increased drug use. Personality changes such as impulsivity and rebelliousness may be early warning signs of drug misuse. This has been labeled by some as the amotivational syndrome.[2] A combination of two or more of the following symptoms in students may be a predictor of future drug misuse: failure in any area of education; difficulty in social functioning; failure to find humor in one's life; frequent use of mood-altering drugs; irregular class attendance; and friction with more than one professor.

Physicians and other health workers may be even more vulnerable to substance abuse than their patients. Prophylaxis and early diagnosis should be practiced not only with the patients but within the health professions.[3,6]

Prescription-drug misuse or dependence as illustrated by nonbarbiturate compounds such as benzodiazepines may be associated with mild withdrawal symptoms of anxiety, insomnia, dizziness, headaches, and anorexia with rapid weight loss. In one series of 24 cases, 22 patients reported that they had tried but were unable to give up diazepam on their own initiative.[9]

Failure of response to treatment should alert the clinician to the possibility of drug dependence. Typical examples are diabetics who cannot be managed by careful insulin regimens, depressed patients who do not respond to tricyclic medication, patients whose infections do not respond as expected to antibiotics, seizure patients who do not respond to anticonvulsants, or surgical patients whose wounds do not heal. Drugs of abuse also affect the actions of prescribed drugs; this can alert the physician to possible drug dependence. For example, acute and chronic alcohol abuse can interact with other drugs as follows[13,17]:

- Anesthetics: decreased effect at usual dosages in chronic alcoholics who are not currently intoxicated (due to enzyme induction).
- Antihypertensive agents: hypotension in hypertensive alcoholics when not drinking (due to presence of hypertension when drinking).

- Anticoagulants: hemorrhage when given to chronic alcoholics (due to changes in prothrombin as a result of drinking).
- Anticonvulsants: increased drug metabolism and seizure in chronic alcoholics.
- Antihistamines: increased lethargy from acute alcohol intake (due to synergistic CNS effects).
- Antidiabetic agents: hypoglycemia and disulfiramlike reactions from acute alcohol intake (due to buildup of acetaldehyde).
- Antimicrobials (e.g., chloramphenicol, furazolidone, griseofulvin, isoniazid, quinacrine): disulfiramlike reactions from acute alcohol intake (due to accumulation of acetaldehyde).
- Barbiturates and other sedatives: lethargy, coma, and decreased lethal dose (LD_{50}) from acute alcohol intake (due to synergistic CNS effects).
- Lithium: fluctuating blood levels in chronic alcoholics, toxic effects from acute alcohol intake (partially due to endocrine changes and irregularity of fluid and electrolyte intake).
- Neuroleptics: lethargy and hypotension from acute alcohol intake (due to synergistic CNS effects).
- Opioids: lethargy, coma, and decreased lethal dose (LD_{50}) from acute alcohol intake (due to synergistic CNS effects).

5. Laboratory Testing and Screening

Laboratory examination can help the clinician in two ways. First, it can contribute important information to the total assessment so that the physician has greater confidence in diagnosing and assessing the patient. Second, in some cases laboratory data can aid in early diagnosis before severe or irreversible damage has taken place.

Laboratory tests that contribute to the diagnosis and assessment of drug dependence are of two kinds. First, drugs may be measured directly in serum, urine, or exhaled air. Second, biochemical and physiological functions affected by drugs can be assessed. No one laboratory measure is pathognomonic of drug dependence. Laboratory tests complement but cannot replace history and physical examination in the diagnosis of drug dependence.

Many drugs can be detected in the urine for 12–48 hr after their consumption. A few drugs may be detected for even several days to a few weeks in heavy users (e.g., cannabis, certain alkaloids). Drugs detectable by urine screening include the opioids, sedative/hypnotics, stimulants, and hallucinogenics. The blood and urine detection measures today are primarily of two types: those which employ immunoassay methods and those which depend on chromatography. Urine screening for drug abuse is more widely employed than determinations that use whole blood or plasma. The latter are used more for quantitative analysis.

Urine- and blood-screening tests may be appropriately used in several situations where they may aid in detection of drug dependence. Some of these uses are (1) screening for detection of hidden drug-dependent persons; (2) differential diagnosis in the patient who is comatose or who exhibits bizarre or psychotic behavior; (3) monitoring patient progress during drug abuse treatment programs; (4) assessing patients at high risk to drug dependence (e.g., inpatients on orthopedic, psychiatric, medical wards); (5) assessing patients in whom drug dependence is especially dangerous (e.g., during pregnancy, preoperative evaluation).

Urine screening presents certain problems because of the drug-dependent person's ability to manipulate physicians. The patient may claim an inability to void, drink large amounts of liquids to dilute the urine, or substitute another person's urine.

The specificity of urine screening is dependent on several variables. Some substances interfere with the interpretation of the test (e.g., a nicotine spot may be mistaken for an opioid spot on the chromatography plate). False negative or false positive tests may be reported. A second determination may be indicated for forensic reasons, or when the laboratory data and clinical status of the patient do not seem to agree.

A blood alcohol level (BAL) of more than 0.15 g% without gross evidence of intoxication indicates tolerance. The nonalcoholic person with a BAL of about 0.13 g% would show evidence of intoxication.

The naloxone challenge test for persons suspected of, or claiming to be, abusing opioids is simple, quick to administer, and inexpensive. It detects those persons who are physically dependent on opioids. Challenge by naloxone has been used in screening persons at high risk to opioid dependence and for legally certifying former addicts as being free of opioid dependence.

Elevated γ-glutamyl transferase or γ-glutamyl transpeptidase (GGT) is a sensitive indicator of heavy, chronic alcohol intake.[8] About 80% of both males and females who have been drinking heavily have elevated GGT values. Considerable acute alcoholic hepatitis damage can occur before the GGT becomes elevated, however, so that negative GGT tests do not rule out alcoholism. An abnormally elevated mean corpuscular volume of the red blood cells and an elevated GGT are the two most sensitive markers of alcoholism.[1,12]

An effective screening measure for drug abuse lies in testing blood and urine for drugs in hospitals and clinics.[4] Of 1476 patients screened at the University Hospital of Basel, Switzerland, 12% of admissions to the surgical service, 9% of admissions to the medical service, and 2% of outpatients had blood alcohol levels higher than 0.10 g%. Other laboratory data that may be associated with alcoholism are an increase of GGT (it was positive in 63% of inpatient alcoholics), an SGOT increase (48% positive), macrocytosis without anemia (26% positive), elevated serum triglyceride (28% positive), alkaline phosphatase (16% positive), bilirubin increase (13% positive), and an increase in uric acid (10% positive).[11] Routine posteroanterior and lateral chest X-rays may show rib and/or thoracic vertebral fractures in as many as 30% of the alcoholic male patients while nonalcoholic male patients will show only a 2% incidence ($p < 0.0001$).[7]

6. Self-Rating Scales

The clinical database can be augmented by the use of one or more of the self-rating inventories. These self-rating scales can be used to obtain information such as the following: patients' dependence, both psychological and physiological; their feelings about dependence or impaired control; and drug-dependence problems that are biomedical, occupational, interpersonal, or related to the criminal justice system. They can be employed to further substantiate the diagnosis and its severity. They also permit a quantitative measure to be assigned. Self-rating scales may be incorporated as a part of a general health questionnaire that the patient fills out prior to the initial visit to the physician. These data can provide direction for the physician to pursue additional data in this area of the history.

Several self-rating scales are described here. While most of them concern alcoholism, they can be readily adapted to other drug dependence.

A brief self-rating inventory is the CAGE Inventory.[5] It consists of four questions that are asked during the medical history: (1) Have you ever felt you should *C*ut down on your drinking? (2) Have you been *A*nnoyed by a criticism of your drinking? (3) Have you ever had *G*uilty feelings about your drinking? (4) Do you ever take an *E*ye-opener (i.e., drink in the morning)? Affirmative answers to these questions have assisted in identifying alcoholics who show these percentages of positive responses:

- 90% of alcohol-dependent persons report "Guilty feelings."
- 66% of alcohol-dependent persons report "Annoyed by criticism."
- 66% of alcohol-dependent persons report "Eye-opener drinking in the morning."

The more CAGE questions answered positively, the greater the probability is that the physician is dealing with an alcohol-dependent person. Positive responses to any of the CAGE questions can serve as an entree to further discussion. For example, the patient endorsing a need to cut down drinking might be asked, "Why do you feel you should cut down?" This then aids in eliciting any alcohol-related problems.

Another widely used self-report measure is the MAST (Michigan Alcohol Screening Test), developed by Selzer[14] and revised both by the original author and by others. This is shown in Table I. There is also a SMAST (Shortened Michigan Alcohol Screening Test) with 16 questions. Questions in both forms are weighted (i.e., some positive responses are scored as 1, others are 2 or 5). If

Table I
Michigan Alcoholism Screening Test (MAST)[a]

	Questions	Scoring points Yes	Scoring points No
1.	Do you feel you are a normal drinker?	0	2
2.	Have you ever awakened the morning after some drinking the night before and found that you could not remember a part of the evening before?	2	0
3.	Does your wife (or parents) ever worry or complain about your drinking?	1	0
4.	Can you stop drinking without a struggle after one or two drinks?	0	2
5.	Do you ever feel bad about your drinking?	1	0
6.	Do friends or relatives think you are a normal drinker?	0	2
7.	Do you ever try to limit your drinking to certain times of the day or to certain places?	0	0
8.	Are you always able to stop drinking when you want to?	0	2
9.	Have you ever attended a meeting of Alcoholics Anonymous (AA)?	5	0
10.	Have you gotten into fights when drinking?	1	0
11.	Has drinking ever created problems with you and your wife?	2	0
12.	Has your wife (or other family member) ever gone to anyone for help about your drinking?	2	0
13.	Have you ever lost friends or girlfriends/boyfriends because of drinking?	2	0
14.	Have you ever gotten into trouble at work because of drinking?	2	0
15.	Have you ever lost a job because of drinking?	2	0
16.	Have you ever neglected your obligations, your family, or your work for two or more days in a row because you were drinking?	2	0
17.	Do you ever drink before noon?	1	0
18.	Have you ever been told you have liver trouble? Cirrhosis?	2	0
19.	Have you ever had delirium tremens (DTs), severe shaking, heard voices or seen things that weren't there after heavy drinking?	2	0
20.	Have you ever gone to anyone for help about your drinking?	5	0
21.	Have you ever been in a hospital because of drinking?	5	0
22.	Have you ever been a patient in a psychiatric hospital or on a psychiatric ward of a general hospital where drinking was part of the problem?	2	0
23.	Have you ever been seen at a psychiatric or mental health clinic, or gone to a doctor, social worker, or clergyman for help with an emotional problem in which drinking had played a part?	2	0

(continued)

Table I. (*Continued*)

	Questions	Scoring points Yes	No
24.	Have you ever been arrested, even for a few hours, because of drunk behavior?	2	0
25.	Have you ever been arrested for drunk driving or driving after drinking?	2	0

[a]From Selzer.[14] Copyright 1971, American Psychiatric Association. Reprinted with permission.

the total score exceeds 20 points, there is a high probability that the patient is alcohol dependent.

The Adolescent Alcohol Involvement Scale[10] is a 14-item questionnaire for adolescents. The instrument was not primarily designed to detect adolescent alcoholism, but rather to identify young people who are misusing beverage alcohol.

The Spare Time Activities Questionnaire, formulated by Wilkins[18] at the University of Manchester, England, has been used to detect alcohol dependence in general practice. The Mayo Clinic Questionnaire, an adaptation of the Michigan Alcoholism Screening Test, presents 34 questions that have proven useful in detecting alcohol-dependent persons in clinical practice.[16]

7. Collateral Informants and Family Assessment

The behavior of the identified patient usually has a profound and adverse affect on the family and other significant persons (e.g., extended family, friends, employer, clergy). Information about the severity, duration, and course of the problem should be sought from the people who are in close association with the patient. Such data can assist in validating the clinical impression of drug dependence and assessing its severity. Additionally, interviewing the family members and significant others can assist the physician in planning intervention and therapeutic endeavors.

Another cogent reason for interviewing family members is that they may be so profoundly affected by the behavior of the identified patient that they may be, or perceive themselves as being, more distressed than the patient. Consequently, the family members may be more open to accepting assistance than the patient, who may be so deeply mired in the denial of the problem as to not perceive the need for help.

The clinician should have the clinical competency to secure a thorough family history: to conduct, individually or collectively, a family interview; to observe and evaluate the family dynamics; to be able to involve the family members in therapeutic efforts; and to understand the phases of the drug-dependence problem and its impact on the family constellation.

Adaptive consequences of drug dependence can occur in the family.[15] The following possibilities should be considered in a family assessment:

1. Drug dependence is a symptom of a dysfunctional family, that is, one in which the essential family functions are distorted by drug dependence. For example, spouses who prefer being antagonistic to each other can quarrel over drug usage.
2. Drug dependence may have an adaptive function for the family, or for some family members. For example, a spouse may have more power or influence in the family if the husband or wife is drug dependent.
3. If the drug user becomes abstinent, the family's pathological equilibrium may be seriously threatened until a new and hopefully healthier equilibrium can be established. For example, a drug-dependent son may become more independent of parental influence during recovery.

Assessment of the family makes it possible to move from the old equilibrium (which perhaps needed or benefited from the patient's drug dependence problem) to a new equilibrium.

Let us assume the clinician's data acquisition has led to the diagnosis and assessment of drug dependence. Next, the diagnosis and the assessment must be conveyed to the patient and family.

8. Communicating the Diagnosis

Clinicians are often reluctant to communicate their diagnosis of drug dependence to the patient and family members. Deterrents to conveying the diagnosis are based on mutual feelings of ignorance, fear, and beliefs in both the patient and the physician. Dynamics of these resistances to communicating the diagnosis are delineated in Table II.

These resistances to confronting the patient with his or her drug-dependence problem are mainly in the emotional or feeling realm. Clinicians not only must be sensitive to patients' feelings, but must also be aware of their own feelings. Making the emotional component an integral part of the communication process enhances the ease of communicating the diagnosis, as well as the likelihood of the patient's acceptance of the diagnosis.

Conveying the diagnosis to the patient requires that the physician has validated the diagnosis by being certain that it meets accepted diagnostic criteria. Making this diagnosis with an inadequate database that fails to satisfy diagnostic standards invites failure because the physician's uncertainty is readily perceived by the patient. Drug-dependent patients are typically sensitive and alert to their physician's uncertainty and ambivalence.

At times the patient will have several minor symptoms of early drug dependence, but these symptoms may be insufficient to warrant a diagnosis. In such cases the clinician can express concern that the patient's current use may pro-

Table II
Patient–Physician Communications Regarding Drug Dependence

Patient generated	Behavior manifested	Physician generated
Lack of factual knowledge about drug dependence and its pervasive effects	Ignorance	A narrow and biased perception of drug dependence
1. Fear of rejection (based on past experience) 2. Fear of being incurable or hopeless 3. Fear of surrendering the drug dependence	Fear	1. Fear of rejection (wants patient's approval) 2. Fear of ability to manage the drug-dependent patient
1. Overt hostility: openly aggressive, challenging 2. Covert hostility: passive–aggressive behavior	Hostility	1. Overt hostility: "I don't treat drug dependents" 2. Covert hostility: subtle, judgmental, punitive
Has a large, ingenious repertoire of reasons for drug use	Rationalization	May be persuaded by the rationalizations of the patient
Feelings of anger, guilt, shame, and remorse are projected onto others	Projection	May project feelings of hostility and frustration at inability to engage the patient in a treatment plan
Perceives the physician's ambivalence of the proper time to initiate confrontation	Communicating the diagnosis	Attempting to communicate too soon or waiting too long
All the foregoing feelings and behaviors are incorporated in an entrenched denial that the current problems are related to drug dependence	Denial	The clinician can be taken in by the patient's denial because of: 1. Stereotypic perception of the patient (i.e., derelict, skid-row type) 2. Own heavy or abusive use of drug

gress to psychoactive dependence. The patient should also be invited back after some weeks or months to reassess the drug use status over time.

If diagnostic certainty is assured, then the physician should communicate this knowledge to the patient at once. Premature communication (i.e., before the diagnosis is certain) or delaying the communication (i.e., after it is certain) can undermine the patient's trust in the physician.

The clinician's ability to communicate the diagnosis can be enhanced if the problem is given the proper name (i.e., drug dependence). The patient must know the reasons for the diagnosis. For example, the physician might say to the patient, "From what you have told me and from my physical examination and the laboratory tests I believe your problem is due to your dependence on alcohol [or tobacco, coffee, opioid, cannabis]. Let me explain in detail why I believe this is your diagnosis.'' This should be followed by an explanation in detail to sustantiate the diagnosis. The physician should solicit questions from the patient (and spouse and family members if present) and take the appropriate amount of time to answer them.

Both the therapeutic recommendations and the prognosis depend on assessing the severity of drug dependence in the particular patient. Any number of phases can be arbitrarily assigned, but most investigators describe early, middle, and late stages along a continuum. Of course, any one patient may present manifestations that fall into more than one category, such as predominantly middle-phase behavioral problems with the late-phase biomedical problems (or vice versa). Younger or recent drug dependents often have relatively more social or behavioral problems, while older or more chronic drug dependents tend to have relatively more biomedical problems—but with much overlap in both categories. Patients and their families should be informed about the severity of the problem in its various manifestations.

Diagnostic labels (e.g., alcoholic, junkie, drug addict) are potent means to generate feelings, either positive or negative, in the physician–patient relationship. The shock value of such frank terms in the communication of the diagnosis may be judiciously employed only after a relationship of trust has been generated. If used prematurely, the patient may interpret this frank communication merely as condemnation. Such direct aggressive communication by the physician may be appropriate if the physician perceives that the patient is making continued use of denial, rationalization, and projection. The clinician must avoid being cautious and timid to the degree that honesty suffers. Clinicians may conceal the proper diagnostic terms with vague statements ''Maybe you should cut down on your drug usage'') or use an acceptable biomedical term (e.g., gastritis) without assigning the primary etiological diagnosis of drug dependence. Honesty and objectivity combined with empathy are necessary.

Communicating the diagnosis to the person with drug dependence requires the following:

Attitudes

1. Empathy toward and advocacy for the patient.
2. Nonpossessive warmth and concern.
3. Nonjudgmental and nonmoralistic approach (clinicians make clinical, not moral, judgments).
4. Acceptance of the patient as a person, with firm and consistent behavior by the clinician.
5. Introspective self-awareness: clinicians need to be aware of their own feelings.

6. Realistic hope: hope is a potent motivating factor.
7. Maturity and equanimity to deal with the patient's response upon receiving the diagnosis.

Knowledge

1. Be able to inform the patient about the physiological and psychological effects of drug being used.
2. Understand what the patient with a drug-dependence problem brings to the physician–patient interaction (i.e., feelings, resistances, defense mechanisms).
3. Know the process of forming a therapeutic alliance with the drug-dependent patient.
4. Have the concepts for utilizing a here-and-now, supportive, goal-focused approach.
5. Understand the process of recovery and the steps necessary to accomplish recovery.

Skills

1. To sense the critical moment for communication, including skills in crisis intervention.
2. To possess a variety of ways to break through the patient's resistance.
3. To assist, lead, facilitate the patient's assuming responsibility for accepting the diagnosis, admitting that help is needed and making a commitment to a therapeutic program.
4. To be able to help the patient devise and accept a therapeutic program, including skill in clinical problem solving.
5. To help the patient change to a life-style more adaptive than dependence on drugs.

Knowledge of the patient and the family provides insight for the best and most effective strategy. Sometimes this is *interrogative,* as follows: "Have you ever thought that you might be an alcoholic?" Or it may be *direct:* "I believe from my exam that you have a real problem with drugs." Or alternatively, the approach could be *subtle and incremental:* over a series of office visits the patient is led to a realization of the drug-dependence problem by providing increments of data and repeated questions that focus on the problem from several directions (e.g., ways in which the drug may be interfering deterimentally to the various dimensions of life: family, occupation, health, leisure, and recreation).

Typical patient responses are as follows:

- Anger—overt hostility to cover anxiety.
- Yes, but—"I can handle it."

- Denial—"No, my drug use is not a problem."
- Ambivalence—"Perhaps you are right, Doctor. There may be a problem about which I should do something."
- Acceptance—"Doctor, can you help me?"

Therapeutic responses by the clinician have the following characteristics:

- Flexible: avoid an inflexible, rigid approach.
- Perceptive: realize that overt hostility often hides anxiety, that ambivalence is asking for help.
- Firm: without being accusatory, moralistic, or judgmental.
- Persistent: don't stop with one denial or ambivalent attitude.
- Tolerant: accepting of the patient as a person.
- Hopeful: perceiving the disorder as treatable.
- Responsible: identifying the physician's responsibilities as distinct from the patient's.
- Sensitive: to one's own attitudes—which implies having honesty about one's own use of drugs and dealing with one's own feelings about this.
- Helpful: offering to help the patient with treatment alternatives.

Forming a therapeutic alliance with the patient is a critical step in treatment. It should include the following:

- Therapeutic contract: Spell out physician and patient expectations and responsibilities.
- Treatment plan: Establish mutually agreed-upon comprehensive therapy plan.
- Family involvement: Agree on involvement for family, spouse, friends, employer, and others.

In clinical practice the diagnostic process inevitably overlaps with therapeutic intervention (unless assessment is done for some nontherapeutic purpose, such as forensic evaluation). Thus, conveying the diagnosis to the patient and family serves concurrently as the final step in the assessment process and the first step in the therapeutic process.

Immediately following communication of the diagnosis, a treatment plan should be offered. Whether the patient agrees with the physician's diagnostic assessment or rejects it, the clinician is obliged to offer a plan of treatment for the patient's problem. Preliminary statements should indicate that, while the patient's condition is not instantly curable, it can be managed. The patient needs to hear emphatically that the problem is not hopeless. Often patients believe that drug dependence is hopeless. Life without dependence on drugs is possible, but not without effort and commitment to a treatment program.

The management of patients with drug-dependence problems can be frustrating. Therefore, the physician should decide about his or her own degree of commitment to a management plan. Clinicians may choose not to work intensively with people with drug dependence, but they should be able to make the diagnosis, communicate it to the patient, and refer the patient for treatment with some comfort, tact, and respect. It helps to realize that the drug-dependent person's experience is alien to that of the ordinary person. Consequently, most people underrate the problem of drug dependence, not realizing that it is overwhelming to the drug-dependent patient.

The physician should be able to work collaboratively to formulate a treatment plan that is comprehensive and has continuity. The key elements are as follows:

- *Collaboration*—working with others
- *Comprehensive*—implies a knowledge of resources and the ability to make appropriate use of them; since drug-dependence problems are often chronic and relapsing
- *Continuity*—ongoing care and monitoring of the treatment plan

The family interview and assessment should define the family strengths and resources, the dysfunction within the family, and the family forces that enable the drug dependence to continue. This information can provide direction for assisting the family in its efforts to move to a new and more adaptive homeostasis.

A treatment plan for the patient must be negotiated. The clinician must clarify those responsibilities which treatment staff can assume as well as those responsibilities which the patient must assume. The expectations of the patient must be explored. If these expectations are unrealistic, they must be challenged with the facts of the situation. It is best to tell the patient early in the treatment planning process that painless paths to recovery are not appropriate in a realistic treatment plan.

The specific terms of the therapeutic agreement may involve individual and family counseling, medication, education, group sessions, and referral to self-help groups. The patient needs to know that the physician will maintain contact throughout treatment.

The family of the drug-dependent patient needs to be motivated toward an active participation in and commitment to a treatment program. The family should be educated about the nature of the patient's illness, its genesis, evolution, course, and its tendency to relapse. They, like the patient, must be directed to a new and more healthy relationship. The family members need to be offered a program that acknowledges their individual needs. They, too, need to hear that life without drug dependence is possible. This process has been aptly called *therapeutic education*.

References

1. Beresford T, Low D, Hall RCW, Adduci R, Goggans, F: A computerized biomedical profile for detection of alcoholism. *Psychosomatics* 1982; 23:713–720.
2. Cohen S: Cannabis: Impact on motivation, Part I and Part II. *Drug Abuse Alcoholism Newsletter* 1980, 1981; ix(10), x(1).
3. Cohen S: *The Substance Abuse Problem.* New York, Haworth Press, 1981.
4. Dubach UC, Schneider J: Screening for alcoholism. *Lancet* 1980; 29:1374.
5. Ewing J: Recognizing, confronting and helping the alcoholic. *Am Family Physician* 1978; 18(5):107–114.
6. Golstein JN, Sappington JT: Personality characteristics of students who became heavy drug users: An MMPI study of an avant-garde. *Am J Drug Abuse* 1977; 4:401–412.
7. Israel Y, Orrego H, Holt S. Macdonald DW, Meema HE: Identification of alcohol abuse: Thoracic fractures on routine chest X-ray as indicators of alcoholism. *Alcoholism: Clin Exp Res* 1980; 4:420–422.
8. Lewis K, Paton A: ABC of alcohol: Tools of detection. *Br Med J* 1981; 283(5):1531–1532.
9. Maletzky BM, Klotter J: Addiction to diazepam. *Int J Addict* 1976; 11:95–115.
10. Mayer J, Filstead W: The Adolescent Alcohol Involvement Scale: An instrument for measuring adolescent use and misuse of alcohol, in *Galanter M (ed): Currents in Alcoholism. Recent Advances in Research and Treatment.* New York, Grune & Stratton, 1980, vol VII, pp 169–181.
11. Morse RM, Heest RD: Screening for alcoholism. *JAMA* 1979; 242:2687–2690.
12. Ryback RS, Eckardt MJ, Pantter CP: Biochemical and hemotolgic correlates of alcoholism. *Res Commun Chem Pathol Pharmacol* 1980; 27:533–550.
13. Seixas FA: Alcohol and its drug interactions. *Ann Intern Med* 1975; 83:86–90.
14. Selzer M: The Michigan Alcoholism Screening Test (MAST): The quest for a new diagnostic instrument. *Am J Psychiatry* 1971; 127:1653–1658.
15. Steinglass P: Experimenting with family treatment approaches to alcoholism, 1950–1975. A review. *Family Process* 1976; 15:97–123.
16. Swenson W, Morse R: The use of a self-administered alcoholism screening test in a medical center. *Mayo Clin Proc* 1975; 50:204–208.
17. Weller RA, Preskorn SH: Psychotropic drugs and alcohol: Pharmacokinetic and pharmacodynamic interactions. *Psychosomatics* 1984; 25:301–309.
18. Wilkins R: The use of a questionnaire to detect the alcoholic in general practice. University of Manchester, Darbishire House Health Centre, 1972.

Further Reading

Feurlin W: Early detection and diagnosis of alcoholism. *Bull Schweiz Akad Med Wissenschaft* 1979; 35:173–186.

Porter L, Arif A, Curran WJ: *The Law and the Treatment of Drug- and Alcohol-Dependent Persons.* Geneva, WHO, 1986.

Woodrull R, Clayton R, Cloninger R, Guze S: A brief method of screening for alcoholism. *Dis Nerv Syst* 1976; 37:434–435.

World Health Organization: Final Report of the Working Groups on the Application of Laboratory Methods in the Surveillance/Epidemiology of Drug Dependence. Manila, WHO, 1979.

9

Detoxification and Management of Medical Emergencies

1. Introduction

Most drug-related conditions can be managed safely and effectively if they are recognized early. Effective management depends on prompt initiation of specific treatment based on accurate diagnosis.

2. Intoxication

Only a small percentage of untoward drug reactions come to medical attention.

2.1. Acute Pathological Intoxication

Violent behavior sometimes ensues from intoxication, more likely with alcohol, but also with stimulants, hallucinogens, and phencyclidine (PCP). The individual may destroy property or attack people, or both. Acute pathological intoxication occurs among a variety of users: naive users, users taking more drug than usual, and users with recent loss or emotional crises.

Treatment essentially consists of preventing the intoxicated person from harming self or others and waiting for the effects to wear off. Management consists of the following:

1. Adequate, well-trained personnel to restrain the patient without injury to staff or patient.

2. Adequate, but modulated sensory input (e.g., soft light, soft speech).
3. Observation for signs of overdose, withdrawal, associated medical or surgical emergency (e.g., subdural hematoma).
4. Physical restraints may be necessary, but they can contribute to the patient's fear and panic and can lead to dehydration or hyperthermia if struggles against the restraints persist.
5. Frequent reassurance should be offered that everything is all right and no harm will come to the patient.
6. Neuroleptic medication may be necessary, but should be avoided if possible.

2.2. Acute Anxiety, Panic Attack

Tachycardia, dyspnea, and fear of impending death may occur with intoxication from any psychoactive drug, but are most common with stimulants (including cocaine), cannabis, and hallucinogens. Confusion and suspiciousness may be present. Drug-induced hallucinations or delusions may give rise to anxiety symptoms: the clinician should inquire whether these are present. In most cases general supportive measures, as outlined in Section 2.1, are sufficient.

2.3. Toxic Psychosis

Drugs may produce illusions (i.e., misperceptions or alteration of perceptions), but the intoxicated person can usually recognize the drug effect and separate it from reality. In rare cases, the intoxicated person may be unable to distinguish drug-induced hallucinations and delusions from reality. This appears most likely to happen if an excessive dose is taken, or if the person has a constitutional or situational tendency to psychosis. Confusion may be present, but often sensorium is clear. Cannabis, stimulants (including cocaine), and hallucinogens are most likely to produce a toxic pychosis.

Delusions in toxic psychosis can be dangerous. For example, a patient might try to destroy some part of the body (e.g., eyes, genitalia, a hand) due to a belief that the affected organ is harming self or others. Or a paranoid patient may launch a lethal attack in a delusional attempt to eliminate a presumed enemy.

Toxic psychosis usually clears in several hours to several days. Typically, improvement is uneven, with variation from hour to hour. Consistent improvement can usually be noted on a day-to-day basis.

Supportive milieu management (as outlined) is usually adequate. If hallucinations are quite frightening or if delusions are potentially dangerous, neuroleptic medication in low to moderate doses is warranted (i.e., haloperidal, 1–10 mg q.d. to b.i.d.; chlorpromazine, 25–100 mg q.d. to t.i.d.). An anticholinergic crisis may be precipitated by adding neuroleptic medication to toxic levels of belladonalike compounds.

2.4. Drug-Precipitated Psychosis

Psychosis may persist beyond several days. In such cases one sees continuing or worsening psychotic symptoms, rather than gradual improvement. Sensorium is typically clear, but may be difficult to assess if mental functions are severely impaired. Symptoms may assume various features of mania, psychotic depression, or schizophreniform psychosis.

Management follows accepted psychiatric practice for psychosis. Depending on the clinical picture and the severity of symptoms, treatment may include neuroleptics, lithium, and/or antidepressants. Rarely, electroconvulsive therapy may be helpful in cases that do not improve with medication. Many psychiatrists attempt to discontinue medications earlier in these cases (i.e., after several weeks or a few months, rather than several months or a few years), since it is believed that such patients with drug-precipitated psychosis may not have constitutional factors as pathological as other psychotic patients. Of course, medication should be discontinued gradually and the patient followed closely in order to assess whether medication should be resumed.

2.5. Special Problems Associated with Intoxication

Pulmonary edema associated with opioid use can occur immediately or be delayed for as long as 24 hr after the last dosage. Most victims probably die before they can reach medical care. Treatment is symptomatic, consisting of oxygen and—as indicated—intubation and a respirator. Recovery or death occurs within a day or two. Narcotic antagonists do not reverse the edema.[18,27]

Fluid and electrolyte imbalance are especially likely to occur following alcohol intoxication and may endure several days or weeks. Low magnesium, sodium, and potassium are especially common. Overhydration may occur particularly with beer drinking, while dehydration can occur as a result of vomiting, diarrhea, heavy perspiration, or inadequate fluid intake. Fluid and electrolyte replacement must be carefully managed, since overly vigorous correction can cause cerebral edema, herniation of the cerebrum below the tentorium, and ischemia to the midbrain. Emergency laboratory tests should guide replacement therapy. If these tests are not available, vital signs, neurological status, and hydration signs (i.e., skin turgor, body weight, oral mucous membranes, urine output) should be followed frequently during replacement.

Numerous medical problems common to drug-dependent persons can mimic or exacerbate intoxication. These problems include cerebral or lung abscess, subacute bacterial endocarditis, septicemia, pneumonia, urinary tract infection, meningitis, malaria, hepatitis, nephrosis, nephritis, occult gastrointestinal hemorrhage, depressed skull fracture, subdural hematoma, anaphylactoid shock (from injected materials), myocardiopathy, beriberi, Wernicke–Korsakoff psychosis, diabetes, pancreatitis, occult fracture (especially of the femur or pelvis), anemia, and myoglobinuria.[8,21,25] Certain folk treatments for severe intoxication (such as pouring fluids into the person's mouth) may further exacerbate the patient's condition.

Anesthesia may be necessary for the intoxicated patient with a surgical emergency (e.g., upper gastrointestinal hemorrhage). In such cases the anesthetist must be careful not to overmedicate the patient.[13]

Accidental ingestion may occur. A child may consume an adult's drug, or an innocent victim may be given a drug as a practical joke. This is usually quite alarming to the patient, so that confusion or panic may occur. Unintended deaths and prolonged, even disabling psychiatric conditions have occurred under these circumstances.

2.6. General Treatment Measures

It is important to approach the acutely intoxicated person in a subdued manner. The clinician should not speak in a loud voice, move quickly, or approach the patient from behind. Touching the patient should be avoided unless assessment shows that it is safe to do so. Repeated orientation to time and place is usually helpful. A nightlight helps to prevent nighttime misperceptions and panic. Some modified stimuli are helpful, but intense stimuli can agitate or excite the patient. Frequent reassurance regarding the temporary nature of the condition is useful. The nurse or physician should try to focus the patient's attention on objects in the room, music, or simple tasks.

2.7. Specific Treatment Measures

2.7.1. Stimulant Intoxication

Stimulant intoxication (particularly with amphetamine and cocaine) may produce hyperactivity, hyperpyrexia, dilated pupils, tremor, increased pulse and blood pressure, excessive sweating, and a paranoid-type psychotic picture. Stimulants with potential for abuse include amphetamine and its derivatives, methylphenidate, various diet pills, and cocaine. Even milder drugs, such as caffeine, can produce intoxicating effects if taken in sufficiently high doses or by individuals sensitive to their effects.

Treatment of amphetamine intoxication includes acidification of the urine with ammonium chloride.[4] Haloperidol is useful in treating acute psychotic reactions.

2.7.2. Hallucinogen Intoxication

Symptoms of hallucinogen intoxication include distortion and intensification of sensory perception. For example, the patient may hear colors or feel sounds. Other common symptoms include dilated pupils, nausea, decreased appetite, headaches, dizziness, polyuria, rambling or incoherent speech, and toxic psychosis. The most significant characteristic of a hallucinogen-precipitated psychiatric crisis is fear. Most acute confusional states alone are short lived and can be handled without medication. It may be difficult at times to distinguish between an acute confusional state and an acute psychotic reaction, but with observation over time and mental status examination by an experienced clinician, this distinction can usually be made. The hallucinations associated with drug use are predominantly visual, whereas a psychotic reaction is typically associated with auditory hallucinations. If hallucinations or delusions persist for more than a few days, a hallucinogen-precipitated mental disorder should be suspected.

When an acute confusional state is being treated, it is important to make person-to-person contact with the patient, for example by talking with the patient or holding the patient's hands. The nurse or physician should continually reassure the patient that the condition is temporary and adequate care is being administered. The clinician should try to establish contact with the patient during the patient's lucid intervals so that this contact can be maintained during the intense period of the drug reaction.

The reactions to hallucinogenic drugs are often cyclical, with periods of lucidity alternating with periods of intense reaction to the drug. If the frequency of these cycles is monitored, the phase of recovery from intoxication can be identified. If the cycles are becoming more frequent, the patient is in the early part of the intoxication and the syndrome has not yet peaked. If the cycles are occurring less frequently, the syndrome has already peaked and is beginning to clear.

If sedation for acute agitation is necessary, diazepam, 10–20 mg, may be administered orally. Neuroleptics should be avoided in the treatment of an acute reaction to hallucinogens because most street preparations of hallucinogens are impure, and it is impossible to ascertain exactly what drug the person has actually taken.[22] The anticholinergic effects of neuroleptics potentiate the anticholinergic agents which are frequent contaminants or adulterants in hallucinogen samples. This can exacerbate the delirium. Of course, neuroleptics, lithium, and/or antidepressants may be necessary if the patient suffers from hallucinogen-precipitated schizophreniform, manic, or depressive psychosis.

2.7.3. Phencyclidine Intoxication

Phencyclidine, often abused alone, is also found as a contaminant in other drugs. In low-dose intoxication, the patient presents with nystagmus, confusion, ataxia, and sensory impairment. When the drug is taken in moderate doses, the patient may present a catatoniclike picture, staring blankly and not responding to any stimuli. In high doses, the drug can produce seizures and severe hypertension. The hypertension should be treated vigorously with diazoxide or nitroprusside because it may cause hypertensive encephalopathy or intracranial bleeding. A contaminant from PCP manufacture, 1-piperidino-cychohexane-carbonitrile, can cause severe abdominal cramps, hematemesis, and diarrhea. Violence against self or others can occur at any dose level.[5]

The effects of PCP intoxication may last several days. During recovery, levels of consciousness may fluctuate rapidly. The patient may manifest hallucinations and delusions.

Urinary excretion is enhanced by acidifying the urine. This can be done by giving ammonium chloride (0.5–1.0 g every 6 hr) or ascorbic acid. The urine pH should be monitored and kept around 5.5.[2] If psychosis persists beyond several days, treatment and rehabilitation like that provided for schizophreniform or affective psychosis may be necessary.

2.7.4. Inhalant Intoxication

Acute intoxication can cause respiratory depression; artificial respiration usually reverses this condition rapidly if it is detected in time. Circulatory support (e.g., fluids, vasopressors) may be needed if the cardiac center has similarly been affected.

3. Overdose

While relatively few cases of intoxication reach medical facilities, many overdose cases do reach emergency centers as a result of the critical, even life-threatening problems that may result.

3.1. General Measures

First, an adequate airway should be established and maintained. In severe cases intravenous fluids should be initiated so that rapid drug administration, fluid replacement, and drug excretion can be facilitated. Vital signs should be monitored frequently. Antihypotensive medication, and sometimes antihypertensive drugs, may be necessary.

The drug should be identified if at all possible. History from the patient and informants, physical examination, and laboratory tests should be carried out rapidly.

Emesis or gastric lavage should be considered if the drug was ingested, unless the patient has ingested hydrocarbons. Emesis of hydrocarbons may lead to pulmonary aspiration and hydrocarbon pneumonitis, a highly lethal condition. For emesis or gastric lavage, the patient should not be comatose; gag reflex should be intact. Most clinicians prefer to administer syrup of ipecac (15 ml) owing to its relative safety. Depending on the amount and contents of the vomitus, the clinician may want to lavage the stomach through a tube of adequate diameter using isotonic saline for lavage.

Activated charcoal (100 g) may also be useful for certain drugs, such as barbiturates and glutethimide, which bind to the charcoal and are then excreted in the stool. Repeated charcoal doses facilitate excretion of those drugs with entero-hepatic recirculation.

Urinary excretion of the drug should be facilitated whenever possible. For drugs excreted in the urine, increased urinary volume may be accomplished by intravenous fluids or increased oral intake. Alkalinization of the urine (with sodium bicarbonate or lactate) enhances barbiturate excretion. Acidification of the urine (by ammonium chloride) hastens amphetamine and PCP excretion.[3]

Dialysis may aid in the removal of drugs not bound to plasma proteins. In cases where the drug is bound to albumin (such as secobarbital), addition of albumin to the dialysis solution may partially remove the offending agent. Peritoneal dialysis is rarely necessary. The clinician should consider dialysis for CNS-depressant overdose under the following conditions: history of a potentially lethal dose; worsening vital signs, mental status, and neurological signs; very high blood levels; prolonged coma; or concomitant major medical or surgical conditions.[9]

3.2. Specific Measures

3.2.1. Opioid Overdose

Pinpoint pupils, depressed respiration, and profound somnolence are the classical signs of opioid overdose. Usually patients in opioid sleep can be easily aroused, but they fall back to sleep unless continually stimulated. Occasionally, coma may be profound. Naloxone, an opioid antagonist, is a specific treatment for opioid overdose. Naloxone is superior to its predecessor, nallorphine, because it has no agonist effects and will not worsen respiratory depression. This absence of agonist effect may be crucial if the overdose was secondary to non-opioids such as barbiturates.[17]

The signs of opioid overdose are not always the same. Meperidine, for example, may cause an overdose with dilated pupils. Pupils may also be dilated if anoxia has been prolonged or if stimulants or phenothiazines have been taken concurrently with the opioid.[17]

Opioid overdose, even in extremely high doses, can be readily overcome with intravenous naloxone. The first dose is usually 0.4 mg in an adult; up to 0.01 mg/kg should be given to children. Doses can be repeated every 10–15 min until the patient is awake. Sometimes two or three doses are necessary. Failure of this regimen to relieve respiratory depression indicates that other drugs or medical conditions besides opioid overdose are present. Excessive naloxone dosage will precipitate withdrawal, so excessive doses should be avoided (although naloxone itself is safe owing to lack of agonist activity). Withdrawal can precipitate agitation or even violence in a disoriented patient. Additional naloxone will be needed every 2–3 hr until the drug is excreted. This may take up to 24 hr or longer, depending on the dose, the type of opioid, and the rapidity of excretion. Later doses can be administered intramuscularly instead of intravenously. Since patients typically become quite alert with the first naloxone dose, there is a danger that the patient will subsequently be neglected. Should this occur, the patient can gradually slip back into coma and die. Frequent checks (i.e., every 15 or 30 min) during the first 24 hr are warranted. Some clinicians prefer an intravenous naloxone drip (4 mg/1000 ml fluid) given over 8–12 hr.[28]

3.2.2. Sedative Overdose

Sedative overdose occurs with barbiturates, benzodiazepines, alcohol, and other nonbarbiturate hypnotics. Signs of sedative overdose include respiratory depression, depressed level of consciousness, nystagmus, hypotension, ataxia, dysarthria, depressed deep-tendon reflexes, confusion, coma, and shock. The clinician must first provide an adequate airway and maintain the cardiovascular system. Once these initial measures have been carried out, treatment should begin with gastric lavage and charcoal instillation (100 g) into the stomach. If barbiturates are the cause of the overdose, sodium bicarbonate should be administered to alkalinize the patient's urine. Alkalinization of the urine increases the rate of excretion of barbiturates; the urine pH should be monitored and kept at about 7.5. Laxatives may be used to induce catharsis. Several of the sedative drugs, particularly glutethimide and methaqualone, are lipophilic, and consequently these drugs are erratically absorbed and stored in body fats. They are metabolized to active substances which have a long half-life. Excretion via bile results in reabsorption through the enterohepatic recirculation. Because of these effects, blood levels of the drug may fluctuate, causing fluctuations in the level of consciousness. It is therefore important to keep patients who have taken overdoses of these drugs under observation for several days.[1] Stimulants were used in former times, but have only a short-lived effect and no demonstrable influence on eventual morbidity or mortality.

Benzodiazepines, particularly diazepam, chlordiazepoxide, prazepam, and chlorazepate, are often metabolized to active long-acting metabolites. Although these drugs produce less respiratory depression than barbiturates, the long-acting metabolites often cause intoxication which lasts for several days.[16]

There are no antagonists such as naloxone for alcohol, barbiturates, and other sedatives. Therefore, removal of the drug from the stomach and enhanced excretion are key elements. A serum level over 3.5 mg% for short-acting barbiturates and 10 mg% for long-acting barbiturates may presage a fatal outcome. In such cases dialysis is indicated.

3.2.3. Overdose with Stimulants, Hallucinogens, and Other Drugs

Stimulant overdose is rarely fatal. Close observation in a hospital setting, monitoring of vital signs and fluid balance, acidification of the urine (for amphetamines), and increased urinary output usually suffice. Severe hypertension responds to alpha-blocking agents such as phentolamine or vasodilators such as nitroprusside. This is especially important for extremely high blood pressure in order to prevent stroke or renal cortical necrosis.

Likewise hallucinogen overdose rarely has a lethal outcome. Some hallucinogens have belladonalike actions, and anticholinergic death rarely ensues. Care must be taken not to exacerbate the anticholinergic effect by administering drugs such as the neuroleptics which have belladonalike activity. Some clinicians use diazepine compounds in these cases when sedation is desired, although sedative drugs can contribute to the patient's confusion, agitation, hyperthermia, and dehydration.[23]

Various drugs besides the hallucinogens can produce an anticholinergic crisis. These include many over-the-counter preparations for asthma, gastritis, and diarrhea. Physostigmine can reverse this effect. Usually 1–2 mg i.m. is given initially, with subsequent titration against clinical signs. Like naloxone, the effect of physostigmine is short (often as brief as 30 min) so that the anticholinergic toxicity may recur. Consequently the patient must be closely reassessed over the first 24 hr.

4. Withdrawal

Mild withdrawal symptoms do not require routine medication. In such cases the patient should feel safe and confident that treatment is available in case of exacerbation. Withdrawal treatment without medication (so-called cold-turkey withdrawal) is adequate in some mild cases. If undertaken in a supportive and humanitarian fashion, withdrawal treatment can lead to a positive therapeutic relationship and continued patient compliance.

4.1. Principles of Withdrawal Therapy

The aim of a sound regimen is to provide a substitute drug-dose level which will reduce suffering to a tolerable degree, and then subsequently withdraw it. The clinician builds a regimen by giving a known dose and then observing its effects. There is no absolute quantitative method for determining the level of drug dependence. This requires gradual titration of dose while observing the patient's clinical condition. Disappearance of withdrawal symptoms indicates the titration end point.

Stimulant withdrawal (primarily due to amphetamine and cocaine) tends to be marked by depressant effects, including insomnia, anergy, and weakness. Conversely, depressant withdrawal from opioids and sedatives is characterized by stimulant effects such as hyperreflexia, insomnia, and agitation. Delusions may occur with either stimulant or depressant withdrawal. Stimulant withdrawal tends to be briefer and milder than depressant withdrawal.

The onset, duration, and severity of withdrawal are related to the pharmacology of the drug. With drugs having a short half-life, withdrawal tends to begin earlier, with more florid symptoms but with a shorter total withdrawal course, as compared to drugs with a long half-life. Heroin among the opioids and alcohol, amobarbital, and secobarbital among the sedatives are examples of drugs with a short half-life.

Withdrawal convulsions are particularly prevalent with the sedative drugs and infrequent with the opioids and stimulants. Withdrawal can be lethal if the dose has been particularly high, or if the patient is elderly or has a serious associated illness. Sedative and alcohol withdrawal is more life threatening than opioid withdrawal.

Withdrawal pharmacotherapy consists of administering the same or pharmacologically similar drug, to suppress withdrawal or produce mild intoxication, followed by gradually decreasing doses. Any opioid drug can be used for opioid withdrawal, and any sedative drug for sedative withdrawal. In general, withdrawal drugs should be long acting; this permits a relatively smooth withdrawal, without cyclical intoxication and withdrawal. (Drug abusers tend to prefer the more rapid-acting drugs with shorter half-life.) Withdrawal drugs should also have a wide margin of safety between therapeutic dose and lethal dose. Longer-acting drugs include methadone and tincture of opium among the opioids and phenobarbital and diazepam among the sedatives.

Duration of withdrawal treatment depends on the drug, the severity of physiological dependence, and the patient's condition. For short-acting drugs, a 4–5-day withdrawal regimen is adequate. In the case of severe withdrawal, the initial doses may need to be given intravenously since oral or intramuscular doses may not be adequately absorbed. In the case of alcohol dependence, a typical withdrawal regimen is as follows:

- Day 1—10 mg diazepam q.i.d. (40 mg total).
- Day 2—10 mg diazepam t.i.d. (30 mg total).
- Day 3—10 mg diazepam b.i.d. (20 mg total).
- Day 4—10 mg diazepam h.s. (10 mg total).

Similarly for heroin, a 5–7-day withdrawal regimen is adequate. For longer-acting drugs, however, withdrawal regimens may be longer (e.g., 10 days for opium, 3–6 weeks for diazepam or methadone dependence). Longer regimens may be necessary if the patient is elderly, debilitated, or has an associated medical or surgical illness.

Withdrawal syndromes also occur with cannabis, cocaine, and amphetamine dependence. Ordinarily these are not life threatening, and they resolve within a few to several days. At times temporary sedation is used for agitated or insomniac patients. Paranoid or hallucinating patients may require a brief course of low-dose neuroleptics. Severe stimulant withdrawal, especially when accompanied by symptoms of major depression, has been treated with tricyclic medication.

Detoxification can be carried out successfully on an outpatient basis or in nonmedical residential facilities if the patient is not acutely ill and if close monitoring and nursing care is available. Costs can be kept down in this way. Patients with delirium tremens, withdrawal seizures, or associated medical problems should be hospitalized for detoxification.

4.2. General Measures

Withdrawal symptoms range from fairly mild to severe and life threatening. It is often not possible to distinguish the severity of the case until withdrawal is underway. The patient requires careful monitoring during the early hours and days of treatment. Behavior, appearance, fluid output, and vital signs must be assessed around the clock for several hours to several days, depending on the patient and the drug that has been abused. In the case of severe withdrawal, a physician must observe mental status and neurological signs, note the nurses' observations, and reconsider the treatment regimen on a daily basis.

The milieu for the patient should be emotionally supportive and provide adequate, but not excessive interpersonal contact and sensory stimuli. A nightlight should be provided, and loud noise avoided. Participation in educational or therapy sessions should be minimal until the patient is oriented and comfortable. Confused patients should be reassured that they will be protected and kept safe. Hallucinating patients should be told that their mental dysfunction is temporary.

Patients should be told that some discomfort and insomnia will occur during withdrawal, but these symptoms will be reduced to a level consistent with good recovery. Initially diet should consist of clear fluids until the patient's condition is improving; then a full liquid diet can be given until all physical signs are normal.

Most physicians prefer to avoid routine orders for medications for symptomatic relief (e.g., analgesics, sedatives, antacids), since this can mask a worsening medical condition and facilitate the type of drug seeking that led to drug dependence. Other physicians prefer to administer medications for symptomatic relief other than the original dependence-producing drug (especially in social or political settings where use of opioid or sedative drugs for withdrawal is opposed by social or political policy). In order to avoid continued drug seeking, medication for withdrawal is given on a routine basis at regular intervals, and not on request by the patient.

Measures to hasten elimination of drugs are generally avoided (i.e., agonists for opiate withdrawal, alkalinization of the urine for secobarbital withdrawal, and acidification of the urine for amphetamine withdrawal). Such measures may exacerbate the patient's withdrawal condition if some drug is still present. Rarely, accelerated withdrawal may be indicated; it should be done under supervision of a clinician experienced in withdrawal treatment.

4.3. Specific Measures

4.3.1. Opioid Withdrawal

Cold-turkey withdrawal in the case of severe withdrawal has no medical rationale. Clinical experience over many decades in all parts of the world has shown that patients do not subsequently avoid readdiction merely because withdrawal is painful and discomforting, and nothing is gained psychologically through a cold-turkey program. Medical stress is severe and occasionally risky in older or medically ill patients. Cold-turkey withdrawal also discourages patients from seeking other treatment and prevents the optimal development of the physician–patient relationship, which can aid in future management and recovery of the patient. Cold-turkey withdrawal also delays postdischarge planning in the hospitalized patient and leads to higher costs and unnecessarily prolonged hospitalization.[24]

Long-acting opioids useful for opioid withdrawal include methadone, tincture of opium, and opium tablets. Medication should not be started until mild signs of withdrawal are present, and the dose should be titrated to suppress all but mild signs. Methadone should be given twice a day for withdrawal, and opium three or four times a day. Morphine therapy produces an uneven withdrawal due to its relatively short duration of action. Codeine, propoxyphene, and similar opioids ameliorate mild withdrawal symptoms, but are inadequate for severe opioid withdrawal symptoms.

Patients and their families should be told that a chronic withdrawal syndrome lasts many months following the achievement of a drug-free state.[20] Attention to this syndrome is a key part of a successful recovery program. This lengthy subclinical syndrome includes sleep disturbance, labile blood pressure, autonomic symptoms, elevated sedimentation rate, and variable responsiveness of the respiratory center to carbon dioxide. Psychophysiological stability may not occur until a year after abstinence is initiated.

α-Adrenergic agonists such as clonidine reverse many of the signs and symptoms of the opioid withdrawal syndrome. Clonidine is the α-adrenergic agonist with which there is the most experience. The dose necessary to reverse opioid withdrawal is substantially higher than the dose used in the treatment of hypertension. Opioid-dependent persons must stop using all opioids because drugs like clonidine have sedative effects which are powerfully potentiated by concurrent use of opioids. The clonidine dose is built up from 0.1 mg/day to 1.5 mg/day over a 10-day period, and then the drug must be tapered. Clonidine's usefulness in treating opioid withdrawal is limited by the fact that tolerance develops to its effects on withdrawal so that withdrawal must be accomplished in 10–14 days. Sedation and hypotension may be troublesome side effects. Hallucinations and confusion have also been reported in patients taking clonidine. Outpatient use of clonidine has been effective in some patients, but a hospital setting often is used because of the need to monitor side effects.[6,7,14,15]

4.3.2. Sedative Withdrawal

Symptoms produced by sedative withdrawal include confusion, nystagmus, tremulousness, agitation and irritability, insomnia, elevated temperature, hyperactive deep-tendon reflexes, convulsion, and weakness.

Any sedative drug may be used to treat withdrawal from any other sedative drug. However, many clinicians prefer longer-acting drugs, such as diazepines for alcohol withdrawal and phenobarbital for barbiturate withdrawal. Initial doses may be given intravenously if the patient is having convulsions or is severely agitated. Once the patient is stable, the drug may be administered orally. Intramuscular injection is not ordinarily employed owing to slow absorption. Duration of treatment is usually 4 or 5 days for alcohol and 10 days for barbiturates. Withdrawal regimens may need to be two or three times longer for very severe dependence, or in the presence of complicating medical conditions. Withdrawal regimens for benzodiazepines, ethchlorvynol, and similar drugs may take a few weeks to a few months, depending on the duration of dependence, amount of drug being used, and condition of the patient.[26]

The classical drug in the treatment of alcohol withdrawal was formerly paraldehyde. Athough this drug is still used in some centers today, some of the disadvantages in its use are (1) fresh supplies should be made up daily because the drug can deteriorate over time; (2) paraldehyde is short acting and has to be given frequently; and (3) sterile abscesses may result from intramuscular injections.

One of the life-threatening aspects of the alcohol and sedative withdrawal syndrome is the onset of delirium tremens. Delirium usually occurs 48–72 hr after alcohol use is stopped, and sooner or later in the case of other sedatives, depending on their half-life. This syndrome is characterized by elevated temperature, tachycardia, elevated blood pressure, diaphoresis, and an acute confusional state. Since the mortality rate with untreated delirium tremens is as high as 10–50%, this condition should be treated immediately. An intravenous line should be established for fluids and medication. Intravenous diazepam, 10 mg, can be given slowly over 3–5 min if the patient is toxic, confused, or hallucinating. Diazepam treatment can be monitored by checking the pulse, and repeated doses of diazepam can be given every 20 min until the pulse falls below 120.

Once a mildly sedating dose has been established, the patient should be started on oral medication and gradually withdrawn over the next 4–5 days. If there is recurrence of the delirium tremens symptoms, the patient should be once again treated with intravenous diazepam. Symptoms may recur if the patient has been abusing longer-acting sedatives along with alcohol or shorter-acting sedatives. Thiamine should be administered prophylactically as a preventive against possible Korsakoff's syndrome.

Seizures in the acute withdrawal state from sedatives or alcohol occur within the first 24–48 hr. These seizures are usually self-limited, but can lead to life-threatening status epilepticus. They can be blocked by administration of any of the sedative agents previously described.

Treatment for withdrawal from barbiturates resembles that for withdrawal from all sedatives, including the minor tranquilizers and alcohol, since all drugs in these categories exhibit cross-tolerance. The first step is to determine the approximate level of drug to which the patient is tolerant, since patients often exaggerate the amount of drug they are taking. Many physicians employ a sedative such as secobarbital or pentobarbital, administering it to the point of mild drowsiness, dysarthria, and ataxia. An initial oral or intravenous starting dose is 200 mg, and an additional 100 mg is administered every 20–30 min until the patient is comfortable or even mildly intoxicated. A total dosage of up to 600 or 800 mg may be necessary. Pentobarbital and secobarbital are relatively short-acting barbiturates, so that if by chance the patient receives too high a dose the effects can usually be slept off without difficulty. Intravenous barbiturates (e.g., sodium seconal) can be slowly administered over 10–15 min in order to achieve the same effect. If the patient becomes sedated with 200 mg or less of seconal, severe physical dependence requiring withdrawal treatment is not present.[29]

After the intoxicating dose is determined, the patient may be switched to a longer-acting sedative, such as phenobarbital (30 mg phenobarbital per 100 mg pentobarbital or secobarbital). This is not critical, however, since pentobarbital or secobarbital regimens provide a smooth withdrawal. The dose is then reduced by 10% of the initial starting dose each day.[26]

4.3.3. Maternal Drug Dependence and Neonatal Withdrawal

The pregnant opioid-dependent patient presents a therapeutic dilemma. If she is suddenly withdrawn from opioids, there is a significant possibility that her fetus may die in withdrawal. Maintaining the pregnant opioid-dependent woman with high doses of opioid is associated with unacceptable morbidity and mortality of the neonate. The path followed by most clinicians is to maintain the opioid-dependent female on a dose of methadone of 20 mg or less per day. At this level of maintenance, the neonate will have an easily treatable withdrawal syndrome, athough many neonates of mothers maintained on such low doses frequently do not require any specific pharmacological treatment. If the patient is reliable and can be closely followed, gradual withdrawal and abstinence throughout the remainder of the pregnancy is the optimal course of action. Even less-reliable patients can often be gradually withdrawn later in their last trimester prior to delivery.[11]

Infant withdrawal syndromes have not been reported with stimulant drugs, but do occur with opioids and sedatives, including alcohol. Signs include agitation, high-pitched cry, hyperactivity, pulling legs up to the abdomen with apparent cramps, and anorexia. Tremulousness or convulsions are relatively frequent in neonatal withdrawal. Due to immaturity of the neonatal liver, withdrawal therapy must be carefully monitored. Many clinicians prefer tincture of opium or phenobarbital since their use in neonates is well known, although methadone, morphine, and diazepam have also been employed.[30]

4.3.4. Multiple Simultaneous Dependence

Occasionally a patient may be encountered who is concurrently dependent on opioids and on sedatives or alcohol. These complicated clinical problems may be approached by substituting long-acting members of the various classes of the drugs involved. For example, a patient who has been taking heroin intraveneously six times a day and also using over 3 g of barbiturates daily for many weeks could be managed as follows:

1. Methadone for management of the opiate dependence with discontinuation over 15–30 days.
2. Phenobarbital, 600–1200 mg daily in divided doses to cover the barbiturate dependence with discontinuation over 10–20 days.

After a period of stabilization the patient's withdrawal can be accomplished either concurrently or in sequence. The withdrawal should be slow, with withdrawal symptoms kept to a minimum. Some clinicians advocate withdrawing the sedatives first and then withdrawing the opioids; other clinicians prefer the reverse.[24]

4.3.5. Stimulant Withdrawal

Over the years it has been stated that there is no withdrawal syndrome with stimulants. Today, however, the severe depression, somnolence, and increased appetite that frequently occur after cessation of stimulant drug use are generally considered to be a withdrawal syndrome. During this withdrawal phase, the drug-dependent person frequently attempts to resume stimulant use.

If the depressive symptoms persist longer than a week, the patient should be evaluated to determine whether a major depression exists. If depression persists or a depression emerges, the patient should be treated with an appropriate antidepressant regimen. Although amphetamines are usually withdrawn abruptly from chronic users, gradual withdrawal with tricyclic antidepressants over several days can be effective in reducing withdrawal symptoms.[10]

5. Other Acute Conditions

5.1. Wernicke–Korsakoff Encephalopathy

The Wernicke syndrome consists of paralysis of eye movements, ataxia, and disturbances of the state of consciousness. Korsakoff described a similar syndrome with an emphasis on mental confusion, disorientation, loss of recent memory, and a tendency to confabulate. The recent memory loss is due to atrophy of the mamillary bodies of the brain. Usually this syndrome is described as the Wernicke–Korsakoff syndrome.

Wernicke–Korsakoff's encephalopathy can occur in any condition as a result of thiamine deficiency, but is especially likely to occur as a complication of thiamine deficiency in alcohol dependence. Prompt parenteral administration of thiamine can reverse the neurological damage and prevent permanent dementia. This potential outcome is so disastrous that many clinicians routinely administer thiamine to alcohol-dependent persons admitted to the hospital in a confused condition, even though they may have another disorder besides Wernicke–Korsakoff's psychosis (e.g., delirium tremens, head injury). If thiamine administration is delayed, the patient may survive, but in a demented condition. An initial dose of 100 mg thiamine should be administered parenterally, particularly in the toxic or severely ill patient whose gastrointestinal absorption may be compromised.

5.2. Management of Medical or Surgical Problems

A patient requiring hospitalization for a medical or surgical problem should not undergo the stress of drug withdrawal treatment from opioids or sedatives concurrent with the stress of medical or surgical illness. Maintenance with methadone or benzodiazepines, for example, is indicated until the medical or surgical crisis has passed.[12]

Analgesic need in an opioid-dependent patient is independent of the opioid being administered to control the dependence. It is curious but true that a methadone maintenance patient taking 80 mg of methadone daily does not derive any clinically significant analgesia from the dose and requires additional analgesics, in the usual doses. Pentazocine, or other agonist–antagonists, is contraindicated for analgesia in anyone who is opioid dependent because it will produce withdrawal and exacerbate pain.[19]

In the event of surgery or other procedure requiring general anesthesia, the anesthesiologist should be made aware of the patient's drug dependence. Alcohol and sedative dependence can greatly alter general anesthesia. For example, alcohol- or sedative-dependent patients require greatly increased doses of short-acting barbiturates for general anesthesia. In some instances anesthesiologists have made the initial diagnosis of sedative dependence based on the patient's lack of response to the usual doses of general anesthetic drugs. During the postoperative period, the opioid-, sedative-, or alcohol-dependent patient should be kept comfortable and out of withdrawal until the medical or surgical condition is stable. At that point a gradual detoxification regimen can be initiated. Under these circumstances the detoxification period should be two or three times longer than usual.

References

1. Arieff AT, Friedman EA: Coma following non-narcotic drug overdosage: Management of 208 adult patients. *Am J Med Sci* 1973; 266:405.
2. Arnow R, Done AK: Phencyclidine overdose: An emerging concept of management. *J Am Coll Emergency Physicians* 1978; 7:56.
3. Beckett AH, Rowland M: Urinary excretion kinetics of amphetamine in man. *Pharm Pharmacol* 1965; 17:628–639.
4. Beckett AH, Rowland M, Turner P: Influence of the urinary pH on excretion of amphetamines. *Lancet* 1965; 1:303.
5. Besson HA: Intracranial hemorrhage associated with phencyclidine abuse. *JAMA* 1982; 248:585.
6. Brown MJ, Salmon D, Rendell M: Clonidine hallucinations. *Ann Intern Med* 1980; 93:456–457.
7. Charney DS: Iatrogenic opiate addiction: Successful detoxification with clonidine. *Am J Psychiatry* 1980; 137:989–990.
8. Cherubin CE: Infectious disease problems of narcotic addicts. *Arch Intern Med* 1971; 128:309.
9. Cronin RJ, Klinger EL, Avasthi PS, Lubash GD: The treatment of nonbarbiturate sedative overdosage, in Bourne PG (ed): *Acute Drug Abuse Emergencies: A Treatment Manual.* New York, Academic Press, 1976, pp 105–112.
10. Ellinwood EH: Emergency treatment of acute adverse reactions to CNS stimulants, in Bourne PE (ed): *A Treatment Manual for Acute Drug Abuse Emergencies.* National Clearinghouse for Drug Abuse Information. Rockville, Maryland: NIDA, 1975, pp 63–67.
11. Finnegan LP (ed): *Drug Dependence in Pregnancy: Clinical Management of Mother and Child.* Washington, DC, Service Research Monograph Series, DHEW Publication no. (ADM) 69-678, 1979.
12. Fultz JM, Senay EC: Guidelines for the management of the hospitalized narcotic addict. *Ann Intern Med* 1975; 82:815–818.
13. Giuffrida JG, Bizzarri DV: Intubation of the esophagus: Its role in preventing aspiration pneumonia and asphyxial death. *Am J Surg* 1957; 93:329–334.
14. Gold MS, Redmond DE Jr, Kleber HD: Clonidine in opiate withdrawal. *Lancet* 1978; 1:929–930.
15. Gold MS, Pottash AC, Sweeney DR, Kleber HD: Opiate withdrawal using clonidine. *JAMA* 1980; 243:343–346.

16. Hollister L: Clinical pharmacology of psycotherapeutic drugs, in *Monographs in Clinical Pharmacology*, ed 2. New York, Churchill Livingstone, 1983, (Monographs in Clinical Pharmacology, Vol 1.)
17. Jaffee JH, Martin WR: Narcotic analgesics and antagonists, in Goodman LW, Gilman A (eds): *The Pharmacologic Basis of Therapeutics*. New York, MacMillan, 1975, pp 245–283.
18. Kjeldgaard JM, Hahn GW, Heckenlively JR, Genton E: Methadone-induced pulmonary edema. *JAMA* 1971; 218:882–883.
19. Kreek MJ: Medical mamagement of methadone-maintained patients, in Lowinson JH, Ruiz P (eds): *Substance Abuse: Clinical Problems and Perspectives*. Baltimore, Williams & Wilkins, 1981, pp 660–673.
20. Martin WR, Jasinski DR: Physiological parameters of morphine dependence in man: Tolerance, early abstinence, protracted abstinence. *J Psychiatr Res* 1969; 7:9–17.
21. Most H: Falciparium malaria among drug addicts: Epidemiology and studies. *Am J Public Health* 1940; 30:403.
22. Schnoll SH, Vogel WH: Analysis of ''street drugs.'' *N Engl J Med* 1971; 284:781.
23. Schwarz CJ: Paradoxical responses to chlorpromazine after LSD. *Psychosomatics* 1967; 8:210.
24. Senay EC: *Substance Abuse Disorders in Clinical Practice*. Littleton, MA, John Wright PSG, 1983.
25. Siegel H, Helpern M, Ehrenreich T: The diagnosis of death from intravenous narcotism. *J Forensic Sci* 1966; 11:1.
26. Smith DE, Wesson DR: Phenobarbital technique for treatment of barbiturate dependence. *Arch Gen Psychiatry* 1971; 24:56–60.
27. Steinberg AD, Karliner JS: The clinical spectrum of heroin pulmonary edema. *Arch Intern Med* 1968; 122:122–127.
28. Waldron VD, Klint CR, Seibel JE: Methadone overdose treated with naloxone infusion. *JAMA* 1973; 225:53.
29. Wikler A: Diagnosis and treatment of drug dependence of the barbiturate type. *Am J Psychiatry* 1968; 125:758.
30. Zelson C, Rubio E, Wasserman E: Neonatal narcotic addiction: 10-Year observation. *Pediatrics* 1971; 48:178.

Further Reading

Bourne P (ed): *Acute Drug Abuse Emergencies: A Treatment Manual*. New York, Academic Press, 1976.

10

Medical Complications

1. Introduction

Drug dependence often presents to clinics and hospitals by virtue of medical, surgical, and psychiatric complications. Drug dependence can also mimic a wide variety of medical conditions. Unless the clinician remains alert to the possibility of drug dependence, the patient may obtain treatment for the secondary complication while the primary problem, drug dependence, goes untreated.

2. Nonspecific Complications

2.1. Malnutrition

Drug dependence can lead to malnutrition in various ways. If the drug is relatively costly, and the patient's financial resources are relatively limited, the person may choose to buy the drug rather than purchase food. This is especially true with strongly addicting substances, such as the opioids and alcohol.

Another cause for malnutrition can be the suppression of appetite. Opioid and amphetamine drugs are especially notable as anorexiants but nicotine and caffeine also have this effect. Malabsorption due to alcoholism can result in malnourishment, since excessive alcohol can produce intestinal changes that impede absorption.[15,49,59,79] Consumption of large amounts of alcohol also causes difficulty by supplying so-called empty calories. Alcohol contains 7 cal/g (as compared to 4 cal for carbohydrates), but is devoid of essential vitamins, minerals, fats, and protein. A heavy drinker may easily consume 1000–2000 cal/day in alcohol alone and thus have a much reduced intake of other foods. Chronic alcohol consumption is especially associated with deficiences in thiamine, folate, pyridoxine, magnesium, and zinc,[10,109] as well as abnormalities of iron absorption and deposition.[21,27] Drug-induced nausea, vomiting, diarrhea, anorexia, and hyperthermia can lead to severe depletions of fluid, potassium, sodium, and chloride.

2.2. Infectious Disease

Infectious disease may similarly have several causes in a drug-dependent person. One cause may be the general effect of substance abuse on lifestyle. The patient may have inadequate clothes, lack of shelter for protection against the climate and elements, and inadequate diet.[110] An unstable lifestyle, exposure to infectious companions, and a high rate of upsetting life changes have also been shown to correlate with increased rates of medical and psychiatric disease.

Lack of body defenses against infectious disease may also predispose to infectious diseases.[18,43,66,69] Hepatitis B, septicemia, bacterial endocarditis, and acquired immune deficiency syndrome (AIDS) occur in those who abuse drugs by parenteral means. Even those who ingest their drug have been shown to be prone to a variety of infectious diseases, including tuberculosis, bronchopneumonia, lobar pneumonia, and urinary tract infections.[71,72] Chronic alcohol dependence leads to leukopenia and immunosuppression, with increased infections. Suppression of the cough reflex and of ciliary movement in the bronchial tree may lead to the development of respiratory infection, including aspiration pneumonia.

Venereal diseases and venereal spread of AIDS also occur among drug-dependent persons. To some extent this may be due to the fact that individuals who exercise poor judgment regarding their drug use may also exercise poor judgment with regard to sexual partners. Those likely to be discerning in their sexual behavior while sober may not be so discerning while intoxicated. In later stages, the drug-dependent person may seek out prostitutes or casual sex partners because of inability to sustain a stable sexual relationship.[123]

2.3. Trauma

Physical injuries are especially prevalent among those abusing drugs. Injuries can occur by several mechanisms.

Drug-related vehicular accidents[40,50] result from driving too fast, not anticipating dangers, taking risks that would not otherwise be taken, or being unable to react in a rapid, coordinated manner to a sudden emergency. In a previous era when slower means of transportation prevailed, drug-related vehicular accidents posed less of a risk. In an era of high-speed motor vehicles, trains, boats, and airplanes, these problems are increasing in frequency. Intoxicated pedestrians are at risk when ordinary caution is not exercised in proximity to dangerous traffic. Sober drivers, passengers, and pedestrians are also at risk to the intoxicated driver.

Violence is another complication of drug dependence. A person is more likely to be engaged in fights, to assault others, or to become the victim of an assault while intoxicated. Some rape victims have not exercised judicious protectiveness as a result of being intoxicated. Children, spouses, and even elderly parents are sometimes physically abused by intoxicated relatives.

Drug-dependent persons are prone to a wide variety of other injuries from their immediate environment. These injuries include frostbite (from exposure to extreme cold) or hyperthermia (from exposure to extreme heat), burns from cigarettes or fires, drowning by falling out of boats or off of bridges, and falls. Frequently falls occur in environments that are not normally dangerous (e.g., a kitchen or bathroom, the curb of a street). So common are these nonvehicular accidents that chest X-rays that reveal numerous old rib fractures can serve as a diagnostic clue to possible drug dependence. Subdural hematoma and depressed skull fracture must be considered in obtunded drug-dependent patients.

Suicidal attempts and completed suicides may occur as a result of losses and decreased self-esteem associated with drug dependence. The drug-dependent person may commit suicide even while sober. A despondent person, although ordinarily inhibited from self-destruction, may become sufficiently disinhibited while intoxicated to commit suicide.

Interpersonal and group violence, in the form of assault and homicide, are common in the criminal underworld which conducts illicit drug trade. Such violence is prevalent especially among the high-profit cannabis, cocaine, and opioid trades. Lower-socioeconomic addicts may resort to mugging and burglary as a means of obtaining funds for drugs, with subsequent violent victimization of innocent persons.

2.4. Psychiatric Disorders

Drugs can lead to a variety of specific psychiatric syndromes as a result of their pharmacological actions. These syndromes are discussed in greater detail in later sections. However, there are also a number of nonspecific psychiatric disorders that can occur with drug dependence.

Repeated drug-related problems can lead to loss of job, loss of friends, alienation from family members, financial crises, health and social disability, and legal problems. As one attempts to maintain control over use of the drugs, and repeatedly fails at this, loss of self-esteem and self-confidence results. A recent decrease in the social network and loss of material resources are frequently present. These losses can lead to a variety of psychiatric manifestations, including adjustment reactions, generalized anxiety, somatiform disorders, major depression, schizophreniform psychosis, and panic disorder. These psychiatric manifestations may then persist when the individual ceases drug use or become temporarily worse when the drug is no longer available.

Chronic drug dependence often leads to personality changes. These vary from person to person, but typically include traits such as manipulation of others, passive–aggressiveness in interpersonal relationships, and sociopathic behavior (e.g., lying, stealing, breaking commitments). These personality changes are probably due to a variety of factors, including central nervous system effects of regular intoxication, preference for the drug experience over other experiences and commitments, and the need to obtain the drug continuously despite financial or societal constraints. These attitudinal and behavioral changes can greatly distort the patient's usual character structure.

2.5. Psychosomatic Disorders

General physicians encounter a wide variety of symptoms associated with drug dependence, depending on the drugs as well as the individual. Common symptoms include tension headaches, insomnia, fatigue, weakness, myalgia, abdominal pain, migraine, dyspareunia, impotence, amenorrhea, and similar disorders. A vicious cycle may ensue, in which the person takes even more drug to relieve these symptoms, which leads to further exacerbation of the symptoms.

While extensive physiological testing may sometimes reveal a particular cause for symptoms (such as vitamin deficiency or depression), the symptom may be related to the stresses and losses associated with drug dependence. Generally these symptoms clear as the person recovers from drug dependence, although occasionally they may persist even during abstinence. As with psychiatric disorders, the now-sober patient may become more aware of the disturbing symptoms and interpret the problem as becoming worse.[85] This awareness may lead to resumption of drug dependence.

3. Mode of Administration

3.1. Ingestion

Oral ingestion of drugs can lead to problems by the directly irritating properties of the substance. Perhaps the greatest offender in this regard is alcohol, which can cause inflammation of the pharynx, esophagus, stomach, and duodenum. Laryngitis, esophagitis, and gastritis are frequent complications.[57] Indigestion and occult gastrointestinal blood loss are common findings. If abuse continues over years, neoplasms of the hypopharynx, larynx, and esophagus can result.[67,117]

With depressant drugs such as opioids, alcohol, and sedatives, overdose can lead to emesis and aspiration of saliva or vomitus into the lungs. Aspiration may be directly life threatening by shutting off the airway. The individual may develop aspiration pneumonia or lung abscess.

3.2. Chewing

Many plant substances around the world are chewed, including tobacco, tea, betel-areca, and khat. These dependency-producing substances are often used throughout the day. Over a period of months and years, the individual is exposed to hours of an altered oral environment with the chewing cud.

Chronic chewers manifest a variety of nonspecific oral pathologies regardless of the substance. These include gingivitis, inflammation of the oral structures (such as the uvula), pyorrhea, and—in advanced cases—oral cancers. Certain added substances (such as the lime used with betel-areca) can cause direct damage to the teeth by dissolving the calcium.

3.3. Nasal Insufflation

Chronic snuffing of drugs leads to changes in the nasal mucosa similar to changes in the oral mucosa. Inflammation appears early. Later complications include epistaxis, acute and chronic sinusitis, benign and malignant neoplasms of the paranasal sinuses, atrophy of the nasal mucosa, and perforation of the nasal septum.[78]

3.4. Smoking

In recent decades smoking has beome increasingly prevalent in many areas of the world. Drugs that are smoked include opium, heroin, morphine, cannabis, tobacco, cocaine freebase, and phencyclidine. Smoking has the advantage of producing immediate high blood levels of the drug without the risk of infection from parenteral injection. Materials for smoking (e.g., a pipe, paper for cigarettes) are more readily available than injection paraphernalia (e.g., syringe, needle).

Early changes with chronic smoking include tracheitis and acute bronchitis. Chronic smoking over several years or longer often leads to chronic bronchitis, emphysema, cor pulmonale, and neoplasms of the respiratory system.[9]

Certain drugs may cause respiratory complications because of their pharmacological effects. For example, oral opioids and alcohol ingestion may suppress cough and impair ciliary movement in the tracheobronchial tree.[11,48] Withdrawal in chronic opiate smokers may present with acute asthmalike conditions, similar to bronchiolitis in children. Care must be taken to rule out cardiac asthma, since administration of opioids under such conditions can depress the respiratory center. On the contrary, bronchiolitis in withdrawing opium addicts may be relieved by opioid drugs.

3.5. Parenteral Injection

Parenteral injection can lead to a variety of complications. One of these is overdose, since a large amount of drug can be rapidly and widely distributed throughout the body. Other routes require smaller doses or have slower absorption.

Another risk of intravenous administration is anaphylactoid allergic responses, with hypotension and occasionally death. It is likely that these allergic responses are the result of fillers that have been added to illicit opiate drugs. Such fillers include milk powder, talcum, and quinine. Laboratory analysis of street drugs has revealed a large number of extraneous materials, including arthropod feces.

Intravenous administration of drugs can also lead to microemboli which travel from the venous site of injection to the right side of the heart. From there the microemboli produce capillary occlusion in the lungs. Intravenous administration can cause death, especially in the chronic parenteral drug user who has repeatedly injected microemboli over years. It can also lead to chronic pulmonary problems by producing cor pulmonale and physiological venous–arterial shunts in the pulmonary bed.

An extremely common problem associated with parenteral injection is infection. *Staphylococcus* is probably the most common bacterial cause of such infections, but other bacterial and fungal infections also occur. Many of these infections are due to enteric or saprophytic organisms with low pathogenicity. This is probably due to the impaired immune defense system which often occurs in drug-dependent persons. Infections occur in those who take their drugs by subcutaneous injection as well as in those who use intravenous injection. When subcutaneous injection produces cellulitis or abcess, the result is a characteristic stellate subcutaneous scar which is virtually pathognomonic of the subcutaneous injecting or skin-popping addict.

Intravenous injection may lead to AIDS, acute phlebitis, and thrombophlebitis, with subsequent linear scars. Linear scars along thrombosed veins are sometimes referred to as tracks. The latter are typically seen on the hand and forearm, but may also be present in the lower extremity. Conversely, the stellate scars from subcutaneous injection are usually present over areas of the body covered by clothing. These areas include the thighs, buttocks, and lower abdomen. Inadvertent tattoos may result when drugs containing pigment are injected into the subcutaneous or paravascular tissues. Hyperpigmented areas can result from repeated inflammation and scarification.

Bacterial and fungal infections can be distributed widely throughout the body directly from injection of unsterile drug solutions. Right-sided endocarditis is especially characteristic of parenteral injection, but left-sided endocarditis may also occur. From that nidus of infection, subsequent abcesses can appear in widely distributed areas of the body, including the lung, skin, brain, kidneys, bone, muscles, and other tissues. Additional problems may result as clots form on the diseased mitral valve. Large clumps of fibrin and bacteria can then break off from the mitral valve, releasing septic emboli to the brain, kidneys, intestines, and other vital organs.

4. Drug-Specific Complications

4.1. Opioids

Medical complications associated with opioid use relate primarily to the mode of administration. Smoking heroin over many years, or injecting it under unsterile conditions, or repeatedly administering it by nasal insufflation results in the type of problems described previously. Nonspecific drug problems include malnutrition, poor hygiene, and secondary infections.

Opioids do not produce as extensive tissue toxicity or organ damage as do alcohol and amphetamines. The principal physical effects from chronic use are long-lasting neuroadaptive changes in the nervous system, which may persist for several months or longer following cessation of drug use. Since opioids cross the placental barrier, administration in the pregnant woman near term can produce life-threatening respiratory depression in the newborn. Newborn children of addicted mothers undergo opioid withdrawal in the days following birth. Among chronic opioid addicts, a number of endocrine effects have been noted. Addicted men experience loss of libido and impotence in association with decreased levels of testosterone. Among addicted women, amenorrhea and sterility are frequent complaints.

In the tolerant individual, withdrawal causes severe morbidity, but little mortality in younger healthy addicts. Overdose is a danger especially in non-tolerant individuals. Opioid drugs produce surprisingly little tissue damage in the chronic user when compared to alcohol. Many of the infrequently reported complications, such as transverse myelitis, may be due to complications of parenteral administration, since they are usually reported in parenteral users, and not in opium smokers or patients maintained on oral methadone.

4.2. Alcohol

Despite its rather simple chemical structure, no drug produces such a variety of physiological disturbance and tissue damage as alcohol. Alcohol influences all cell membranes, altering transport across the membrane. Neurotransmitter and neuroreceptor activity in the brain are also affected by alcohol, which increases acetylcholine and endorphin levels in the brain.[83,103,112,113] Hormone production is affected, and cell replication slowed.

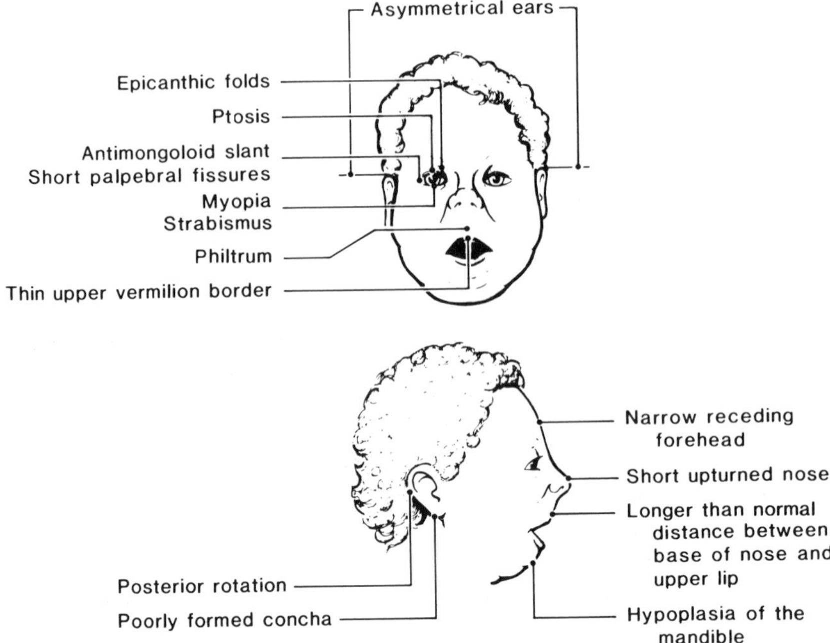

Figure 1. Features of the fetal alcohol syndrome. (From Ref. 123. Copyright by Praeger Publications, a division of Greenwood Press. Reprinted with permission.)

Exposure of the unborn child to high doses of alcohol can produce the fetal alcohol syndrome. This syndrome, shown in Figure 1, is marked by microcephaly, mental retardation, a long upper lip, and railroad track ears.[24,32,56,62,89] It appears that manifestations of this syndrome are most severe with greater alcohol intake, so that even mild alcohol drinking during pregnancy may cause subclinical damage. Many clinicians advise no drinking during pregnancy, or at least small, infrequent volumes (e.g., 2 oz of alcohol or less weekly).

Chronic administration of alcohol over a period of years increases the risk of certain cancers. Heavy smoking in alcohol users probably contributes to this risk. These cancers arise in the mouth, pharynx, larynx, esophagus, liver, and lungs. Daily doses of more than three drinks may increase the risk of such cancers.[67]

Daily drinking over a decade or two in doses as small as four or five drinks per day in females and six to eight drinks per day in males can produce damage to the cerebellar vermis, with subsequent dysarthria, ataxia, and imbalance.* Larger doses can produce toxic effects in much shorter periods (i.e., over days or weeks if tolerance develops and massive doses are consumed). Neuropathologies

*One drink equals 360 ml of beer (3.5% alcohol), 120 ml of wine (10% alcohol), or 30 ml of 80-proof distilled beverage alcohol (40% alcohol). Each drink contains about 12 ml of alcohol.

are often reversible in early stages, but may be irreversible in later stages, leading to such complications as permanent impotence or coordination difficulties.[75,76] Certain problems, such as Wernicke–Korsakoff syndrome due to thiamine deficiency, are due to the malnutrition associated with chronic alcoholism. Other alcohol-related neurological conditions include peripheral neuropathy, cerebellar and cerebral atrophy, alcohol amblyopia, central pontine myelinolysis, and Marchiafava–Bignami disease (a rare disorder resembling progressive dementia). Peripheral neuropathies are usually symmetrical in a stocking-glove distribution, affecting the sensory more than the motor fibers. Hepatic encephalopathy and cerebral atrophy can produce pictures of delirium and dementia, as can delirium tremens—a severe form of the alcohol withdrawal syndrome. Since head injuries may occur, acute or chronic subdural hematoma must be considered when an alcoholic becomes demented.[46] Reversibility of these conditions varies, but early diagnosis, adequate treatment, and abstinence from alcohol can lead to gradual recovery over several weeks to several months. Damage from many years of alcohol dependence may become permanent; cerebral atrophy may be apparent on computerized axial tomography.

Endocrine and metabolic dysfunctions result in hyponatremia, hypokalemia, a diabetic glucose tolerance picture, hypoglycemia, ketoacidosis, abnormal thyroid tests, hypercholesterolemia, various kinds of triglyceride abnormalities, positive dexamethasone suppression test, or pseudocushionoid syndrome. Mild endocrine abnormalities are seen in early cases.[22,28,36,39,63,77]

Inflammation and cancer of the mouth, pharynx, esophagus, and stomach increase with chronic alcohol dependence, especially when combined with cigarette smoking. Upper abdominal pathologies include gastroenteric, hepatic, and pancreatic problems. Esophagitis, gastritis, and peptic ulcer produce pain and occasionally bleeding or perforation. Small intestinal mucosa shows a nonspecific, reversible change which can result in malabsorption.

A variety of hepatic problems include alcoholic hepatitis, fatty liver, and cirrhosis. Once cirrhosis is established, continued drinking leads to a high mortality. Bleeding esophageal varices from portal vein hypertension frequently cause death. Superimposed infection, hepatic encephalopathy progessing to coma, hepatic failure, and hepatorenal failure are also common final events.[20,92] Hepatoma is an unusual, but fatal complication.

Both acute and chronic pancreatitis may ensue, with pancreatic pseudocyst and calcification of the pancreas. Diabetes mellitus and malabsorption can occur in advanced stages when little pancreatic tissue remains.[80,102,126] Four to six drinks per day (depending on body weight and gender), if continued over a decade or two, put one at risk to gastroenteric, hepatic, and pancreatic disease.[34]

Alcohol dependence produces a wide variety of sleep disturbances. Even small doses of alcohol can produce a reduction in rapid-eye-movement (REM) sleep, although this effect tends to disappear with repeated doses over time. Chronic alcoholics have reduced REM sleep. Upon withdrawal from alcohol, alcoholics have more arousal during the night—an effect that can last for many months despite abstinence. Even small or moderate doses of alcohol can reduce sleep latency, but increase wakefulness later in the night. Sleep time tends to increase during intoxication and decrease during withdrawal. Frightening dreams and hallucinations, sometimes called night terrors, affect alcoholics during withdrawal from large doses.[45,55,58]

Infections have been reported among alcoholics to a greater extent than in the general population. These include infections and abscesses of the lung, urinary tract, brain, and even peritoneum.[26] Organisms include not only *Staphylococcus,* pneumococcus, and *Streptococcus,* but also other organisms such as *Hemophilus influenzae, Klebsiella pneumoniae,* and *Legionella pneumophila.* Pulmonary tuberculosis, as well as other forms of tuberculosis (such as tuberculous peritonitis and tuberculous prostatitis), occurs more frequently among alcoholics. Causes for increased infection include leukopenia, suppressed immunological response, aspiration, and trauma. The acquired immune deficiency syndrome occurs among alcoholics in association with promiscuous sexual habits, although alcohol-induced damage to the immune system may perhaps also play a role.

Readily observable skin and oral conditions often accompany chronic alcoholism. Around the head and neck these include glossitis, cheilosis, acne roacea, skin flushing, parotid enlargement, thinning of hair, and facial edema. Body stigmata include spider nevi, atrophic skin, loss of axillary hair, feminine hair pattern and gynecomastia in males, and breast atrophy in women.[74,129]

Myopathies can be due to direct alcohol toxicity. They may also be neuropathic or nutritional in origin, the result of various metabolic changes.[98,130] Acute myolysis, myoglobinuria, and elevated blood levels of skeletal muscle enzymes (such as aldolase) can occur. Mineral from bone can be lost, especially in older alcoholics.[29]

Alcohol affects the bone marrow by directly reducing the red cells. The associated anemia may be macrocytric or microcytic. Macrocytic anemia or macrocytosis without anemia occurs in association with folate deficiency. Macrocytosis is often a sign of alcoholism. An elevated white blood count may occur in association with various toxic and infectious states, although neutropenia and thrombocytopenia from bone narrow suppression are frequent in chronic stages.[64] Less frequent conditions include sideroblastic anemia, hemolytic anemia, and various iron storage abnormalities.[21,27,35,82,84,120,121]

Chronic alcoholism has numerous effects on both the male and female reproductive systems. In men the effects include decreased libido, impotence, testicular atrophy, infertility, female escutcheon, and gynecomastia. Even acute alcohol consumption can produce morphological abnormalities in spermatazoa; this may lead to defective offspring. Chronic alcoholism in women can lead to menometrorrhagia, amenorrhea, infertility, repeated miscarriages, and the fetal alcohol syndrome. Ethanol suppresses uterine contraction, and so has even been used to inhibit threatened abortion.[23,65,118,119,127,132]

Other problems associated with alcoholism include hypertension, alcoholic cardiomyopathy, cardiac arrhythmias, vascular abnormalities, and cerebral vascular accidents.[8,14,93,94,97] Cardiomyopathy can be due to thiamine deficiency, but cardiomegaly may also be the result of direct alcohol toxicity. Either obesity (especially of the central-type distribution, with muscle wasting in the extremities) or cachexia may be present. Surgery as well as acute medical conditions in chronic alcoholics can lead to serious complications (e.g., atelectasis, infection, poor healing). General anesthesia in alcoholics tends to be especially difficult owing to the need for higher levels of drug to produce analgesia.[90,122]

At low blood alcohol levels the experienced social drinker has a low probability for vehicular accidents, but young or less-practiced drinkers run an increased accident risk even at quite low blood alcohol levels. For more complex perceptuomotor tasks, such as flying an airplane or steering a large boat in close quarters, the risk to accident is increased at even low blood alcohol levels.

In the chronic alcoholic, blackout or amnesia for behavior while drinking may result in accidents or violence that the individual cannot recall. There is considerable variability in this blackout phenomenon, with some patients encountering it fairly readily and others not encountering a blackout even long after developing tolerance to high doses of alcohol. In some cases there may be an hysterical component in which the drinker forgets painful or embarrassing events.

Delirium tremens, a toxic condition with hallucinosis and sometimes convulsions, ensues when the dependent drinker either ceases drinking or cannot drink more owing to a medical or surgical condition. Hallucinosis with a clear sensorium may occur during intoxication in association with organic brain damage or with psychiatric conditions such as paranoia or schizophrenia. Illusions (i.e., misperceptions of actual sensory stimuli) can accompany intoxication or withdrawal.

4.3. Sedative–Hypnotics, Anxiolytics

Acute or chronic sedative–hynotic intoxication can lead to many of the behavioral problems associated with alcohol dependence. These include vehicular accidents, falls, drowning, exposure to the elements (with frostbite or heat stroke), and development of various infections. With the short-acting drugs, such as most of the short-acting barbituates, withdrawal in the dependent person can lead to delirium or seizure similar to alcohol withdrawal. Withdrawal occurs within a few days of the last dose.[130] With the longer-acting drugs or those which are sequestered in body stores for a long period (such as the longer-acting benzodiazepines or ethchlorvynol) the withdrawal phenomenon may not begin for several days or a few weeks after the last dose.[38] Unexpected onset of confusion or acute psychotic delirium is prominent in this late-onset syndrome; withdrawal seizure is infrequent.[107]

Most of the symptoms associated with sedative–hypnotic dependence are directly related to the drug and the development of tolerance, rather than to tissue damage. Symptoms include anxiety, tremors, nightmares, insomnia, fever, emesis, and loss of appetite. Tissue damage, such as fractures from falls or burns inadvertently sustained in smoking or cooking while intoxicated, results from the secondary effects of the barbiturate. Acute or chronic organic brain syndromes can occur from repeated episodes of hypoxia and/or head injuries from falls.

4.4. Amphetamines

The opioids, alcohol, and sedative–hypnotics produce delirium or dementia only indirectly (such as by overdose, vitamin deficiencies, head injuries) or after prolonged usage (alcohol dementia, dementias secondary to hypoxia and head trauma). While there is some variability in the apparent sensitivity among individuals to delirium, dementia, and convulsions from the sedatives and alcohol, the interindividual variation with these drugs does not appear large. Amphetamine complications are markedly different from those of opioids, alcohol, and sedatives. Amphetamine can be psychotoxic, sometimes inducing delirium and psychosis in ordinary doses taken recreationally. Considerable variation exists among individuals regarding liability to psychotoxic effects. Some people can take amphetamines in high doses for years before encountering amphetamine psychosis. Others may suffer psychosis within hours or days.[7]

There appear to be two general types of amphetamine-related psychosis. One of these is the acute psychosis, which clears within hours, days, or weeks. In some patients this short-lived psychosis mimics acute anticholinergic psychosis with delirium, while in other patients it resembles schizophreniform psychosis with a clear sensorium. In yet other cases the drug precipitates a chronic psychosis, which persists over months and cannot be distinguished from schizophrenia, manic psychosis, or paranoid psychosis. Tissue damage may result indirectly from these psychotic episodes: self-injuries, burns, falls, and other injuries have been reported. These injuries have resulted from delusional thinking in many cases (i.e., thinking that one could fly like a bird or could kill people merely by looking at them).[125]

Most of the somatic concomitants of the amphetamines are the result of their direct pharmacological effect. These include anorexia, constipation, dry mouth, flush with pruritus, tachycardia, insomnia, weight loss with chronic use, mydriasis, hyperreflexia, hypertension, tachycardia, seizures, and cerebral vascular accident. Withdrawal does not manifest severe neurological toxicity, but depression and suspiciousness may progress to suicidal intent or paranoid psychosis.

4.5. Cocaine

Like amphetamine, cocaine can produce toxic psychosis. This typically occurs after binge usage or after prolonged use of the drug, although it may ensue more acutely in vulnerable individuals.[91]

Tissue complications result from the route of administration. These complications include nasal septum perforation, septicemia, and various lower-respiratory disorders. Preparation of cocaine for smoking can involve the use of solvents; serious burns and death by fire have occurred. Self-injury can occur from secondary psychosis.[105] Depression following cessation of the drug may be severe.

Direct tissue damage from the drug itself is minimal. Since the effect of the drug readily wears off, direct pharmacological effects (other than those on the central nervous system) are not usually disabling.[95]

4.6. Hallucinogens

As with the stimulants, hallucinogens can produce a short-lived psychosis, with either delirium or a clear sensorium. Panic reactions may also occur, particularly in those who unknowingly consume a hallucinogen. Such reactions are often short lived. In vulnerable individuals, however, these drugs can precipitate long-lasting psychosis similar to schizophrenia, manic–depressive psychosis, or paranoid psychosis. Since many of these drugs have an anticholinergic effect, dry mouth, blurred vision, gait and speech incoordination, and disturbances in swallowing may accompany acute intoxication or overdose.[53]

4.7. Phencyclidine

Phencyclidine (PCP) can produce the psychiatric disturbances described for the hallucinogens, with the special addition of perseveration. In addition, there are other serious acute side effects. These include hypotension and hypertension, hyperpyrexia, horizontal nystagmus sometimes with vertical nystagmus as well, decreased corneal reflex, perspiration, lacrimation, and salivation. Agitation has been so severe that even patients in physical restraints have fractured long bones in attempts to fight against the restraints. Since preparation of this drug in nonprofessional laboratories generally results in toxic by-products, the latter may also produce severe and toxic side effects. Less frequent complications include hypertensive crisis, seizure, acute dystonias, and acute renal failure secondary to hypertension or myoglobinuria. These effects may occur with the first dosage, or they may supervene only after the patient has used the drug repeatedly for a long time.

Other subacute effects are more common in the chronic user. These include weight loss, trouble with memory, poor concentration, blocking, and illogical thinking. Stuttering or poor speech articulation can appear. A variety of psychological complications may occur, including anxiety, panic disorders, depression, social withdrawal, and personality changes. Many clinicians have observed aggression, violence, random or stereotypic behaviors, paranoia, and catatonia in association with PCP use. These changes may persist for several months to a year even after the drug is discontinued.[53]

4.8. Cannabis

High doses of cannabis in vulnerable persons or prolonged high doses even in nonvulnerable people can lead to psychiatric syndromes similar to those described for the stimulants, hallucinogens, and PCP. These syndromes range from short-lived anxiety, panic reaction, or paranoia to long-lasting schizophrenia or manic–depressive psychosis. There is considerable variability among individuals to such complications.[116] Despite its potential to mimic the psychotoxic effects of the stimulants, hallucinogens, and PCP, regular episodic use of cannabis in small doses affects a smaller percentage of individuals as compared to the synthetic hallucinogen and stimulant drugs.[3]

Tissue effects outside the central nervous system are mainly related to the mode of administration, so that chronic respiratory problems can complicate prolonged smoking. Acute symptoms such as restlessness, confusion, disorientation, problems judging time, conjunctival injection, and increased appetite occur during acute intoxication. These symptoms clear within a few to several hours of the last dose.[19]

4.9. Nicotine/Tobacco

Nicotine use in the form of tobacco presents another model for medical complications attending drug dependence. Tobacco dependence does not cause disabling intoxication even in the presence of obvious nicotine dependence. People can use the drug for years, even decades, without evident psychological or social impairment, although nicotine does have metabolic and endocrine effects.[51,128]

Several major medical complications attend prolonged tobacco dependence.[47,96] These complications begin to occur after about 20 pack-years; that is, the smoking of one pack of cigarettes per day over a 20-year period, or an equivalent amount of tobacco usage (say half a pack over 40 years, or two packs over 10 years). The problems of chronic tobacco dependence include cancer of the lung and coronary artery disease. Heavy chronic tobacco usage causes laryngitis, tracheitis, chronic bronchitis, and emphysema. Oral hygiene is often adversely affected, with gingivitis, glossitis, and pyorrhea. On abrupt cessation of smoking, dependent persons experience craving for tobacco, irritability, agitation, trouble concentrating, headache, and pulse, blood pressure, and gastrointestinal changes.[99] These symptoms are relieved by nicotine.[17,100]

Although a certain amount of irreversible damage occurs after 20 pack-years of smoking or more, stopping smoking at any age can decrease the complications of tobacco dependence.

4.10. Caffeine

Caffeine produces its effects by releasing catecholamines, such as norepinephrine.[12,13] Clinical studies and surveys indicate that most caffeine users do not encounter problems with caffeine in doses of less than 500 mg/day. This is the equivalent of about three to five cups of brewed coffee. Above this level, tolerance and symptoms of caffeinism develop.[16,25,44] These include tachycardia, arrhythmias, hyperstimulation with intrusiveness or volubility, gastric irritation, abdominal cramps, diarrhea, muscle twitching, dry mouth, polyuria, insomnia, headache, migraine, excessive perspiration, and nausea. Withdrawal effects may also occur, with lethargy and headache.[31]

In sensitive individuals, such as those with a history of manic-depressive disorder, caffeine can precipitate hypomanic or manic symptomatology.[37,41,111] Extremely high doses, such as 1000 mg taken acutely or larger doses taken over several hours, have been known to precipitate delirium. Massive doses have been lethal. Drug interactions with other common social intoxicants have so far received little attention.[73]

4.11. Volatile Inhalants

These drugs rarely produce the long-lasting psychiatric syndromes described. Intoxication tends to be fairly short-lived. Both acute and chronic tissue damage can be serious, even life threatening.

Pathological effects vary from drug to drug. Especially the aerosols can cause sudden death from cardiotoxic effects.[42,70,115] Volatile hydrocarbons, from gasoline and paint thinners to industrial solvents, may produce hepatic damage, renal impairment,[114] and central nervous system deterioration.[5,33,81,86] The effects are generally reversible if diagnosed early, but chronic use may lead to hepatic or renal failure and permanent dementias. If dependence becomes repetitive, these patients may have the same difficulty abandoning inhalant abuse as do other drug-dependent persons.[4]

Problems associated with specific inhalant chemicals are as follows:

- Toluene—hepatorenal damage, neuropathy.[1,88]
- Benzene—pancytopenia, possibly leukemia.
- Nonsolvent additives such as lead—cerebellar damage, neurological problems, or death (sometimes associated with high blood lead levels).[104]
- Hexane—neuropathies, cerebellar damage, spinal cord degeneration, cerebral deterioration, neuropathy.
- Ketones—neuropathies, neurotoxicity to the central nervous system.
- Heptanes—seizure.
- Chlorohydrocarbons—neurological problems, disulfiramlike response to trichloroethylene.[2,54]
- Fluorocarbons—cardiotoxicity.
- Nitrous oxide—hematopoietic effects, seizures, anoxia, neuropathies.[6,30,101]
- Alkyl nitrates (amyl nitrite, butyl nitrite)—neuropathy, methemoglobinemia, possible cardiotoxicity.[52,61,106]

Often inhalant dependence occurs in epidemic fashion among certain subgroups. Reports have included halothane dependence by hospital personnel,[108] glue and thinner and gasoline dependence in children,[60,78,87] and the volatile nitrates as sexual adjuncts in some groups.[68]

4.12. Designer Drugs

Rogue chemists have synthesized new compounds with special effects, and often great potency. These compounds can have opioid, sedative, stimulant, and/or hallucinogenic properties. In some cases these drugs, or unintended side products associated with their manufacture, can produce temporary, permanent, and even lethal damage. A permanent form of severe parkinsonism has resulted from one chemical synthesis. These modern chemists resemble yesterday's bootleggers, whose illicit alcohol could cause palsies, blindness, dementia, or death (from methyl alcohol or plumbism) through dangerous distillation practices.

References

1. Akiguchi I, Fujiwara T, Iwai N, Kawai C: A case of chronic thinner (toluene) intoxication with myeloneuropathy and EEG abnormality. *Rinsho Shinkeigaku* 1977; 17:586.
2. Alapin B: Trichloroethylene addiction and its effects. *Br J Addict* 1973; 68:331.
3. Allentuck S, Bowman KM: The psychiatric aspects of marihuana intoxication. *Am J Psychiatry* 1942; 99:248.
4. Altenkirch H: Sniffing addiction: Chronic solvent abuse with neurotoxic effects in children and juveniles. *Deutsch Med Wochenschr* 1979; 104:935.
5. Amaducci L, Arfaioli C, Inzitari D, Martinetti MG: Another possible precipitating factor in multiple sclerosis: The exposure to organic solvents. *Boll Inst Sieroter (Milan)* 1978; 56:613.
6. Amess JAL, Burman JF, Rees GM, Nancekievill DG, Mollin DL: Megaloblastic haemopoiesis in patients receiving nitrous oxide. *Lancet* 1978; 2:339.
7. Angrist BM, Gershon S: The phenomenology of experimentally induced amphetamine psychosis. *Biol Psychiatry* 1970; 2:95.
8. Ashley MJ, Rankin J: Hazardous alcohol consumption and diseases of the circulatory system. *J Stud Alcohol*, 1980; 41:1040–1069.
9. Auerbach O, Hammond EC, Garfinkel L: Changes in bronchial epithelium in relation to cigarette smoking, 1955–1960 vs. 1970–1977. *N Engl J Med* 1979; 300:381.
10. Baker H, Frank O, Zetterman RK, Rajan KS, Ten-Hove W, Leevy CM: Inability of chronic alcoholics with liver disease to use food as a source of folates, thiamin and vitamin B_6. *Am J Clin Nutr* 1975; 28:1377–1380.
11. Banner AS: Pulmonary function in chronic alcoholism. *Am Rev Respir Dis* 1973; 108:851.
12. Bellet S, Roman L, DeCastro O, Kim KD, Kershbaum A: Effect of coffee ingestion on catecholamine release. *Metabolism* 1969; 18:288.
13. Berkowitz BA, Tarver JH, Spector S: Release of norepinephrine in the central nervous system by theophylline and caffeine. *Eur J Pharmacol* 1970; 10:64.
14. Berthelot P, Walker JG, Sherlock S: Arterial changes in the lungs in cirrhosis of the liver-lung spider nevi. *N Engl J Med* 1966; 274:291.
15. Bode JC: Factors influencing alcohol metabolism in man: Alcohol and the gastrointestinal tract. *INSERM Symp Ser* 1980; 95:65–92.

16. Boyd EM, Dolman M, Knight LM, Sheppard EP: The chronic oral toxicity of caffeine. *Can J Physiol Pharmacol* 1965; 43:995–1007.
17. Brantmark B, Ohlin P, Westling H: Nicotine-containing chewing gum as an anti-smoking aid. *Psychopharmacologia* 1973; 31:191.
18. Brayton RG, Stokes PE, Schwartz MS, Louria DB: Effects of alcohol and various diseases on leukocyte and mobilization phagocytosis and intracellular killing. *N Engl J Med* 1970; 282:123–128.
19. Bromberg W: Marihuana intoxication: A clinical study of Cannabis sativa intoxication. *Am J Psychiatry* 1934; 91:303.
20. Buffet C, Chaput JC, Abuisson F, Subtil E, Etienne JP: La macrocytose dans l'hepatite alcoholique chronique histologiquement prouvee. *Arch Fr Med Appl Diag* 1975; 64:309–315.
21. Charlton RW, Jacobs P, Seftel H, Bothwell TH: Effect of alcohol on iron absorption. *Br Med J* 1964; 2:1427–1429.
22. Cicero TJ: Neuroendocrinological effects of alcohol. *Annu Rev Med* 1981; 32:123–142.
23. Cicero TJ, Bell RD, Meyer E: Effects of ethanol on testicular steroidogenesis: Mechanism of action. *Drug Alcohol Depend* 1980; 6:50–51.
24. Clarren SK, Alvord EC Jr, Sumi SM, Streissguth AP, Smith DW: Brain malformations related to prenatal exposure to ethanol. *J Pediatr* 1978; 92:64–67.
25. Colton T, Gosselin RE, Smith RP: The tolerance of coffee drinkers to caffeine. *Clin Pharmacol Ther* 1968; 9:31.
26. Conn HO, Fessel JM: Spontaneous bacterial peritonitis in cirrhosis: Variations on a theme. *Medicine* 1971; 50:161–197.
27. Conrad ME, Barton JC: Anemia and iron kinetics in alcoholism. *Semin Hematol* 1980; 17:149–163.
28. Cooperman MT, Davidoff F, Spark R, Pallotta J: Clinical studies of alcoholic ketoacidosis. *Diabetes* 1974; 23:433–439.
29. Dalen N, Lamke B: Bone mineral losses in alcoholics. *Acta Orthop Scand* 1976; 47:469.
30. DiMaio VJM, Garriott JC: Four deaths resulting from abuse of nitrous oxide. *J Forensic Sci* 1978; 23:169.
31. Dreisbach RH, Pfeiffer C: Caffeine-withdrawal headache. *J Lab Clin Med* 1943; 28:1212.
32. Dreosti IE, Ballard FJ, Belling BG, Hetzel BS: Ethanol, DNA synthesis, and fetal development. *Alcoholism: Clin Exp Res* 1981; 5:357–362.
33. Easson W: Gasoline addiction in children. *Pediatrics* 1962; 29:250.
34. Edwards G: *Alcohol and Alcoholism: The Report of a Special Committee of the Royal College of Psychiatrists.* New York, Free Press, 1979.
35. Eichner ER, Hilman RS: The evolution of anemia in alcoholic patients. *Am J Med* 1971; 50:218–232.
36. Ellis FW: Effect of ethanol on plasma corticosterone levels. *J Pharmacol Exp Ther* 1966; 153:121.
37. Erhardt E: Psychic disturbances in caffeine intoxication. *Acta Med Scand* 1929; 71:94.
38. Flemenbaum A, Gunby B: Ethchlorvynol (Placidyl) abuse and withdrawal. *Dis Nerv Syst* 1971; 32:188.
39. Frajria R, Angeli A: Alcohol-induced pseudo-Cushing's syndrome (letter). *Lancet* 1977; 1:1050.
40. Freisen G: Vancouver Island traffic fatalities, 1966–1970. *J Trauma* 1974; 14:791.
41. Furlong FW: Possible psychiatric significance of excessive coffee consumption. *Can Psychiatr Assoc J* 1975; 20:577.
42. Garriott J, Petty CS: Death from inhalant abuse. Toxicological and pathological evaluation of 34 cases. *Clin Toxicol* 1980; 16:305.
43. Gluckman SJ, Dvorak VC, MacGregor RR: Host defense during prolonged alcohol consumption in a controlled environment. *Arch Intern Med* 1977; 137:1539–1543.
44. Greden JF: Anxiety or caffeinism: A diagnostic dilemma. *Am J Psychiatry* 1974; 131:1089.

45. Gross MM, Hastey JM: Sleep disturbances in alcoholism, in Tarter R, Sugerman A (eds): *Alcoholism*. Reading, Massachusetts, Addison-Wesley, 1976.
46. Gross MM, Lewis E, Hastey J: Acute alcohol withdrawal syndrome, in Kissin B, Begleiter H (eds): *The Biology of Alcoholism, Clinical Pathology*. New York, Plenum Press, 1974, vol 3.
47. Hawthorne VM, Fry JS: Smoking and health: The association between smoking behaviour, total mortality, and cardiorespiratory disease in West Central Scotland. *J Epidemiol Community Health* 1978; 32(4):260–266.
48. Heineman HO: Alcohol and the lung: A brief review. *Am J Med* 1977; 63:81–85.
49. Hilman RW: Alcoholism and malnutrition, in Kissen B, Begleiter H (eds): *The Biology of Alcoholism: Clinical Pathology*. New York, Plenum Press, 1974, vol 3.
50. Holczabek W: The alcoholized pedestrian as a victim of fatal traffic accidents. *Wein Klin Wochenschr* 1976; 88:206.
51. Husain MK, Andrew GF, Ciarochi F, Robinson AG: Nicotine-stimulated release of neurophysin and vasopressin in humans. *J Clin Endocrinol Metab* 1975; 41:1113.
52. Israelst AMS, Lambert S, Oki G: Poppers, a new recreational drug craze. *Can Pyschiatr Assoc J* 1978; 23:493.
53. Jaffee JH: Drug addiction and drug abuse, in Gilman AG, Goodman LS, Gilman A (eds): *The Pharmacological Basis of Therapeutics*. New York, MacMillan, 1980, pp 535–584.
54. James WRL: Fatal addiction to trichloroethylene. *Br J Ind Med* 1963; 20:47.
55. Johnson LC, Burdick JA, Smith J: Sleep during alcohol intake and withdrawal in the chronic alcoholic. *Arch Gen Psychiatry* 1970; 22:406–418.
56. Kaminski R, Rumeau-Rouquette C, Schwartz D: Consommation d'alcool chez les femmes enceintes et issue de la grossesse (Alcohol consumption among pregnant women and outcome of pregnancy). *Rev Epidem Sante Publique* 1976; 24:27–40.
57. Kaufman SE, Kaye MD: Induction of gastro-esophageal reflux by alcohol. *Gut* 1978; 19:336–338.
58. Knowles JB, Laverty SG, Kuechler HA: Effects of alcohol on REM sleep. *Q J Stud Alcohol* 1968; 29:342–349.
59. Korsten MA, Lieber CS: Nutrition in the alcoholic. *Med Clin North Am* 1979; 63:963–972.
60. Lawton J, Malmquist C: Gasoline addiction in children. *Psychiatr Q* 1961; 35:551.
61. Layzer RB, Fishman RA, Schafer JA: Neuropathy following abuse of nitrous oxide. *Neurology* 1978; 28:504.
62. Lemoine P, Haronsseau H, Borteryu JP, Menuet JP: Les enfants de partents alcoholiques: Anomalies observees a propos de 127 cas (Children of alcoholic parents: Anomalies observed in 127 cases). *Quest Med* 1968; 25:476–482.
63. Lieber CS, Jones DP, Mendelson J, De Carli LM: Fatty liver, hyperlipemia and hyperuricemia produced by prolonged alcohol consumption, despite adequate dietary intake. *Trans Assoc Am Physicians* 1963; 76:289–300.
64. Lindenbaum J, Hargrove RL: Thrombocytopenia in alcoholics. *Ann Intern Med* 1968; 68:526–532.
65. Lindholm J, Fabricius-Bjerre N, Bahnsen M, Boiesen P, Bangstrup L, Pedersen ML, Hagen C: Pituitary-testicular function in patients with chronic alcoholism. *Eur J Clin Invest* 1978; 8:269.
66. Louria DB, Almy TP: Susceptibility to infection during experimental alcohol intoxication. *Tran Assoc Am Physicians* 1963; 76:102–112.
67. Lowenfels AB: Alcohol and cancer: A review and update. *Br J Alcohol Alcoholism* 1979; 14(3):148–163.
68. Lowry TP: The volatile nitrites as sexual drugs: A user survey. *J Sex Educ Ther* 1979; 1:8.
69. Lundy J, Raaf JH, Deakins S, Wanebo HJ, Jacobs DA, Tsung-dao L, Jacobowitz D, Spear C, Oettgen HF: The acute and chronic effects of alcohol on the human immune system. *Surg Gynecol Obstet* 1975; 141:212–218.
70. Lupke H, Gerchow J, Schmidt K: On two cases of lethal trichloroethylene intoxication. *Z Rechtsmed* 1978; 81:237.

71. Lyons HA, Saltzman A: Diseases of the respiratory tract in alcoholics, in Kissin B, Begleiter H (eds): *The Biology of Alcoholism: Clinical Pathology*. New York, Plenum Press, 1974, vol 3.
72. MacGregor RR, Gluckman SJ, Senior JR: Granulocyte function and levels of immunoglobulins and complement in patients admitted for withdrawal from alcohol. *J Infect Dis* 1978; 138:747–753.
73. Marbach G, Schwertz MT: Effects physiologiques de l'alcohol et la caffeine au cours du sommeil chez l'homme. *Arch Sci Physiol* 1964; 18:163.
74. Margolis J, Robert DM: Frequency of skin lesions in chronic drinkers. *Arch Dermatol* 1976; 112:1326–1327.
75. Mawdsley C, Mayer R: Nerve conduction in alcoholic polyneuropathy. *Brain* 1965; 88:335–356.
76. Mayer R: Peripheral nerve conduction in alcoholics: Studies of the effects of acute and chronic intoxication. *Psychosom Med* 1966; 28(part 2):475–483.
77. Mendelson JH, Mello NK, Ellingboe J: Effect of acute alcohol intake on pituitary gonadal hormones in normal human males. *J Pharmacol Exp Ther* 1977; 202:676–682.
78. Merry J, Zachariadis N: Addiction to glue sniffing. *Br Med J* 1962; 2:1448.
79. Mezey E: Intestinal function in chronic alcoholism. *Ann NY Acad Sci* 1975; 252:215–227.
80. Mezey E, Jow E, Slavin RE, Tobin F: Pancreatic function and intestinal absorption in chronic alcoholism. *Gastroenterology* 1970; 56:657–664.
81. Mikkelsen S, Gregersen P, Klausen H, Dossing M, Nielsen H: Presenile dementia as an occupational disease following industrial exposure to organic solvents: A review of the literature. *Ugeskr Laeger* 1978; 140:1633.
82. Morin J, Porte P: Macrocytose erythrocytaire chez les ethyliques. *Nouv Presse Med* 1976; 5:273.
83. Muller P, Britton RS, Seeman P: The effects of long-term ethanol on brain receptors for dopamine, acetylcholine, serotonin and noradrenaline. *Eur J Pharmacol* 1980; 65:31–37.
84. Myrhed M, Berglund L, Bottiger LE: Alcohol consumption and hematology. *Acta Med Scand* 1977; 202:11–15.
85. Nolan JP: Alcohol as a factor in the illness of university service patients. *Am J Med Sci* 1965; 249:135–142.
86. Normura N, Mitani K, Terao A, Shirabe T: A case of myeloneuropathy induced by chronic exposure to organic solvents. *Rinsho Shinkeigaku* 1978; 18:259.
87. Nylander I: Thinner addiction in children and adolescents. *Acta Paedopsychiatr* 1962; 29:273.
88. O'Brien ET, Yeoman WB, Hobby JAE: Hepatorenal damage from toluene in a "glue sniffer." *Br Med J* 1971; 2:29.
89. O'Shea KS, Kaufman MH: The teratogenic effect of acetaldehyde: Implications for the study of the fetal alcohol syndrome. *J Anat* 1979; 128:65–76.
90. Orkin LR: Addiction, alcoholism, and anesthesia. *South Med J* 1977; 70:1172–1174.
91. Post RM: Cocaine psychosis: A continuum model *Am J Psychiatry* 1975; 132:225.
92. Ratnoff OD, Patek AJ: The natural history of Laennec's cirrhosis of the liver. *Medicine* 1942; 21:207–268.
93. Regan TJ: Alcoholic cardiomyopathy, in Feldman EB (ed): *Nutrition and Cardiovascular Disease*. New York, Appleton-Century Crofts, 1976.
94. Regan TJ, Ettinger PO, Haider B, Ahmed S, Oldewurtel HA, Lyons MM: The role of ethanol in cardiac disease. *Annu Rev Med* 1977; 28:393–409.
95. Resnick RB, Kestenbaum RS, Schwartz LK: Acute systematic effects of cocaine in man: A controlled study by intranasal and intravenous routes. *Science* 1977; 195:696.
96. Rolleston H: Medical aspects of tobacco. *Lancet* 1926; 1:961.
97. Rubin E: Alcoholic myopathy in heart and muscle. *N Engl J Med* 1979; 301:28–33.
98. Rubin E, Katz AM, Leiber CS: Muscle damage produced by chronic alcohol consumption. *Am J Pathol* 1976; 83:499–575.

99. Russell MAH: Cigarette smoking: Natural history of a dependence disorder. *Br J Med Psychol* 1971; 44:1.
100. Russell MAH, Wilson D, Feyerabend D, Cole PV: Effect of nicotine chewing gum on smoking behavior and as an aid to cigarette withdrawal. *Br Med J* 1976; 2:391.
101. Sahenk Z, Mendell JR, Couri D, Nachtmen J: Polyneuropathy from inhalation of N20 cartridges through a whipped-cream dispenser. *Neurology* 1978; 28:485.
102. Sarles H: Chronic calcifying pancreatitis—Chronic alcohol pancreatitis. *Gastroenterology* 1974; 66:604–616.
103. Schulz R, Wuster M, Duka T, Herz A: Acute and chronic ethanol treatment changes endorphin levels in brain and pituitary. *Psychopharmacology* 1980; 68:221–227.
104. Seshai SS, Rajani KR, Boeckx RL, Chow PN: The neurological manifestations of chronic inhalation of leaded gasoline. *Dev Med Child Neurol* 1978; 20:323.
105. Siegel RK: Cocaine smoking. *N Engl J Med* 1979; 300:373.
106. Sigell LT, Kapp FT, Fusaro GA, Nelson ED, Falck RS: Popping and snorting volatile nitrites: A current fad for getting high. *Am J Psychiatry* 1978; 135:1216.
107. Smith DE, Wesson DR: Benzodiazepine dependency syndrome. *J Psychoactive Drugs* 1983; 15:85–95.
108. Spencer JD, Raasch FO, Trefny FA: Halothane abuse in hospital personnel. *JAMA* 1976; 235:1034.
109. Spivak JL, Jackson DL: Pellagra: An analysis of 18 patients and review of the literature. *Johns Hopkins Med J* 1977; 140:295–309.
110. Stiehm EF: Humoral immunity in malnutrition. *Fed Proc* 1980; 39:3093–3097.
111. Stillner V, Popkin MK, Pierce CM: Caffeine-induced delirium during prolonged competitive stress. *Am J Psychiatry* 1978; 135:855.
112. Syntinsky IA, Guzikov M, Gomanko MV, Eremin VP, Konovalova NN: The gamma-aminobutyric acid (GABA) system in brain during acute and chronic ethanol intoxication. *J Neurochem* 1975; 15:43–48.
113. Tabakoff B, Melchior C, Urwyler S, Hoffman PL: Alterations in neurotransmitter function during the development of ethanol tolerance and dependence, in Idestrom CM (ed): *Alcohol and Brain Research.* Copenhagen, Acta Psychiatrica Scandinavica, 1981, vol 62.
114. Taher SM, Anderson RJ, McCartney R, Popovtzer MM, Schrier RW: Renal tubular acidosis associated with toluene "sniffing." *N Engl J Med* 1974; 290:765.
115. Taylor G, IV, Harris W: Cardiac toxicity of aerosol propellants. *JAMA* 1970; 214:81.
116. Treffert DA: Marihuana use in schizophrenia: A clear hazard. *Am J Psychiatry* 1978; 135:10.
117. Tuyns AJ: Epidemiology of alcohol and cancer. *Cancer Res* 1979; 39:2840–2843.
118. Van Thiel DH, Gavaler JS, Eagon P, Lester R: Effect of alcohol on gonadal function. *Drug Alcohol Depend* 1980; 6:41–42.
119. Van Thiel DH, Gavaler JS, Lester R: Ethanol: A gonadal toxin in the female. *Drug Alcohol Depend* 1977; 2:373–380.
120. Wallenstedt S, Cederblad G, Korsan-bengtsen K, Olsson R: Coagulation factors and other plasma proteins during abstinence after heavy alcohol consumption in chronic alcoholics. *Scand J Gastroenterol* 1977; 12:649–655.
121. Waters AH, Morley AA, Rankin JG: Effect of alcohol on haemopoiesis. *Br Med J* 1966; 2:1565–1568.
122. Watson TD, Lee JF: Preanesthetic care, intoxication and trauma. *Clin Anesth* 1976; 11:31–38.
123. Westermeyer J: *A Clinical Guide to Alcohol and Drug Problems.* New York, Praeger, 1986, pp 270–271.
124. Whalley LJ: Sexual adjustment of male alcoholics. *Acta Psychiatr Scand* 1978; 58:281–298.
125. Whitlock FA, Charalampous KD, Lynn EJ, et al: *Amphetamines: Medical and Psychological Studies.* New York, MSS Information Corp, 1974.
126. Williams RB, Russell RM, Dutta SK, et al: Alcoholic pancreatitis: Patients at high risk of acute zinc deficiency. *Am J Med* 1979; 66:889–893.

127. Wilson GT, Lawson DM, Abrams DB: Effects of alcohol on sexual arousal in male alcoholics. *J Abnorm Psychol* 1978; 87:609–616.
128. Winternitz WW, Quillen D: Acute hormonal response to cigarette smoking. *J Clin Pharmacol* 1977; 17:389.
129. Woeber K: The skin in diagnosing alcoholism. *Ann NY Acad Sci* 1975; 252:292–295.
130. Wolff MH: The barbiturate withdrawal syndrome: A clinical and electroencephalographic study. *Electroencephalogr Clin Neurophysiol* 1959; 14 (suppl):11–173.
131. Worden RE: Pattern of muscle and nerve pathology in alcoholism. *Ann NY Acad Sci* 1976; 273:351–359.
132. Ylikahri RH: Hormonal changes during alcohol intoxication and withdrawal. *Drug Alcohol Depend* 1980; 6:42–43.

Further Reading

Lieber CS: *Medical Disorders of Alcoholism: Pathogenesis and Treatment.* Philadelphia, Saunders, 1982.

Lieber CS, Jones DP, Losowsky MS, et al: Interrelation of uric acid and ethanol metabolism in man. *J Clin Invest* 1962; 41:1863–1870.

Roberton RJ, Khan I: Designer drugs. *Bull WHO* 1986; 64(6):801–805.

11

Psychosocial Management

1. Introduction

A positive, ongoing physician–patient relationship is especially important in the early stages of treatment. Patients often pursue psychosocial treatments if they are recommended by a physician. These treatment approaches are not always administered by a physician, although many primary care physicians and psychiatrists are skilled in these modalities. Nurses, social workers, counselors, and psychologists may also acquire these treatment skills. All of these approaches are not applied concurrently in a ritualized fashion for every patient. Nonetheless, many of these modalities may be employed in various phases of treatment. Individualized patient and family assessments are key to selecting appropriate therapies. Coordinated treatment using a team approach maximizes treatment resources and therapeutic efficacy.

2. Principles of Psychosocial Treatment

2.1. Individual Assessment Prior to Treatment

For purposes of treatment, drug dependence may be thought of as a group of syndromes each with different symptom clusters. These syndromes manifest varying severity for shorter or longer periods of time. Each patient should to be evaluated to determine which pathological processes are active and should be addressed by treatment. Not all patients have all clusters of symptoms. The physician considers the phase of the disorder (whether early or late) as well as the patient's psychological assets and social resources.

Differences among individual patients can be approached by distinguishing conditions to be addressed in treatment:

1. Conditions existent before the onset of the drug dependence (e.g., other disorders, personal and social factors).
2. Complications produced by drug dependence in the patient, especially those which block recovery (e.g., hepatitis, dementia).
3. Factors that favor continued drug use (e.g., collusion by family members).
4. Disturbances produced by stopping drug use, entering treatment, or beginning recovery (e.g., depression, separation from friends or family).

It is also important to consider available resources that favor the patient's eventual recovery. These include training, employment, family, and community. Positive personality features that may reappear as morbid personality characteristics secondary to drug abuse gradually recede.

2.2. Building a Therapeutic Alliance

The clinician sometimes senses that the clinical observations do not match the patient's reports, and that the patient resists looking at the problems associated with drug use. Supportive interviewing can minimize these inconsistencies. At times the clinician attempts to convert an adversarial situation into a collaborative one.

Failure to engage the patient in treatment is a considerable obstacle to recovery. If the clinician can help the person enter treatment, the prognosis improves. As a result of denial and fear, patients and physicians may both be reluctant to work together to address the drug dependence.

The clinician tries to behave in such a way that the patient chooses to remain in treatment. The physician–patient alliance is based on the patient's discomfort or crisis, as well as the shared belief that treatment can help. Powerful forces at work in drug-dependent patients repeatedly threaten to disrupt the physician–patient relationship and prematurely terminate treatment. The alliance is most fragile when the patient's distress is greatest.

Numerous events commonly precipitate the patient's departure from treatment. One is an increase in discomfort, an inevitable concomitant of treatment. Another is a disappointed hope of immediate or rapid relief. Two useful therapeutic approaches in early treatment are acknowledgment of the patient's suffering and anger, and instillation of hope. These approaches can be communicated by statements such as "I think your drug use is hurting you" and "I see no reason why you cannot overcome your dependence on drugs and get well."

Clinicians can be supportive even in the face of a dubious prognosis by containing their own skepticism. A positive attitude is easier to maintain by keeping in mind that many addicted people do recover. The question should not be whether the patient can recover, but how can the patient recover? If the therapist can instill hope, the patient can often devise a recovery mechanism that the therapist has not yet considered.

Not all patients realize that the physical and emotional symptoms that ensue when they stop using drugs are temporary. It is important for the clinician, the patient, and the family to realize this, as well as the fact that treatment for drug dependence is not brief, easy, or comfortable.

Taking a drug history may be educational for the patient and the family, but it may lead to feelings of shame or remorse. The patient and family need support and empathy during this process. After establishing good communication with the patient, the physician employs the usual medical methods: taking a history, performing an examination, making a diagnosis, conveying the diagnosis to the patient, supporting the patient through the response to the diagnosis, and recommending treatment.

An important therapeutic tactic lies in gathering data about the drug dependence. This is accomplished by maintaining a persistent focus on the sequelae of drug use, not merely on the amounts consumed. Patients repeatedly shift away from the painful subject of drug use. They need the help of a clinician to become aware of the connection between symptoms and the drug use.

It is acceptable for the clinician to agree with patients that they are suffering and need help. However, the clinician may have different explanations for the cause, given the patients' tendency to project blame onto others. One should not insist that patients label themselves as drug dependent at this early point. This change in self-identity may take time. Too rapid a change in identity can even be detrimental. It is important initially to accept the patient, since at this stage most patients feel that they should be deprived, rejected, or punished. This distortion must be clarified. A position of optimistic helpfulness can be maintained by telling patients that they deserve relief, that treatment works, and that the physician can help.

Patients also need to be given credit for everything they are currently doing or trying to do to consolidate their gains and move on to the next task of recovery. Initial assessment should not only identify defects and symptoms, but also identify strengths and resources. Information regarding previous strengths may be elicited by asking about previous problem-solving efforts, past attempts to use treatment, and successes to date in stopping or controlling drug use. One can ask such questions as "When your drinking began to cause trouble, what did you do?" If the patient says, "I stopped drinking for 2 weeks," the clinician can say, "Excellent! How did you do that?" He has just reported that he has the capacity to become sober and maintain sobriety, at least for a time. Patient and clinician both need to be reminded of previous successes. Either therapeutic pessimism or minimizing the problem blocks recovery.

Forging a clinician–patient relationship and fostering a beneficial alliance are inseparable from the therapeutic actions of helping the patient. Establishing a collaborative environment may include

1. Treatment of medical complications.
2. Detoxification if needed.
3. Treatment of social and psychological emergencies.
4. Establishing a therapeutic relationship.
5. Helping the patient stop drug use.

The physician attempts to engage not only the patient, but also responsible members of the patient's social network. A mutual definition of the problem should be worked out by all concerned during resolution of the crisis. Otherwise the patient may leave treatment as soon as the crisis has subsided. Failure to retain a patient long enough for treatment to bring about a change wastes valuable resources and perpetuates chronicity.

2.3. Early Abstinence

Drug use must stop for recovery to begin. The patient ceases drug use so that

1. The craving for drugs will fade.
2. Cerebral impairment from drug effects will decrease, and the patient can think clearly and learn new behaviors.
3. Injury to self-esteem, relationships, and health caused by drug use can stop.

The physician may suggest a therapeutic trial of abstinence. One can usually ask the person to stop for a definite period (say 12 weeks). This may be easier than trying to stop indefinitely. If the patient agrees to begin a trial of stopping drugs, and does not need detoxification, one can schedule a return appointment on the following day, then in a half-week, and weekly thereafter. Intensive early support is essential.

Newly abstinent drug-dependent patients can expect to experience mild, subclinical withdrawal for several months, with trouble sleeping, intense depression, irritability, anxiety, and sometimes craving. These symptoms improve with time. Relapse may occur if the patient cannot tolerate or obtain relief from these symptoms.

Establishing a safe, drug-free environment is a crucial basis for subsequent recovery. Drug use blocks the learning of new behavior and the thought processes necessary to establish natural recovery. Stopping drug use allows the traumatic effects of intoxication to stop and neurophysiological healing to begin.

Although establishment of a safe, drug-free environment is a necessary condition of recovery, it is not sufficient. Unless other changes also take place, abstinence will remain precarious.

2.4. Facilitating Recovery

Drug-dependence treatment programs teach principles of behavior change. For example, self-help groups suggest: go to self-help meetings, join a group, get a sponsor (a mentor or helper), ask for help, do not use intoxicants. Some also use slogans such as HALT: don't get too *H*ungry, *A*ngry, *L*onely, or *T*ired. Members are urged to look after themselves and their recovery carefully.

A new member of a self-help group, awake at 3 A.M. and wanting to drink, might contact a sponsor and be told: "Take a warm bath, drink some tea, go back to bed, and try to sleep for an hour or so. If the desire to drink doesn't pass, then come and get me." The patient needs a method for not acting on impulse and needs help with the compulsive feelings.

Since denial is frequent among drug-dependent persons, they often believe that they do not have a drug problem. On the contrary, they believe that they can use drugs and that they do not need help. To sustain abstinence, drug-dependent persons have to reconceptualize a large part of their experience and their relationship to drugs in order to grasp the idea that intoxication has negative consequences. They must be reassured that there is help, and that recovery is possible.

The clinician can help the drug-dependent person change drug-centered thinking toward healthy goals. Drug-dependent persons become less likely to use drugs when they think in the following way:

1. "I can't regulate my drug use. If I use drugs, I am going to have trouble."
2. "If I use drugs, it will feel good for a while, but in the long run it will be destructive and dangerous."
3. "I don't have to use drugs, even if I desire them. Treatment works. I know where and how to get help."

Prior to relapse, the person's thinking slips back toward denial, exemplified by statements like

1. "Maybe I can use drugs without trouble. I'll figure a way to control it. I'll just have one dose."
2. "I want to use drugs because I feel bad and deserve relief, and drugs bring relief, at least for a while."
3. "There's nothing else I can do. I can't stand life this way another minute. Treatment is no good. I've tried everything."

In treatment, clinician and patient both need to identify premonitory stages of relapse. Clinicians try to abort relapses at the warning stage before they become relapses to actual drug use.[12]

2.5. Helpful Approaches for the Clinician

Several attributes are needed for the clinician to work successfully with drug-dependent patients. These include the following: (1) a clear treatment philosophy and rationale; (2) capacity to understand the patient's discomfort, fear, denial, and impediments to recovery; (3) therapeutic optimism based on seeing patients recover; (4) support from colleagues with a shared value system and a shared sense of professional identity.

Once assessment is completed, a treatment plan is developed. The plan details the responsibilities of the patient, the family, the treatment team, and perhaps others. Alternatives must be listed in case the patient relapses or complications from treatment occur. Communication among team members is needed when more than one person is involved in implementing the treatment plan.

Primary health care resources can serve the patient during recovery. For example, the physician can provide a safe, drug-free environment in a clinic or hospital. Where specialized detoxification centers do not exist, patients can be detoxified in a general hospital unit, an emergency room, or an outpatient department. Patients with mental or emotional symptoms may be hospitalized on psychiatric units during the early recovery period.

Religious institutions can sometimes help. For example, a dependent person might move into a religious community that prohibits drug use. This can function like a halfway house.

Areas with limited formal resources often have rich informal ones. In many rural areas, although there are few physicians or institutional treatments for drug dependence, there are strong extended-family networks and intense regional pride. Such families and communities are often able to help patients with symptoms that would lead to rejection in other communities. Instead of using a halfway house, a newly abstinent patient might move in with a family that has a recovered drug-dependent member.

Formal drug-dependence treatment facilities offer many advantages. They are especially helpful for those with mental disorders, physical handicaps and disorders, family alienation, employment disability, or social deterioration.

Successful treatment often involves more than one therapeutic modality. Matching treatment approaches to specific needs and stages of illness is critical.

2.6. Phasing Therapeutic Priorities and Tasks

Conditions that are immediately life threatening (such as overdose, some withdrawal syndromes, or medical complications) are addressed first. Next follows treatment of nonemergency life-threatening conditions, such as the patient's leaving treatment or continuing to use drugs. After that the clinician pursues conditions which, though less dangerous, impede recovery. These conditions include denial of drug dependence or central nervous system impairment with inability to learn new behavior. Only later can one attend to grief work, psychological maturation, family reintegration, and social issues.

The therapeutic changes that must be made for most people to recover are as follows:

1. Establishment of an alliance with a therapist or therapeutic group.
2. Establishment of an environment of safety from easy drug availability.
3. Learning how to become drug free.
4. Learning alternatives to drug use.
5. Addressing the problems and conditions that ensue from stopping drug use.
6. Grieving about the losses incurred from the drug dependence.
7. Remodeling psychological patterns and social life-style.

If at any point in treatment the patient relapses, one must discontinue the more sophisticated forms of later recovery and return to the fundamental steps of early recovery.

3. Individual Treatment Approaches

3.1. Physician–Patient Relationship

Individual treatment for drug dependence serves an important function in the recovery process for many patients. Local cultural and value systems determine the style for such treatment.[5] Yet few patients move through all the recovery stages without individual help and guidance, though their own discomfort and energy provide the fuel for the process.

Individual treatment of drug dependence is based on a relationship between two people, one of them in distress as a result of drug dependence, the other trying to help the recovering person. They meet together with the goal of relieving the discomfort and problems caused by drug dependence. Abstention from drug use and repair of damage caused by drug use are the usual goals. The process is interpersonal. This technique rarely works with people who continue drug use. The reasons someone started using drugs are not the same as the reasons for continuing drug use.[13]

3.2. Behavior Therapy

This application of learning principles concentrates on the behavior itself and attempts to attack deviant behavior directly. It focuses primarily on current behavior patterns rather than on etiological dynamics from the past. Basic to this approach is the theory that all behavior is subject to psychological principles of learning. Since the emphasis is on behavior rather than underlying dynamics, these principles are not specific to a particular culture. They can be applied anywhere regardless of literacy, psychological sophistication, or indigenous value system. Each culture has its own definition of what is desirable behavior and what is deviant behavior.

Within the context of the behavioral approach, excessive drug use (regardless of how it is defined) is seen as a learned response which is acquired according to the same principles as any other response and which is shaped and maintained because of its rewarding consequences. The aim is to change behavior rather than necessarily to understand it.

Behavioral techniques have many similarities with other forms of therapy. These techniques are based on the relationship between physician and patient. They require acceptance by the patient, as well as suggestion, persuasion, and encouragement by the physician. In addition, behavioral techniques require a precise and detailed behavioral analysis of the immediate circumstances that relate to drug use, carefully graded training programs, and specific schedules of positive or negative reinforcement. The behavioral schedule must be discussed extensively with the patient. Behavioral modification programs are carried out as a joint venture between clinician and patient, rather than imposed on the patient.

While the principles underlying behavioral modification are largely psychological, the application may be somatic. These somatic forms are reviewed elsewhere. Here we describe only the psychological application of these techniques. These techniques include aversion therapies, one of which is verbal aversion or covert sensitization. Contingency contracting (also called contingency management or therapeutic contracting) is another behavioral technique which may or may not involve somatic treatment (such as disulfiram, naltrexone, or methadone).

3.2.1. Verbal Aversion (Covert Sensitization)

In covert sensitization, the noxious stimulus is aversive verbal imagery rather than somatic stimuli, such as electrical shock or emetic chemical agents. The patient is first taught self-relaxation and then is asked to visualize clearly drugs and scenes involving their use. As each scene is visualized, the patient is instructed in graphic and explicit terms to imagine step by step the onset of violent nausea and vomiting, so that the scenes involving drugs become strongly associated with nausea.

Practically, there seem to be advantages to using covert sensitization as a form of aversion therapy since it does not require elaborate equipment, is less painful than electrical aversion, and does not involve the possible serious consequences to health that may accompany chemical aversion techniques. Then too, patients are taught a technique that may be practiced and used outside the treatment situation and thus may be self-administered. However, the powerful visual imagery required and the necessary intensity of emotional response may be difficult for some patients to create at will. When covert sensitization is used as a treatment technique, repeated booster sessions should be included as part of the treatment program. This may be a more appropriate technique for patients who are highly motivated or are early into their drug problem. The latter group (i.e., motivated and early) may be more suitable for eventual return to controlled-usage goal (e.g., involving moderate use of licit substances) than a complete lifelong abstinence goal.[11]

3.2.2. Relaxation Training

Relaxation training is designed to relieve anxiety, particularly when associated with certain contexts. The training is often undertaken by giving graded exercises in which the patient is taught to relax his entire body and achieve a comfortable state. At this time the patient may be shown how to introduce the relaxed state into certain situations that have been fraught with anxiety. Since this approach will enable the patient to neutralize anxiety-provoking situations, it is often used in the treatment of phobic anxiety. These situations can act as cues which would otherwise precipitate drug use.

3.3. Contingency Contracting (Contingency Management, Therapeutic Contracting)

Contingency management procedures are based on the assumption that the consequences of any given behavior govern the probability of continuing or discontinuing that behavior. The first step is to identify the target behavior to be modified or eliminated. The second is to find effective reinforcers that are sufficiently powerful not only to modify that behavior, but also to diminish the value of the reinforcers that are maintaining that behavior. Essentially, this is a scientific reiteration of the simple principle that people act in such a way as to maximize the rewards and minimize either the punishments or loss of rewards in their lives.

Prior to entering treatment, drug-dependent persons have usually been subject to powerful contingencies associated with their drug-taking behavior. However, they typically do not link these outcomes with drugs. It is surprising how ineffective such serious consequences as marital breakdown, loss of job, social isolation, and even imprisonment can be in the modification of drug dependence. With contingency contracting, the consequences are linked in an explicit and direct way to the drug-taking behavior.

Treatment can include specific behavior training focused on the improvement of long-standing vocational, interpersonal, and family problems. Role playing, rehearsing behavior, and teaching patients to restructure perceptions, attitudes, and beliefs about the appropriateness of certain behavior are among the techniques used. Successful use of contingency management procedures can be developed into a community reinforcement program. Clinicians can contract with patients in setting specific goals, helping them to regain jobs or lost affiliations with family, and undertaking marital counseling or other means of improving family relationships. The patient finds that dealing more effectively with family, job, and friends is a rewarding experience. Then these new experiences can become reinforcers which can be incorporated into the contingency management program. During latter phases of treatment, return to home or job, access to treatment facilities, or other resources can be made contingent on sobriety.[6]

An early-warning system can be introduced. This system may consist of the patient, family, friends, and employers reporting to the clinician if drug use resumes. A neighborhood support person (e.g., clergy, visiting health worker, clan elder, local community leader) may provide continuing social support before and after professional care has stopped. To reduce the amount of professional time involved, small follow-up groups can be set up to include several patients and families. The health worker can then meet with these groups all at one time.

One method of behavioral contracting has required outpatient drug-dependent persons to deposit funds with a clinic. Patients are repaid in small installments when they attend the clinic.

Contingency contracting has even proven successful with chronic, debilitated drug dependents. Social services may be provided if the patient can demonstrate continued improvement. Urine, blood, or breathalyzer tests may be used to document decreasing drug dependence. If the tests indicate increasing drug dependence, the services can be withheld for a period of time (usually days or weeks). The rendering and withholding of services contingent on drug use is far more effective than supplying these services without making them contingent on drug behavior.[6]

Spouses, family members, and employers of drug-dependent persons rarely adhere to the contingencies as rigorously or consistently as they should for maximum therapeutic effectiveness. Contingencies are effective only when they are specifically articulated, based on mutual agreement between all parties (including the patient and the clinician), carefully observed, and rigorously carried out.

4. Family Treatments

4.1. Principles of Family Treatment

Family treatment must address both the drug-dependent behavior of the drug-dependent member, as well as the preceding (primary) or consequential (secondary) family operations. The first goal of family treatment is to achieve an interruption of the current drug-using pattern. When intoxicated, the family member may not attend family therapy sessions or may be unable to participate if present. Faced with acute drug episodes, family members are preoccupied with the acute crisis, do not engage in problem analysis, and cannot undertake change.

The family may be able to monitor detoxification under the physician's direction. The drug-dependent member should be included in family sessions, if possible, so that the family strategies for handling the drug-dependent member can be observed and corrected in the family session. Clinicians must avoid alliances with the family against the drug-dependent member, as well as alliances with the drug-dependent member against the family. The therapeutic task is to teach the family to neither rescue nor reject, but rather interact with and respond in adult terms to the realities of the situation. Therapists identify the dysfunctional interactions of the family members and attempt to guide the family members into more fruitful patterns through actual practice in the family therapy sessions. Psychodynamic motivations and underlying conflicts are not the first priority of family treatment. Rather the focus is placed on the immediate communications and behavioral interactions.

Clinicians should be aware of the tendency to take sides with different family members. Family members often split into a rescuing faction and a rejecting faction, thus leading to internal family conflict. Scapegoating the patient as the presumed cause for all family problems may occur. Therapists must identify for the family which problems are caused by the patient and which problems are inherent in the family system with its particular styles of operation.[14]

Cultural factors may affect family treatment. Especially in traditional societies accustomed to folk methods of problem solving, the young or single clinician may meet considerable resistance. This can be ameliorated if the family understands that an older person (who might appear occasionally during therapeutic sessions) is involved in or supervising the treatment.

4.2. Treating Particular Family Types

In most functional families with a drug-dependent member there is minimum overt conflict. These families usually manifest considerable denial of any member's drug dependence. Family education sessions are often helpful in such circumstances. Exploration of family roles and responsibilities can lead to identification and redefinition of role conflict, role ambiguity, and family rules. New family interactions and new methods of family rule setting may be accomplished. These families are psychologically defensive and maintain marginal homeostasis. They often resist psychodynamic treatment, which may make them uncomfortable and anxious. Educative and behaviorally oriented techniques may be acceptable. Adjunctive use of medication such as disulfiram can be useful.

In the treatment of the enmeshed family system the therapist usually addresses the problem of converting the family to a drug-free system. These families usually require much initial support, encouragement, and gentle guidance from the therapist because all family members are experiencing demoralization, failure, and hopelessness. The therapist needs to take an active role in defining and assigning family tasks and specifying new family role behaviors. Short-term contracts with the family to achieve some success in immediate yet modest family tasks is helpful in restoring family competency and family self-esteem. The next major step requires a refocusing of the family problems, so that the drug dependence does not remain the primary focus. The family has usually lost sight of the importance of other family functions—such as home maintenance, education, recreation, and religious worship—in their overconcern with the patient. The clinician must help reframe or redefine the problems of the family to include, but not be limited by, the drug-generated problems. The needs of other family members have typically been sacrificed and ignored. The therapist must help each family member reclaim his own needs, rights, and responsibilities. New boundaries for individual roles must be defined and reinforced in actual behavior in family sessions. The enmeshment of the family in the addictive behavior often leads to family withdrawal from other social relations. Therefore, the therapist should actively encourage reinvestment in neighborhood, work, recreation, and church activities. Participation in self-help groups for family members is usually helpful in this redirection of family linkages to the external world.

Disintegrated families cannot reconstitute during the early phases of treatment. Here treatment should begin with the individual patient. Drug-dependent individuals must face their responsibility for the family situation without inordinately blaming themselves. At the same time they must not be allowed to scapegoat their spouse, children, employer, relatives, or friends, as the reason for their social alienation. Often 2–3 months of drug-free life is necessary before cognitive and affective stability can be achieved so that these patients can begin to effectively reevaluate their family alienation. The treatment program must provide substitute support systems during this initial treatment phase. Potential ties to spouse, family, kin, and friends should be explored early in treatment, and staff should initiate contacts with them. There should be neither explicit nor implicit assumptions that such family ties will be fully reconstituted. When sobriety and personal stability have been achieved over several months, more substantive family exploration can be initiated to reestablish parental roles and family and kin relations, but still without full reconsititution. These exploratory family sessions can be used to discuss family relations or to reconcile the family. In either case, it is important for both the patient and the family system to renegotiate new roles and relationships on the basis of a new patient identity as a rehabilitated drug-dependent person. Some families may not wish to or cannot achieve reunion, but can achieve a healthy family separation. Family reunion will require new family relationships.

The problem in the absence of a family is not reconstitution of a family system, but rather creating viable social support systems as in a halfway house or other residential facility. Domiciliary care is often the only viable social system for patients who lack the psychological capacity to create and maintain any marital or family system of their own. Among some younger patients in this group, progressive resocialization, with the acquisition of independent vocational skills, may lead to psychological growth and social adaptation. Subsequently they may develop the ability and interest later to establish marriage and family along with a life-style of sobriety.

Cultural or religious rules sometimes dictate to family members behavior patterns different from those of the physician. For example, in certain African and Asian populations it would be unthinkable for a woman to express to a therapist her feelings about her husband while in his presence. However, she may readily express the feelings in his absence. Clinicians insisting on culture-alien expressive behavior may create confusion and serious interpersonal disturbance. In certain North American Indian tribes, it is considered improper for men to express their feelings in the presence of an outsider, especially a female, including a female clinician. Such behavior might be misconstrued by a culturally naive physician as a lack of motivation to improve family relations in therapy.

5. Group Treatment

5.1. Psychodrama, Social Skills Learning

Psychodrama or role playing has been useful in a variety of mental health settings. As applied to drug dependence, the patient usually role-plays a particular situation that may lead to drug craving or drug use. Later, during recovery, this approach may be used to learn new social behaviors (e.g., applying for a new job). A group of patients may be asked to create a certain interchange so as to allow them to better understand their fellow patients, others in their lives, and themselves. This approach may be helpful in the treatment of drug dependence because certain conflicts are difficult to address directly. Denial of illness, for example, may be removed when the patient observes a situation enacted in which a spouse expresses suffering over the drug problem. Empathy for authority figures who have been seen as enemies might be elicited when, for example, a physician's problems in managing a refractory patient are dramatized. The technique is particularly useful in a group context, but may also be used in individual or family exchanges.

5.2. Group Psychotherapy

Several patients (usually about 6 to 10) may meet with the clinician for one to one-and-a-half hours. Patients may be grouped by age (e.g., teenagers), gender (e.g., all men or all women), diagnosis (e.g., opioid-dependent patients who are also depressed), or treatment modality (e.g., patients on disulfiram).

Several therapeutic advantages occur with group treatment. Patients usually develop positive attachments not only to the therapist, but to other group members as well. They are often better able to understand the nature of their own problems by seeing them occur in others. Patients can learn from other patients about methods to maintain abstinence and to find alternatives to drug use. There may also be disadvantages. One uncooperative patient may retard the recovery of other patients. A sociopathic patient may manipulate other patients for personal reasons.

Group therapy differs with the skills of the therapist and the needs of the patients. Typically it involves several therapeutic elements, including the following:

1. Educating the patients regarding drug dependence.
2. Facilitating the patients' discussion of their drug dependence and their recovery.
3. Therapist support and mutual patient support for continued recovery.
4. Early identification of signs or behaviors that may signal recurrence of drug dependence (e.g., irritability, social withdrawal).
5. Identification of common problems during recovery (e.g., marital problems, depression).

6. Inpatient and Residential Treatment

6.1. Indications for Inpatient or Residential Care

The decision to admit the patient is generally made on the basis that treatment will be more effective in a hospital setting than in the patient's natural environment. This decision must be made on positive clinical grounds rather than merely as a routine procedure.

Admission may be necessary to effect drug withdrawal, particularly if severe dependence on alcohol or other sedative drugs carries the likelihood of developing a life-threatening abstinence syndrome. Admission may also be essential to enable a general assessment and sorting out of the complicated medical and social problems. Occasionally it may be helpful for stabilizing medication dosage (e.g., disulfiram, naltrexone, lithium, antidepressants, methadone, neuroleptics) in patients who have major psychopathology or inability to abstain from drugs.

Underlying psychiatric and physical problems may also require assessment and treatment. Infrequently, patients may need protection from committing violence either against themselves or against others. In some remote communities the lack of local follow-up care and difficulties in travel to the health centers may mean that stabilization and abstinence can only be achieved in a residential treatment setting. An exhausted, bewildered family ready to eject the patient may be the cause for hospital or residential admission. Patients likely to produce considerable risk to others if even mild drug dependence persists (e.g., airline pilots, physicians) may best be treated for a time in a residential setting to minimize the chances for relapse.

6.2. Hospital Units for Drug Dependence

Specialized drug hospital units have been developed, either as free-standing hospitals or as drug units in general or psychiatric hospitals. Their primary tasks involve acute medical care, careful assessment, early stabilization, and postdischarge planning. The daily schedule may also include health lectures, psychodrama or social skills learning, recreational time, exercise activities, and group discussions. Patient self-government may exist if the average stay is more than a few weeks. Individual and family counseling sessions may be available. Self-help meetings are often included. Alumni evening meetings, in which former patients visit, help to bridge the transition back to the home community.

6.3. Therapeutic Communities

Some drug-dependent persons are unable to cope in their home community, or have been extruded from their community, or require more social rehabilitation than can be accomplished in other treatment. For them, the therapeutic community provides

1. A supportive and protective asylum.
2. Time out from usual social responsibilities.
3. Promoting self-awareness, often by confrontation methods.
4. Training in more effective social coping skills.
5. Social reentry on a gradual basis.

Therapeutic communities are replacement communities for those who have lost or cannot participate in their home community. They do not simply offer individual treatment in a safe setting; rather the therapeutic social system is organized to provide treatment through its social processes.

6.3.1. Self-Help Houses

Self-help houses define drug dependence as a result of individual pathology which can be changed through self-help and reeducation in a highly organized community of recovering individuals. Within a rigid philosophical concept and a strict hierarchical structure, the newcomer progresses according to work, attitudes, and behavior. A variety of group techniques are also employed, including encounter, sensitivity, and social skills groups. Although the evaluation of such communities is not easy, it is apparent that those residents who complete the course and remain within the community for more than 6 months gain considerably and are more likely to remain abstinent than those who drop out within the first 2–3 months. In some communities the dropout rate may be as high as 80% within 3 months, so that it is not clear if it is the length of stay that improves prognosis, or if it is only the group with a better prognosis that can endure the course of rehabilitation. In an attempt to improve the retention rate some houses have modified their programs, introducing a less rigid structure with a wider range of individual and group activities.

6.3.2. Religion-Based Centers

The religion-based centers, like the concept houses, isolate the individual from the problems of daily life in the outside world. These centers exist in Buddhist temples, Islamic mosques, and Christian churches. Often based on evangelical or fundamentalist movements, religious conversion usually becomes part of the goal of rehabilitation. There are various centers with different therapeutic styles. Most centers offer work with the community, training opportunities, and some group counseling. Because of their contact with the church, they can offer ex-residents continued support within the community. Formal research into their effectiveness has not been conducted, but religion-based centers can achieve good results with uncomplicated cases when the recovering person adopts the expected religious life-style.

6.3.3. Community Houses

In contrast to the religious hostels and the concept houses, community houses do not separate drug users from the community, but rather try to integrate them into it from the beginning. Residents live in a community together with resident staff and others who are not drug dependent. The importance of drug taking within the community is thus minimized. A variety of therapeutic techniques may also be employed, including individual counseling and group therapy. These houses tend to be more selective in their admissions and have a higher retention rate than the other therapeutic communities. Their residents appear to have a greater motivation to remain drug free, and the rules of the house are less restrictive. As with other therapeutic communities, these houses operate a phased reintegration into the outside world. Some have halfway houses in which the recovering person works outside the house, but returns to the home in the evening.

6.4. Partial Care Residences

In halfway houses the drug-dependent person agrees to participate in a 3-to 6-month rehabilitation program. Residents are given work assignments in the care of the house management, with graded increases in responsibility. There are regular self-help meetings. Group discussions around realities of everyday living may be held. Family contacts may be initiated and vocational retraining may start. Residents begin to work and pay for their own board and room as they gradually make the change to independent living.

Three-quarter-way houses are domiciliary programs for recovering people who do not need the structure of a halfway house, but have no family, kin, or other social networks. These programs, often in old hotels, schools, or churches, provide some minimal social structure, a stable environment, and some friendship networks, while the recovering person is stabilizing an independent existence. Administrative management of the living environment remains in the hands of a program director.

Therapeutic lodges are communal group houses. The recovering inhabitants assume financial and management responsibility for the lodge. They share expenses and group administration and provide a stable living environment. For selected recovering persons this type of milieu is a useful learning and rehabilitation strategy.

Drug-free houses or apartments are more informal. A few to several recovering persons agree to live together in a setting that excludes drug use. They merely share expenses and are not involved in any formal therapeutic activities vis-à-vis one another.

6.5. Emergency Service Centers (Detoxification Stations)

Emergency service centers were originally conceived as alternatives to placing a public inebriate in jail. These centers often function as a triage where a patient may enter a network of treatment services. Staffed by nursing and social work personnel, such facilities offer temporary shelter and observation for a day or two. These centers may be coordinated with the legal system, although not necessarily so. They are less expensive and more humanitarian than jails.

Shelter houses often offer overnight food, bed, shower, laundry facilities, and a receptive social climate for the indigent, homeless, drug-dependent person. These shelters by themselves can facilitate continued drug dependence if the same indigents return time after time. They are humane social resources but may not be rehabilitative if evaluation and referral do not exist. Such shelter programs can be a useful adjunct to outpatient treatment programs which have outreach service for indigent addicts.

A variant of sheltering stations has been developed into nonmedical detoxification programs. Many drug-dependent persons do not need continuous medical supervision of detoxification. These facilities are an entry point for the acutely intoxicated or indigent person. They offer a week or two of shelter and social support, with subsequent referral to a longer-term treatment program. The staff offer initial reality orientation, assessment of the social needs of the addict, and a motivational push toward treatment. Some patients need to be referred for medical care.

The better centers have more highly trained staff. Staff members coordinate their activities with police departments, the legal system, and drug-treatment services. Centers help the patient attain a secure place and enter a relationship with treatment personnel.

7. Day, Evening, and Weekend Programs

Outpatient programs may provide aftercare following inpatient treatment, but can also function as a primary treatment center for patients who do not require inpatient care. Modalities range from ambulatory detoxification, to psychotherapy and behavior therapy, to pharmacotherapy. Depending on the diversity of services offered, clinic staff includes psychiatrists, psychologists, social workers, internists or general physicians, psychiatric nurses, and health visitors. Volunteers from self-help groups may also assist at these clinics.

Since new patients are evaluated by different members of the team, the initial assessment may take a few to several days. The diagnosis–evaluation may include blood or urine tests. Some clinics insist on daily attendance, with repeated urine testing, while others may require only one or two visits per week initially.

Diagnosis of drug dependence does not warrant taking the patient out of the family and community context, unless there are good reasons for doing so. These reasons include medical or psychiatric complications, suicide risk, threat of violence, lack of social supports, or inability to maintain abstinence or reduce drug intake. Even these criteria must be judged as to their appropriateness for the individual, since hospital admission may serve only to alleviate these problems temporarily.

8. Outpatient Follow-up Treatment

Outpatient follow-up consistently enhances patient outcomes. One program was able to achieve an unusually high abstinence rate (51%) among alcohol patients by having them return for booster sessions of the aversive conditioning procedures at 15, 30, 60, and 90 days posttreatment.[15] Outcome was enhanced in another program by continuing to give constructive directives to members of the client's community after discharge.[6] Supportive sessions with a widely dispersed patient group can be maintained through monthly telephone conference calls. Even written reminders or expressions of concern are helpful.

It seems to matter little whether or not follow-up is voluntary. In fact, coercive follow-up may enhance outcome especially in certain populations. The Tai Lam Prison Program, Hong Kong, admitted only convicted drug-dependent persons. Treatment of from 6 to 18 months, in lieu of sentencing, was limited to the 70% of applicants who were deemed optimal candidates and consisted of withdrawal, individual, and family counseling, work, and careful postdischarge planning and placement. Persons failing to cooperate in treatment were returned to prison. Failure to cooperate with postdischarge planning resulted in revocation of probation. At the end of 1 year's postdischarge supervision, 1355 of 2281 persons (59%) had no reconvictions, were gainfully employed, kept their aftercare appointments, and had negative urines. An additional 4% were reconvicted, but had drug-free urines. Considerable confidence can be placed in these figures since similar outcome rates were obtained for each of the years 1969 through 1976 based on the 9783 1-year follow-ups.[4] It can be argued either that probation amounted to an outpatient program, or that probation was artificially maintaining recoveries that would dissipate once probation expired. To address the second potential criticism, a 10% random sample of 452 inmates from the 1977 cohort was followed up 3 years later. Of these inmates, 179 (40%) had no subsequent convictions, were gainfully employed, and had been drug free for the 3 years. Similar findings for compulsory treatment in the United States have been reported.[16]

9. Religious Programs

In Egypt, treatment facilities have been set up in mosques, with emphasis on the role of the sheikh both as a religious leader and as a therapist. A social worker, psychiatrist, and clinical assistants consult the mosque and the patients. Efforts are made to facilitate community links by the use of mass media and by mass religious meetings in which the Imam (leading sheikh) makes special reference to drug dependence and its socioreligious implications, inviting drug-dependent persons to seek medical help and volunteer for treatment. Within the treatment programs provided at the mosque, the religious leader encourages and strengthens social ties among patients, giving advice and social support and holding group meetings. He also explains Islamic teaching on dependence-producing drugs.[1]

In Thailand, Buddhist temples have been used as residential facilities for the treatment of opiate dependence. Although treatment activities are led by a monk, there is also active involvement of former clients and volunteers. Prior to admission, clients are informed that they must abstain completely from dependent drugs, obey the monks, not engage in disruptive behavior, and remain within the temple compound during the entire 7–10 days of treatment. Clients are not admitted unless they are willing to comply with these rules. Religious sessions are conducted by the monks. After the first 5 days, clients are encouraged to help in the daily chores or assist in the treatment sessions for newcomers. On the last day of admission the group is assembled in the shrine, reminded of its pledge, and then is free to leave. Clients who wish to stay on can volunteer to assist in the various activities. Those clients who wish to live as monks for a time must stay in the temple for a longer period to demonstrate their motivation. Between 1963 and 1983, more than 50,000 opiate-dependent persons entered the treatment program.[9]

Numerous Christian groups also provide programs for drug-dependent persons in Europe, North America, and Asia.[3]

10. Self-Help Groups

Over the past 3 centuries, there have been abstemious and teetotaler societies that both promoted avoidance of all drug use and served as rehabilitative societies. These groups have appeared in many countries of the Americas, Asia, and Europe. These self-help groups provide a syncretistic blend of local religion, custom, and culture.[8] Certain groups such as Alcoholics Anonymous (AA) and Narcotics Anonymous (NA) have chapters and meetings all over the world. Where available, AA and NA are an invaluable resource which can provide recovering people as examples and teachers of techniques of recovery. They also offer structure, meetings, sponsors for new members, an abstinence-oriented subculture, and a supportive philosophy. The group decreases shame and isolation and offers mutual assistance. Alcoholics Anonymous has not been very successful among some peoples, until it has been restructured into a culture-congenial therapeutic movement, as among certain North American Indian populations.[8]

Several countries have self-help systems that consist of people recovering from drug dependence helping one another stay drug free. In the U.S.S.R., Anonymous Societies are run by the government, though they are not integrated with inpatient treatment. In Japan there is an extensive network of successful Sobriety Clubs. Yugoslavia has a long history of Alcoholism Clubs in factories; these clubs have also been transplanted to Italy and Germany.

The concept of mutual help or self-help is observed throughout the world in the informal social structure of face-to-face community life. From agrarian villages to urban communities, there are recognized helpers, elders, or senior wise persons, who have informal social sanction to convene family, village, or community members. There are also somewhat loosely organized, but effective social networks that respond to the drug-dependent person experiencing difficulty in community life. Self-identified networks of drug-dependent persons who gather to drink, smoke, or consume drugs together may be more prominent in communal society life than a group of recovering addicts.[7]

Self-help movements have emerged in many urban and industrialized societies as social structure has changed from face-to-face small communal social units to faceless, anonymous, achievement-oriented, impersonal, large urban societal structures. Whereas health care is individual and personal in the communal society, in urban society health care can become a production line of impersonal encounters. Such institutionalized, bureaucratized health care is effective in acute illness, but it may be less relevant to chronic illness that involves psychosocial adaptation. Chronic illness is the typical target for self-help, whether it be for colostomy care, amputees, paraplegics, rape victims, cancer patients, or drug-dependent persons.

The psychological and social dynamics of self-help groups are generally the same, although the specific target illness and accompanying ideology differ. Self-help groups restore a viable social identity and social acceptance to persons with a negative social identity, whether that identity has been undermined by cancer, surgical mutilation, or drug dependence. There is shared group support and group acceptance of the person, with group guidance toward better adaptation and reorganization of a new life. One learns to live life anew with a handicap, but with dignity. Self-help groups follow a general philosophy as follows:

1. We must help ourselves.
2. We have found a pattern or method to help ourselves.
3. We can achieve success in life and overcome our problems through following our method.

This philosophy is important in the relationship between health professionals and self-help groups. There is an inherent antiprofessional bias in the social ethos of many self-help groups. The success of self-help groups is not measured by empirical scientific generalization, but by personal idiosyncratic experience. With the self-help ideology, failure is defined outside the self-help system as the failure of the individual. The professional health care system and the self-help system are based on different conceptual and operating assumptions. They need not be competing systems; they can be complementary. Where mutual understanding exists, these two systems can even collaborate. The Hong Kong and Yugoslavian groups comprise excellent examples of such collaboration.

Few patients enter self-help groups eagerly. Common resistances include statements like:

1. "I'm not that bad." The superiority masks a fear of worthlessness. One can suggest to the patient that treatment works even better when started early.

2. "It doesn't work." The patient is usually in despair about his own recovery. You might respond by pointing out examples of successful rehabilitation.
3. "I went to an alcoholics meeting and it was all young drug addicts. I was scared." Meetings are diverse. Suggest that the patient visit different groups to find a congenial one.
4. "I hate it." Sometimes the patient should be told to put up with it for six to eight visits. "I know, but you need it. Many people do not like the group at first. I think you should go and decide after eight sessions."

Clinicians can negotiate with a patient who is refusing to go as follows: If you end up taking drugs, let us agree that you will attend four meetings a week. If you still take drugs, let us agree that you will attend daily meetings. And if that isn't enough, we'll put you back in the hospital.

Even where no organization of recovering drug-dependent persons exists, former patients, people who have been drug dependent and figured out how to recover, are a major resource. They can be found in one's own practice, or by posting notices or advertising, asking for their help with patients. A recovering drug-dependent physician can often help by identifying resources.

Available research suggests that about 35% of those who try the AA program achieve sobriety, although we have little evidence of the impact of AA on other aspects of life adjustment. Successful AA affiliators tend more than non-successful affiliators to be more compulsive in life-style, to be socially gregarious and socially affiliative, to come from stable middle- and upper-class family backgrounds, and to have a history of successful life achievements.

Certain liabilities may stem from self-help groups, especially for the family. These groups usually exclude family members from their sessions. Time away from family is necessary to attend the meetings. Families often complain that their needs are being ignored. This can be remedied by family counseling and family self-help groups (e.g., Alanon).

It is important that clinicians establish some personal linkage with local self-help resources, if successful referral is to occur. Personal contact with a sponsor who will meet and introduce a prospective member to a local group is initially important. Casual referral to self-help groups usually results in the patient's failure to initiate contact. Specialized self-help groups of doctors, dentists, lawyers, or other occupational groups have been an important strategy. Ethnic self-help groups which are socioculturally compatible are often salutary.[7]

If self-help groups are not available locally, clinicians should consider helping to establish them. Two members are all that is necessary to start a group. Members from nearby groups are usually eager to help.

Self-help groups for the spouses (e.g., Alanon) and the children (e.g., Alateen) of drug-dependent persons have derived from self-help groups described here. These programs began in the late 1940s, but have only spread widely in the last two decades. A major impetus for the growth of self-help groups was the research on social systems in the 1950s. Such groups directly address drug dependence as a family-system problem.

Family groups follow a meeting format similar to self-help meetings, but with a focus on the needs of the non-drug-dependent family members. They provide education, information, behavioral guidance, and emotional support. Major emphasis is given to separation of their problems as family members from the problems of the drug-dependent member. These groups achieve many of the family therapy goals: i.e., role clarification; behavioral role reformulation; and reduction of scapegoating, rescuing, and rejecting of the drug-dependent member.

Referral to these programs is valuable for spouses and children, even though it may not directly influence the dependent family member. Participation in these programs is also a useful adjunct to family therapy. Referral is more successful when a sponsor can bridge the gap between the health professional system and these self-help systems.

11. Multimodality Approach

With the growing realization of the complexities of drug dependence and the recognition that no single modality is going to provide a magical cure, multimodal treatment programs have been developed. These programs include a variety of therapeutic techniques designed to change personal and interpersonal behavior as well as drug use, and to treat associated medical and psychiatric disorders. The community reinforcement program described earlier is one example of this approach. Other concomitant approaches have included the following: aversion therapy; videotape sessions of psychodrama or social skills learning; education sessions to teach basic facts about drug consumption and effects; relaxation training; and various pharmacotherapies and other somatic treatment. Some programs have also included a form of contingency contracting that requires outpatients to pay all treatment fees in advance. This fee may include a sum that can be earned back if the patient adheres to treatment instructions and attends all treatment sessions.[2]

12. Making an Effective Referral

With the help of the spouse and family, if available, and with self-help groups and other community resources, physicians can treat many patients without referral to specialized drug-dependence treatment. Those drug dependents who have had episodes of psychotic reactions should be referred for psychiatric management. Patients with recurrent major depressions despite abstinence should also be referred for psychiatric consultation and possible antidepressant drug management. It is not unusual to see many psychological problems and interpersonal difficulties which occur during the stages of drug dependence gradually resolve as the duration of abstinence from drugs increases. As previously noted, many of the psychological problems associated with drug dependence are consequences of a drug-centered life-style. One important objective during the early interview process is for the clinician to evaluate whether or not the psychological problems preceded the drug dependence or were a consequence of the life-style of drug dependence. This difficult task may require several months during the recovery process.

Specialized rehabilitation programs can be of additional help by immersing the patient in a program concerned with drug dependence and associated problems. These programs are particularly useful to patients who have become unemployed or disabled as a result of drugs. The very depressed patient and the patient who has recently undergone a severe loss, such as loss of job or family, can also profit from such a program which helps the patient to stop and reexamine current life-style and future goals.

Most drug-dependent patients do not like to view themselves as alcoholic or drug dependent. Treatment by the local or family physician may be more acceptable, particularly in the beginning phase of the problem. A too rapid referral of the patient to specialized treatment facilities or to a psychiatrist may only result in termination of the relationship with the physician who is just starting to make progress with the drug-dependence problem.

A key to successful referral lies in communicating to the patient that the physician plans to continue care for the patient into the future. If the patient perceives referral as a rejection by the physician, the referral will probably not be implemented. The patient should be invited to return if the referral is not successful, or following treatment at the referral resource. It also is helpful if the patient understands the reasons for the referral, has some expectations of what will take place at the referral resource, and is sent to a specific person at the referral resource.

References

1. Baasher TA, Abu-el-Azayem GM: The role of the mosque in treatment, in Edwards G, Arif A: *Drug Problems in the Sociocultural Context*. Geneva, WHO, 1980.
2. Chapman RF, Smith JW, Layden LA: Elimination of cigarette smoking by punishment and self-management training. *Behav Res Ther* 1971; 9:255–264.
3. Desmond DP, Maddux JF: Religious programs and careers of opioid users. *Am J Drug Alcohol Abuse* 1981; 8:71–83.
4. Gardner TGP: Rehabilitation of drug addicts in a correctional setting. *Br J Addict* 1978; 73:205–213.
5. Heath DB, Waddell JO, Topper MD (eds): Cultural factors in alcohol research and treatment of drinking problems. *J Stud Alcoholism* 1981; suppl 9:1–256.

6. Hunt GM, Azrin NH: A community-reenforcement approach to alcoholism. *Behav Res Ther* 1973; 11:91–104.
7. Jilek WG: Native renaissance: The survival and revival of indigenous therapeutic ceremonials among North American Indians. *Transcultural Psychiatr Res Rev* 1978; 15:117–147.
8. Jilek-Aall L: Alcohol and the Indian–white relationship: A study of the function of Alcoholics Anonymous among Coast Salish Indians. *Confin Psychiatr* 1978; 21:195–233.
9. Jilek-Aall L, Jilek WG: Buddhist Temple treatment of narcotic addiction and neurotic-psychosomatic disorders in Thailand, in Pichot P, Berner P, Wolf R, Thau K (eds): *Psychiatry, the State of the Art* (Proceedings of the VII World Congress of Psychiatry (1983), Vienna, Austria.) New York, Plenum, 1985, vol 8.
10. Lazarus AA: Towards the understanding and effective treatment of alcoholism. *S Afr Med J* 1965; 39:736–741.
11. Lovibond SH, Caddy G: Discriminated aversive control in the moderation of alcoholics' drinking. *Behav Ther* 1970; 1:437–444.
12. O'Brien JS, Raynes AE, Patch VD: Treatment of heroin addiction with aversion therapy. *Behav Res Ther* 1972; 10:77–79.
13. Soueif MI: Hashish consumption in Egypt: With special reference to psychosocial aspects. *Bull Narcotics* 1967; 19/2:1–12.
14. Steinglass P: Experimenting with family treatment approaches to alcoholism, 1950–1975: A review. *Family Process* 1976; 15:97–123.
15. Stoljikovic S: Conditioned aversion treatment of alcoholics. *Q J Stud Alcohol* 1969; 30:900–904.
16. Vaillant GE: A 20-year follow-up of New York narcotic addicts. *Arch Gen Psychiatry* 1973; 29:237–241.

Further Reading

World Health Organization: *Drug Dependence and Alcohol-Related Problems: A Manual for Community Health Workers with Guidelines for Trainers*. Geneva, WHO, 1986.

12

Pharmacotherapy

1. Introduction

Several treatment modalities for drug dependence require the participation of a physician and other medical personnel. These modalities include pharmacotherapies and other techniques such as electroacupuncture. These treatments must be prescribed by medical practitioners and monitored by well-trained health personnel, including physicians, nurses, pharmacists, and other health care workers who may collaborate in their administration and regular reassessment. These medical treatment methods are rarely used alone, but are ordinarily accompanied by a psychosocial management plan, using approaches described in Chapter 11.

2. Principles in the Pharmacotherapy of Drug Dependence

Several pharmaceutical agents may be efficacious in the treatment of drug dependence. These include tricyclic antidepressants, narcotic-substitution therapy, narcotic-blocking agents, and disulfiram. Prescribing drugs to treat drug dependence requires certain precautions and special procedures.

The use of chemotherapeutic agents should be carried out with attention to the relationship between the drug-dependent patient and the physician. Prescribing drugs without establishment of a physician–patient relationship represents an unprofessional form of medical care. Pharmacotherapy should be carried out by practitioners who know the therapeutic value of establishing rapport and maintaining regular communication with the patient.

The physician must be aware of the risks that can complicate pharmacotherapies and other somatic therapies. These include drug diversion, childhood overdose (if the patient's child should accidentally take the drug), cost efficacy aspects, types of patients who do or do not benefit, and the distinction between acute and maintenance treatments. Complications of medical treatments and their management should be well known.

The clinician needs to work with the patient to develop a somatotherapy treatment plan that reflects the patient's wishes combined with clinical realities. For example, early in the induction phase of opioid substitution therapy, a patient may request change in the dose. The clinician must make a judgment about the need for a change in dose and should discuss the symptoms that the patient hopes will be reduced or eliminated. If insomnia or autonomic symptoms are prominent (e.g., sweating, tachycardia, hypermotility of the gastrointestinal tract), some patients will medicate themselves with nonprescribed drugs. A change of medication may prevent this. If the clinician initially prescribes an excessively high dose, this may produce severe side effects which discourage compliance.[22]

3. Opioid Maintenance (Substitution Therapy)

How long is the duration of withdrawal treatment versus the duration of maintenance treatment? There is no widely accepted time limit to distinguish between withdrawal and maintenance treatment. Regimens under 1 month are universally considered to be withdrawal in nature rather than maintenance. Some clinicians consider 2 or 3 months on opioids to be time-limited maintenance, while others would consider 1 year on declining doses of opioids to be gradual withdrawal treatment. Several months on stable opioid doses, with no definitive date for discontinuation, is generally considered as maintenance treatment.

3.1. Methadone and Opium Maintenance

Substitution of a legally dispensed opiate is a treatment method with a long history. In the nineteenth century, Thailand instituted a legal opium distribution system. At the turn of the century, the Spanish government in the Philippines created a legal opium distribution system which the government of the United States operated for a time after assuming political control in the Philippines. Morphine was distributed to addicts in maintenance clinics in the United States from 1918 to 1924. English physicians were able to dispense whatever opioid they felt indicated to opiate-dependent persons until 1964, when the government sharply reduced the number of physicians who could so treat opiate-dependent patients.[13,15] Opium maintenance has been used in the twentieth century in several countries of South, Southeast, and East Asia.

Experimentation with methadone as a narcotic substitute was carried out initially in 1964.[4,5] Methadone was selected because it is effective orally and is long acting. Once methadone maintenance has been established over several days, one dose will then suppress the abstinence syndrome for 24 hr or more. Methadone maintenance has been instituted in Australia, Canada, Holland, Hong Kong, Italy, Sweden, Switzerland, the United Kingdom, and the United States.[1,3,7–9,16,20]

Over 200,000 opioid-dependent persons in the United States have received methadone maintenance. It has led to reduced crime rates in areas with widespread opioid dependence. For many addicts social and psychological functioning improves as use of illicit opiates substantially decreases. The health status of most addicts in multimodality treatment (of which methadone is a part) improves also.[14] There is the danger that low-cost methadone maintenance may lead to decreased expeditures on nonmethadone treatment alternatives for opioid-dependent patients.

An initial methadone dose of 10–40 mg is administered, depending on clinical estimates of the severity of the dependence. A patient who is using potent heroin or equipotent doses of other opiates five or six times a day, either by injection or by nasal insufflation (snorting) for many weeks, might require an initial daily dose of 40 mg or more of methadone. A patient who injects only once or twice a day and uses poor-quality heroin might receive an initial dose of 10–20 mg. The clinical principle is to determine the dose level by observing the effects of the initial methadone dose on the objective and subjective aspects of the opioid withdrawal syndrome.[22] Twice-daily dosage may be needed for several days to stem withdrawal symptoms, until stable blood levels can be achieved.

Side effects of methadone maintenance include sedation, sweating, constipation, decreased libido, and, occasionally in females, ankle edema. These side effects are usually due to mild overdose and disappear with dose reduction. Such problems can usually be avoided by starting with 20–30 mg daily dosage and gradually increasing the dose over 2 or 3 weeks to a stable level. Constipation can be ameliorated by increasing fluid intake and eating more fruits and vegetables. Most side effects usually disappear after weeks or months without any treatment; it is important to tell patients that this is the case. Some constipation and perspiration may persist even at therapeutic levels. Sedation, analgesic effects, and intoxication disappear within a few days to a few weeks.[12]

Patients in maintenance treatment should be seen weekly until stable, and then at gradually decreasing frequency, with ultimate visits every 1–3 months. One common early complaint is that the methadone effect wears off before the 24-hr period between doses elapses. This complaint usually disappears once the blood levels have reached a plateau after a week or two on a stable dosage. If patients continue to take the methadone and do not alter their degree of dependence by taking additional opioids, their methadone usually will be sufficient to keep them free of withdrawal symptoms for the entire 24 hr. If the patient continues to complain of withdrawal symptoms, it can be helpful to examine the patient for withdrawal signs at 6 and at 24 hr after taking a dose. Autonomic signs of withdrawal at 24 hr may confirm the presence of withdrawal. Repeatedly positive autonomic signs over a few days on a fixed dose suggest that an increase in dose is indicated.

During maintenance therapy psychiatric syndromes, alcohol dependence, or dependence on other drugs (such as cocaine or benzodiazepines) may appear. These are treated in the usual fashion, using the same approaches as if the patient were not on opioid-substitution therapy. Disulfiram, neuroleptics, or antidepressants can be given to methadone-maintenance patients if needed to treat the associated condition.[12]

Opioid-substitution therapy is usually associated with an improvement in the health of the patient. Oral methadone and opium maintenance appear to be benign. Some addicts have taken these drugs daily under medical supervision for more than a decade without complications.[6,10–12]

3.2. Withdrawing the Patient from Maintenance

During periodic medical monitoring the question of withdrawal from methadone should be discussed. Many patients, while grateful for months or even years of improved living made possible by the maintenance regimen, will not want to visit the clinic indefinitely and take any medication regularly. If a patient wants to be withdrawn, the withdrawal should be done at a time when other stresses are at a minimum. The technique of withdrawal should be decided in consultation with the patient. The patient may elect to control the withdrawal or agree to let the doctor control the withdrawal. The withdrawal may be conducted on a blind or open basis. In blind withdrawal, the patient agrees to a regimen in which reductions in dose are made without his or her knowledge. Some patients are fearful about withdrawal, while recognizing that their fear is as much a problem as the actual withdrawal. A blind regimen is indicated in such instances. In open withdrawal, the patient knows the withdrawal dosages. This may be indicated for patients who have a need for control or have difficulty trusting the physician's judgment.

For optimal results, the withdrawal regimen should take many weeks to many months. If the initial dose level is high, the withdrawal period should be longer. A patient stabilized on maintenance opioids (e.g., taking the same dose of methadone or opium for at least 1 month) or on 20 mg of methadone a day (or equipotent doses of any other opioid) should probably take at least 10 weeks to reach zero dose.[21,22]

Once a patient is drug free, further treatment should consist of regular supportive visits, possibly with urine tests for drugs. Patients should be taught that increases or changes in their symptoms persist for many months following the achievement of abstinence and that continued supportive visits (including family members, if possible) are necessary to prevent relapse.[2,11]

Some patients attempting to withdraw from chronic maintenance treatment will not be successful. Indefinite maintenance may be necessary for such patients if they cannot achieve abstinence despite repeated attempts.

Oral opium maintenance has also been successfully used in countries that produce opium (e.g., Burma, Iran). Its long duration of action permits one or two doses per day. Like oral methadone, stable oral opium administration results in fairly stable blood levels with little intoxication or withdrawal.

3.3. Weak Opioid Drugs

Maintenance treatment with weak opioids such as codeine, diphenoxylate HCl, propoxyphene HCl, or propoxyphene napsylate has been attempted. Results have been variable. Weak opioids have proven less effective among young, male, urban, marginally cooperative patients with lengthy dependence or severe craving. On the contrary, many clinicians have found weak opioids effective when used among older or more cooperative patients, particularly if their dependence history is mild or recent, or if craving is absent or mild.

Propoxyphene napsylate has a longer duration of action than propoxyphene HCl. Both drugs generally cost more than codeine. Most clinicians have utilized a twice-a-day dose schedule with the total daily dose not exceeding 1000–1500 mg of propoxyphene or 100–300 mg of codeine. Doses above these levels for propoxyphene are associated with the production of dysphoria and LSD-like effects of an unpleasant nature or, rarely, convulsions.[29]

4. Naltrexone Therapy

A pure opioid antagonist without any agonist effects, naltrexone occupies the opioid receptors in the central nervous system. Consequently, an addict taking ordinary doses of an opioid drug does not experience the desired drug effect. This absence of desired effect causes the drug-taking behavior to be extinguished so long as the person takes naltrexone regularly. Extremely high doses of opioids are required to overcome the naltrexone blockade, with the result that greater-than-usual doses have only limited effects.[18]

Initiating naltrexone maintenance requires that the patient be opioid free. If opioid drugs remain in the system, naltrexone will precipitate an abstinence syndrome which may last a few to several days if long-acting opioids (e.g., methadone, opium) are present in high amounts. Heroin addicts should be drug free for at least 24 hr; methadone or opium addicts should be drug free for longer. A useful procedure consists of administering a naloxone challenge intravenously before naltrexone is started. If an abstinence syndrome is then precipitated, it lasts only a few hours due to the shorter action of naloxone as compared to naltrexone.

Naltrexone can be administered in once-daily dosages. Since naltrexone administration is often supervised, every-other-day dosage has also been used successfully. Supervised administration is usually combined with contingency contracting for a specific purpose (e.g., continued employment, continued residence with family).

Side effects tend to be few. Gastrointestinal side effects occur in a small percentage of patients. Rarely, psychiatric symptoms may ensue in vulnerable individuals, or at high doses. Close monitoring by a physician is needed early in naltrexone therapy, followed by gradually increasing intervals between visits. Naltrexone maintenance is usually employed for at least 1 or 2 years, or longer, until a stable psychosocial recovery has been established.

5. Disulfiram Therapy

Alcohol is converted in the liver to acetaldehyde, which is converted to acetate and then to carbon dioxide and water. Disulfiram blocks the latter step and causes an elevation of blood acetaldehyde levels. These high acetaldehyde levels produce hypotension, sometimes hypertension, severe dysphoria, flushing, headache, nausea, and vomiting. The patient should be free of alcohol for 24 hr before starting disulfiram therapy. If the disulfiram-treated patient drinks any alcohol, or even uses aftershave lotion or a mouthwash with alcohol in it, an alcohol–disulfiram reaction may be precipitated.

Treatment of the alcohol–disulfiram reaction consists of intravenous antihistamines and careful monitoring of vital signs for 24–48 hr. Depending on the nature and severity of the symptoms, further treatment may be necessary for cardiopulmonary symptoms (e.g., oxygen, intravenous fluids, hypotensive or hypertensive agents). While there are virtually no absolute contraindications for disulfiram, it should be administered only in extraordinary situations if the patient has chronic heart or pulmonary disease, hypertension, pregnancy, or a history of stroke. Such extraordinary circumstances include the failure of disulfiram-free outpatient treatment or life-threatening alcoholism problems (e.g., hepatic cirrhosis, esophageal varices, suicide attempts, risk-taking behaviors, family violence). Infrequently a patient may drink through the disulfiram by rapidly taking a large alcohol dose such that alcohol-induced analgesia covers the adversive effects of the alcohol–disulfiram reaction.

The usual disulfiram loading dose is 500 mg/day for 1–5 days followed by 250 mg/day. Infrequently a loading dose of 1000 mg/day and maintenance of 500 mg/day are necessary for patients with a weak alcohol–disulfiram reaction. Loading doses of only 250 or 125 mg may be adequate for small or elderly patients with proportionately lower maintenance doses. Parenteral disulfiram implants have been tried, but frequently result in inflammation, incision breakdown, or implant rejection. Side effects of disulfiram consist of ataxia, rash, sedation, and headache. Occasionally patients taking disulfiram can become confused or psychotic. Confusion and psychosis are most likely to occur if the patient has an underlying psychiatric condition, is taking psychotropic medication (especially neuroleptics or anticonvulsant medication), has a concurrent organic brain syndrome, or has a viremia (as with influenza). Mild side effects can usually be ameliorated with dose reduction while severe side effects may require cessation of the drug. These side effects are reversible.

Disulfiram is given not as punishment for drinking nor as aversive conditioning, but to prevent drinking, since the patient on disulfiram knows that drinking will produce sickness. Given alone, disulfiram is not adequate treatment for alcohol dependence. However, used in conjunction with other approaches (such as regular supportive visits, self-help groups, marital therapy), disulfiram can be helpful. There is no clinical advantage in producing an alcohol–disulfiram reaction as an adversive procedure. Even though a patient may have been abstinent for some time, disulfiram may be given briefly to help the patient through a period of craving or a crisis during recovery. It may also be used as a part of contingency contracting (to be discussed in the next chapter). For example, disulfiram can be administered by a spouse, work supervisor, or probation officer. When a patient stops the drug without discussion, it may warn of impending relapse.

6. Nicotine Maintenance (Substitution Therapy)

Recently nicotine chewing gum and other preparations have been developed for tobacco-dependent persons. These compounds ameliorate the mild tobacco withdrawal syndrome, but have also been used as maintenance drugs. Nicotine-containing compounds have the advantage of avoiding the chronic inhalation of carcinogens into the lungs. Their long-term effects on the cardiovascular system have not yet been assessed.

Tobacco chewing has also been suggested for tobacco-dependent smokers, but there is a risk for developing oral cancers. Some cigarette smokers are told to switch to pipe or cigar smoking, but tobacco-dependent cigarette smokers also inhale the smoke from these other tobacco forms.

7. Tricyclic Antidepressant Therapy

Tricyclic medications have been used to relieve dysphoric symptoms in alcohol-dependent and opioid-dependent patients, at least during the early months of recovery. Several problems attend the routine application of this treatment, however. Some patients do not like the side effects (e.g., dry mouth, constipation) and so discontinue it. Others return to the intoxicating effects of alcohol, opioids, or other drugs. A few patients may combine the tricyclic medication (especially those with more sedating side effects, such as amitriptyline) with drugs of abuse.

These drugs are also relatively expensive and may need to be taken for many months or years. This can be a serious burden for the patient or society. Tricyclics may cause serious side effects, such as sudden death (especially in patients with conduction abnormalities on electrocardiogram). While such cases are rare, a cautious physician would not want to expose patients needlessly to such risks. At this time it is not known which patients are more likely to recover with tricyclics than without them, although it appears that severely depressed patients or those with recurrent panic attacks may be most likely to benefit.

Tricyclics have also been used in the treatment of stimulant abusers (e.g., amphetamine, cocaine). Again, it seems that depressed patients receive the most benefit.

8. Electroacupuncture

Electroacupuncture has been tried in several clinical settings for acute withdrawal as well as maintenance. Its successful use for some acute opioid and sedative withdrawal symptoms has been reported from Hong Kong,[26] Pakistan,[24] and Australia.[19] Electroacupuncture has also been used for alcohol and tobacco dependence.[17]

Clinicians in Thailand discontinued electroacupuncture after extensive experience, in part because it is too time consuming.[25] It was also abandoned for acute withdrawal in Laos, since it did not relieve the symptoms of those in severe withdrawal for more than a brief time and required considerable staff time.[27] Investigators in Hawaii attempted to detoxify eight opiate addicts with electroacupuncture.[23] Of these eight, two had to be switched to a methadone withdrawal regimen and one left before being detoxified. The remaining five who completed acupuncture detoxification were interviewed 1 month posttreatment. Three had resumed opiate abuse, one had returned to nonopiate drugs, and one was lost to follow-up. An aftercare acupuncture clinic was established in Hong Kong to treat addicts in the months following their return to abstinence. The project was dropped because it was no more effective than supportive visits and other modalities which required less staff time and were much less expensive.

Whitehead[28] in Canada has prepared an excellent review article on acupuncture in the treatment of addiction. He cites signs of *fervor therapeuticus* in the literature on this subject, such as 100% recovery rate, permanent cures, and literally thousands of patients reported to have been carefully studied. At this time, electroacupuncture appears to have limited usefulness in selected cases, or as one approach in a multimodality treatment program.

9. Aversion Therapies

9.1. Electrical Aversion

In this form of treatment, a conditioned stimulus, such as a drug, is presented with an unconditioned stimulus, such as electric shock, until a conditioned response, pain, nausea, or anxiety, follows when the conditioned stimulus is presented alone. This procedure is based in the psychological principles of learning, but requires medical or psychiatric supervision in most settings where applied.

There have been several clinical trials using electric shock as the unconditioned or noxious stimulus. Patients are presented with slides or pictures of drug paraphernalia, cigarettes, or alcoholic beverages, or the actual drugs, tobacco, or alcohol, and asked to smell and taste them. Electric shock is administered during the tasting and smelling on the premise that the subsequent smelling or tasting of the drug will become associated with the pain. Other experimenters have used slightly different procedures where the patient is asked to take the drug, but can terminate the shock if he spits it out or in other cases can avoid shock altogether by not taking it.

Electrical aversion therapy originally seemed a reasonable procedure on theoretical grounds. Also, it was technically superior to other forms of aversion therapy. It enabled greater precision in the control of the subjective pain threshold of the patient, and the time between the administration of the drug (usually alcohol) and the subsequent shock could be well controlled. While the superiority could not be demonstrated in the clinical trials using these procedures, some patients who had undergone this form of treatment reported changes in their perception of their problem and their willingness to stop drinking. However, if these cognitive changes are produced in some patients by the use of electrical aversion, it might be better to develop strategies for eliciting these changes in ways other than subjecting patients to the kind of pain and distress inherent in electrical aversion procedures.

Treatment efficacy of electrical aversion has not yet been demonstrated in controlled studies. Ethical objections have also been voiced, especially when patients have been forced to enter or seek treatment. Thus, electrical aversion has been largely discarded as a treatment for drug dependence.

Self-administered pain has been recommended as a means to interrupt craving. However, this procedure has not been scientifically evaluated.

9.2. Chemical Aversion

Chemical agents have also been used as the noxious stimulus in the aversive control of excessive alcohol drinking and tobacco smoking. In contrast to electrical aversion, these drugs present particular problems when applied in the treatment situation.

Emetine, apomorphine, and syrup of ipecac as aversive stimuli are much more difficult to control than electrical shock. Just prior to the expected onset of nausea and vomiting, various forms of alcohol are smelled and tasted by the patients. In order to develop a preference for other beverages, the patients are also given large quantities of nonalcoholic beverages between treatment sessions. However, there is difficulty in controlling the timing between the administration of the drug and the onset of the nausea. Other problems include considerable distress to patients undergoing this form of treatment and undesirable side effects such as cardiac arrest and myocardial failure. These same objections obtain for the use of disulfiram for conditioned aversion to alcohol.

References

1. Craddock SG, Hubbard RL, Bray RM, Cavanaugh ER, Rachal JV: *Summary and Implications: Client Characteristics, Behaviors and Intreatment Outcomes 1980 TOPS Admission Cohort.* Research Triangle Park, NC, Research Triangle Institute, May 1982.
2. Cushman P: Detoxification after methadone maintenance, in Lowinson JH, Ruiz P (eds): *Substance Abuse: Clinical Problems and Perspectives.* Baltimore, Williams & Wilkins, 1981.
3. Dalton MS, Duncan DW: 50 opiate addicts treated with methadone blockade: 8-year follow up. *Med J Aust* 1979; 1(5):153–154.
4. Dole VP, Nyswander ME: A medical treatment of diacetylmorphine (heroin) addiction. *JAMA* 1965; 193:646–650.
5. Dole VP, Nyswander MD: The use of methadone for narcotic blockade. *Br J Addict* 1968; 63:55–57.
6. Finnegan LP (ed): *Drug Dependence in Pregnancy: Clinical Management of Mother and Child.* Services Research Monograph Series, DHEW Publication no. (ADM) 69-678. Washington, DC, DHEW, 1979.
7. Gunne LM: The fate of the Swedish maintenance treatment programme. *Drug Alcohol Dependence* 1983; 11(1):99–103.
8. Hartnoll RL, Mitcheson MC, Battersby A, Brown G, Ellis M, Fleming P, Hedley N: Evaluation of heroin maintenance in controlled trial. *Arch Gen Psychiatry* 1980; 37:877.
9. Henderson IWD: Chemical dependence in Canada: A view from the hill, in Harris LS (ed): *Problems of Drug Dependence.* Proceedings of the 44th Annual Scientific Meeting, the Committee on Problems of Drug Dependence, Inc. NIDA Research Monograph 43. Rockville, MD, NIDA, 1983.
10. Kleber HD, Slobetz F, Mezritz M: *Medical Evaluation of Long-Term Methadone-Maintained Clients.* US Dept. Health and Human Services, DHHS publication (ADM) 80-1029. Rockville, MD, NIDA, 1980.
11. Kreek MJ: Methadone in treatment: Physiological and pharmacological issues, in Dupont RL, Goldstein A, O'Donnell J (eds): *Handbook on Drug Abuse.* Washington, DC, US Govt. Printing Office, 1979.
12. Kreek MJ: Medical management of methadone-maintained patients, in Lowinson JH, Ruiz P (eds): *Substance Abuse: Clinical Problems and Perspectives.* Baltimore, Williams & Wilkins, 1981, pp 660–673.
13. May E: Narcotics addiction and control in Great Britian, in *Dealing with Drug Abuse.* New York, Praeger, 1972.

14. McLellan AT, Luborsky L, O'Brien CP, Woody GE, Druley KA: Is treatment for substance abuse effective? *JAMA* 1982; 247:1423–1428.
15. Musto DF: *The American Disease*. New Haven, CT, Yale University Press, 1973.
16. Newman RG, Whitehill WB: Double-blind comparison of methadone and placebo maintenance treatments of narcotic addicts in Hong Kong. *Lancet* 1979; 11:485–488.
17. Patterson MA: Electro-acupuncture in alcohol and drug addictions. *Clin Med* 1974; 81:9–13.
18. Report of the National Research Council on Clinical Evaluation of Narcotic Antagonists: Clinical evaluation of naltrexone treatment of opiate-dependent individuals. *Arch Gen Psychiatry* 1978; 35:335–340.
19. Sainsbury MJ: Acupuncture in heroin withdrawal. *Med J Aust* 1974; 2(1):102–105.
20. Sells SB: Treatment effectiveness, in Dupont RL, Goldstein A, O'Donnell J (eds): *Handbook on Drug Abuse*. Washington, DC, US Govt. Printing Office, 1979.
21. Senay EC, Dorus W, Goldberg F, Thornton W: Withdrawal from methadone maintenance: Rate of withdrawal and expectation. *Arch Gen Psychiatry* 1977; 34:361–367.
22. Senay EC: *Substance Abuse Disorders in Clinical Practice*. Littleton, MA, John Wright PSG, 1983.
23. Severson L, Markoff RA, Chun-Hoon A: Heroin detoxification with acupuncture and electrical stimulation. *Int J Addict* 1977; 12:911–922.
24. Shuaib BM: Acupuncture treatment of drug dependence in Pakistan. *Am J Chinese Med* 1976; 4:403–407.
25. Suwanwela C, Poshyachinda V, Sitthi-Amorn C, Tasanapradit P, Dharmkrong-At A: *Overview of Drug Dependence in Thailand*. Mimeographed report. Bangkok, Chulalongkorn University, 1978.
26. Wen HC, Cheung SY: Treatment of drug addiction by acupuncture and electrical stimulation. *Asian J Med* 1973; 9:138–141.
27. Westermeyer J: *Poppies, Pipes and People: Opium and Its Use in Laos*. Berkeley, University of California Press, 1983.
28. Whitehead PC: Acupuncture in the treatment of addiction: A review and analysis. *Int J Addict* 1978; 13:1–16.
29. Woody EG, Mintz J, Tennant F, O'Brien CP, McLellan AT, Marcovici M: Propoxyphene for maintenance treatment of narcotic addiction. *Arch Gen Psychiatry* 1981; 38:898–900.

V

Public Health Approaches

13

Public Health Planning

1. Introduction

The World Health Organization and countries throughout the world have set the goal of health care for all by the year 2000. Primary health care is the cornerstone for this plan. Health care has taken on a new outlook, with strong emphasis on social issues. Equity is one of the major goals in this plan, since large sectors of the population of the world do not have even minimal health services. Changes are occurring not just in present health care systems and technology, but also in the perception of the physician–patient relationship. Previously the doctor functioned in the system as the main actor. It is now recognized that to accomplish the goal of health for all in the year 2000 changes must occur in the physician's role. The community should become the main actor. Community responsibility and participation must play a role as important as that of the physician—more like a partner than a dependent client. The health system should support, educate, and motivate the people in their pursuit of better health.

With this changing concept in health care, drug-dependence treatment gains new relevance. It has long been recognized that drug dependence is not merely a medical problem. Traditional medical approaches alone cannot provide adequate frameworks for successful programs, whether in treatment or prevention. The problem of drug dependence thus serves as an excellent vehicle for implementing and testing the new concept of health for all by the year 2000, with primary health care as a key approach.

2. Drug Dependence from a Public Health Perspective

Drug dependence is often perceived as a problem affecting an individual. That can be useful when treating that particular individual. But in treating and preventing drug dependence, one has to look beyond the individual alone. Considering the entire family, community, or nation as the unit of treatment and prevention provides a better perspective for approaching drug dependence. For example, we can assess the extent to which drug dependence has affected an entire country as a unit. Or the unit could be a village, a town, a city, a province, or an entire region of countries.

2.1. Nature and Extent of the Problem

The first step is to consider whether the population has a drug-dependence problem. Use of drugs can occur in a population without becoming a problem. There may not be agreement concerning whether a problem exists as a result of value judgments or social norms within the community. Recognition and awareness of drug-dependence problems has varied greatly from time to time, and place to place.

To assess drug dependence in a population, it is necessary to identify the nature of the problem (its qualitative aspects) and also its extent (its quantitative aspects). Such assessment must be based on information originating from many sources. Epidemiological methods for obtaining qualitative and quantitative data have been described earlier.

2.2. Assessing Etiological Factors

Communities can have many factors leading to drug dependence, just as do individuals. Three elements interact in the genesis of these problems: drug, host, and environment.

Both the type of drug and its availability are important in assessing the community's drug problem. If the drug is prohibited by law, its source is therefore illicit. Law enforcement, drug-related crime, and organized criminals would then be crucial considerations in that community. Outside forces, such as international politics and international trafficking networks, can contribute to the availability of illicit drugs. For example, the widespread presence of opium in China two centuries ago was forced on that country by a treaty after defeat in the Opium War. As a result of the treaty, both imported and domestic opium flooded the country and resulted in a serious epidemic. Today, availability of certain modern drugs depends on pharmaceutical production, either within the country or from foreign imports. For drugs that have therapeutic purposes, total prohibition would deprive patients of needed drugs. Regulatory approaches are therefore necessary so that drugs are available for legitimate medical purposes. Effectiveness of regulatory drug laws can determine the availability of drugs for abusive purposes.

The host factor refers to the population in the community, along with its social organization and culture. Social attitudes and norms greatly influence drug use and drug dependence. For example, in some communities the people do not have social barriers against certain drugs, so that if availability of that drug becomes great, abuse and dependence rapidly ensue. In other communities where social sanctions against use of a drug are strong, drug dependence does not occur, or occurs rarely, despite drug availability. Social attitudes regarding drug dependence can be related to economic, sociocultural, or political situations in the community. For example, corruption in the police or government may play an important role. Discontent among the youth from rapid or inequitable social changes may favor the development of illicit drug use, with subsequent drug problems. With rapid communication and travel today, social attitudes and norms may spread from one country to another just as do sports activities, hobbies, fashionable dress, and music. Wars affect the morale of a people and can result in increased drug use. Some individuals are vulnerable to drug dependence as a result of genetic, situational, or personality factors.

Environment refers to geographical, political, and economic conditions that may favor or impede drug dependence. Such ecological elements include local conditions facilitating drug production or drug smuggling or access to treatment for drug dependence.

2.3. Consequences for the Community

When a community is affected by drug dependence, the effects range from economic loss, to social loss, to health and manpower loss. Economic loss ensues from the money spent on drugs, in both the licit and the illicit markets. Resources expended in the solution of the drug-dependence problem comprise a loss (although these expenditures can be partially recovered if treatment is cost effective). There is an individual economic loss for each drug-dependent person who cannot contribute economically to the society. Economic as well as social loss occurs if there is an increase in crime. Early death during productive years of life and disability from drug dependence can produce major economic losses, to say nothing of the suffering to individuals and families. If the problem is affecting youth, the future manpower of the community, then a long-term, costly, although frequently hidden cost is imposed on the people in both economic and social terms.

3. Public Health Approaches

Drug-dependence problems are dynamic and ever changing. Social coping with these problems depends on many interacting factors with the community, ranging from the local perception of the problem to the available resources for addressing the problem.

3.1. Intervention: Policy

Policy makers influence decisions at many levels, from the village or town to the nation. Policy making depends on the locus of authority, which in turn relates to the formal social and political organization as well as the informal distribution of power. Public opinion often plays a large role in policy setting. In parliamentary systems, the attitude and beliefs of the parliamentarians are major controlling forces. In dictatorships or oligarchies, a single person or group of persons makes the policy. Identification of both the political structure and the ways for affecting policy is essential in setting up effective policy regarding drug dependence.[8,9]

Awareness and understanding of the problem by the policy maker is an essential step both at the community level and at the national level. Often drug dependence is not perceived publicly as being a social problem which warrants group response. This is especially true if the situation is a long-standing one. Misunderstanding and erroneous concepts can contribute to the lack of awareness. Ignorance or simplistic notions may lead to inappropriate measures, which then can create more problems. Controlling polices solely through legal means is an example.[17]

At the national as well as at the community level, policy makers make decisions about the priority of the drug dependence problem. Other problems facing the nation or the community, including economic, social, and political problems, must be considered in making these decisions. Within the health sector the priority of drug dependence vis-à-vis other health problems must also be set.

3.2. Intervention: Strategy

Intervention strategies can be separated into two types: reducing the supply of the drug and reducing the demand for the drug.

3.2.1. Supply Reduction

As is evident from the previous chapters, the availability of drug significantly affects the nature and extent of the problem. Effective control over drug distribution and reduction of drug availability have virtually eliminated drug dependence in some countries (at least for certain types of drugs). Laws and law enforcement may be used by governments to impose a ban on certain drugs. In addition to a complete ban of the drug, partial control is also possible. Partial control strategies consist of limiting the setting, the time, or the amount of use. Examples of partial controls that reduce but do not eliminate drug use include the following:

- Increasing taxes on legal drugs such as alcohol or tobacco.
- Reducing the number of retail outlets (e.g., taverns, cocktail lounges, opium vends, tobacco sellers).
- Licensing producers, distributors, and sale outlets.
- Reducing the hours of sale.
- Forbidding sale on certain days or to persons under a certain age.
- Requiring a physician's prescription for and a pharamacist's recording of the purchase of psychoactive medication.

3.2.2. Demand Reduction

Demand reduction can be divided into prevention and treatment strategies. These topics are covered extensively in other chapters, but their public health, policy, and strategic aspects are reviewed here. The community and its social and political organization have many means for reducing the demand for abusive use of drugs. Mass communication is an effective means for changing the social attitude as well as creating awareness of the problem. Community development may be a critical step in reducing drug dependence. Absence of health care may lead to the self-initiated use of drugs for the treatment of diseases, resulting in drug dependence. Provision of primary health care would then be necessary. In a setting where poverty, economic anxiety, and drug use have created a vicious cycle, economic development would be an essential step. Comprehensive community development depends on economic, social, educational, health, and social welfare elements. The organization can be both public and nongovernmental. The political nature of this process must be appreciated. Change in individual life-style may be involved. China's success in controlling opium dependence depended largely on changes in social organization, political leadership, and the peoples' life-style.

In planning treatment programs in a country or a community one needs to find the people who are in need of help—a process called early case finding or secondary prevention. Provision of appropriate help for each group of people is important. Some national programs aim only toward certain populations and have little effect on the overall extent of the problem. For example, some drug-dependent persons may repeatedly use a detoxification facility only for temporary relief if they run out of funds, are in trouble with the police, or are having serious health problems. This strategy may meet certain limited goals (such as reducing disability while not curing the disorder). However, dedication of all available resources to this treatment approach will eliminate treatment opportunities for other groups whose problem is not yet so severe or recurrent.

Compulsory and/or voluntary nature of treatment must also be considered in planning. Selection of treatment technologies described in previous chapters also depends on the setting of policy and priorities. Funding strategies must also be addressed.

Drug-dependence problems require a multidisciplinary as well multifaceted approach. Shared responsibility and coordination are essential for a successful program. The role of the health sector needs to be identified in the overall strategy.

Strategy for manpower development is also important. At present the various health practitioners do not have the knowledge, attitude, and skill required to cope with drug-dependence problems. The role of the physician in the various strategies needs to be identified. Once this is determined, education and training can be instituted. Continuing education of practicing physicians and other health manpower, such as pharmacists and nurses, must be tailored according to the needs of various programs. When the problem is widespread and intervention activity is required at the community level, education and training for primary health care workers needs to be devised.[18]

Mass detoxification has been undertaken in some countries. This is especially relevant to rural areas, where all or most drug-dependent persons in a village, town, or district are detoxified over a period of days or weeks. This permits access of rural people to well-trained professionals, who can conduct supervised detoxification and initiate the early recovery steps in a group setting. Local health care workers can then conduct follow-up management and monitoring. This approach further facilitates recovery by reducing the availability of drugs in the region and by creating a new subculture of abstinent, recovering persons. It is important to involve local community leaders, health care workers, law enforcement personnel, and other personnel in this process, so that the effort is locally supported and not just externally superimposed on the community. This approach has been successfully employed in several Asian countries (e.g., China, India, Laos, Pakistan, Thailand, Vietnam).

4. Program Planning, Development, and Management

4.1. Characteristics of Treatment Programs

After policy and strategy have been set, one or more programs can then be developed. For each program there should be several steps in the planning, development, and management.

Effective treatment programs have certain basic characteristics in common:

1. A well-articulated treatment philosophy which is implemented in logical and consistent fashion.
2. Facilities for medical care and for rehabilitation.
3. Energetic and vigorous postdischarge outpatient treatment (if inpatient or residential treatment occurs).
4. Provision for involving families in the treatment of the patient and facilities for assisting these families.
5. Vigorous interaction with community resources which serves (a) to bring the patients into treatment and (b) to effect their transition back into the community after treatment.
6. Availability of an array of treatment, including behavioral, verbal, and somatic therapies.

These facilities may be located in general hospitals, psychiatric hospitals, or specialized units set up for the specific treatment of drug-dependent persons.

The long-term treatment of drug dependence is the most important aspect of the treatment process. Although the treatment of an overdose may be lifesaving, it does not ensure that the patient will not return to drug dependence. The acute treatment and withdrawal are only the first steps. Definitive treatment is a long process taking months or years. Drug dependence is a chronic disorder with remissions and exacerbations. A return to drug use should not be looked at as a treatment failure but as an indication to intensify treatment efforts.

4.2. Goal Setting and Treatment Objectives

Goals of treatment may be formulated from the standpoint of the patient (the clinical perspective) or from the standpoint of society (the public health perspective). Ideally, the clinical and public health perspectives generate similar, or at least overlapping, models for the delivery of service. This is not always the case with drug problems. For example, compulsory treatment may be justifiable from the perspective of the state, while individuals experience it as an infringement on their freedom and preferences. Conversely, long-term supportive care of an economically nonproductive patient may enhance that individual's life, but the expense must be borne by the public who might prefer that their resources be invested elsewhere.

Different perspectives among clinicians and policy makers revolve around the best interests of the individual and the best interests of the group or society. This can lead to adversarial positions, but both perspectives represent equally compelling needs, and a balance between them is desirable. Goal setting is the means by which the competing interests of patients, the public, and clinicians can be arbitrated.

A distinction must be made between treatment objectives and national policy goals, though it is desirable for the two to converge. One reason is that treatment is but one resolution strategy available to the governments. The state may pursue prevention via legal controls and education as well as via treatment to resolve drug problems.

The target population, the people for whom the program is designed, must be specified. Criteria for inclusion into the patient population need to be devised. These can be either narrow and specific or broad and general; in either case they may be subject to change. Methods for recruiting potential patients into the program must be devised.

4.3. Operation of the Program

Programs may be limited to certain modalities or phases in the treatment, or a program may be comprehensive involving many modalities and phases of treatment. Even the most limited program usually involves a combination of treatment techniques. Some range of flexibility is required since the patients and their problems are not homogeneous. The setting for the program can be an inpatient, outpatient, or community setting. If a program limits itself to only one or a few treatment phases and modalities, then coordination with other programs is essential. A referral system needs to be established and maintained—a process that requires communication and understanding.

The first step in treatment is often detoxification. This alone infrequently resolves drug problems,[10,16] although it can provide temporary respite. Detoxification is usually considered a first step in a treatment plan, as preparation for further treatment. Medical detoxification can favor development of a physician–patient relationship, which can be therapeutic in subsequent rehabilitation.

Programs which require their patients to make frequent clinic visits show more favorable recovery rates than programs which do not. The key to high recovery rates seems to be regular, ongoing involvement between the patient and staff.

4.4. Program Evaluation

Evaluation is essential to program management. Information obtained by evaluation is required to improve the efficiency, treatment effectiveness, and cost effectiveness of the program.

The evaluative process seeks to find out whether the stated goals of treatment have or have not been achieved, and why certain outcomes did or did not take place. Policies can then be revised on the basis of the feedback.

The first step in the treatment-planning and evaluation process is defining the problem to be resolved. The wisest course of action is to provide for the measurement of both the short-term and the long-term goals. Otherwise there would be no prospect of knowing whether treatment contributed to valued outcomes. The presenting problem (assessment), the process of resolving it (the treatment plan), the desired short-term goals (treatment objectives), as well as the long-term goals (eventual course of the disorder) should be described. They should be described in a way that would allow an independent observer to make the same observations.

Treatment evaluation can also influence social policy in other sections besides health care. For example, if referrals of cases are not being made, social policy changes might be initiated to stimulate such referrals.

Utilization and retention rates are helpful in ascertaining whether the service is needed. Utilization rates are measured by taking the average daily patient census and dividing it by the program's capacity (e.g., number of beds, number of outpatients who could be seen in a day). These rates reflect a program's ability to generate referrals. High utilization rates generally reflect a favorable reputation and efficient management. However, high utilization alone does not assure that the service is efficiently operated. Retention rates consist of the number of patients who remain in treatment. These rates have different meanings depending on the type of service being provided. Retention rates have little relevance for facilities that limit their services to early case finding, assessment, referral crisis intervention, or detoxification. On the other hand, treatment and rehabilitation programs must retain patients for longer periods: several months to a few years.

Retention rates can be demonstrated by the following examples. In Hong Kong 100 chronic heroin addicts were enrolled in a 3-year outpatient program providing medical care, counseling, and supportive social services. One-half of the group, randomly determined, were withdrawn from drugs gradually. The other half received daily doses of from 30 to 130 mg methadone. At the end of 3 years, 20 of the methadone-treated patients had been retained in treatment while only one of the detoxified patients had stayed with the program.[1] Detoxification did not facilitate retention in this program.

Utilization and retention rates are most useful in conjunction with two other pieces of information: patient demographics and outcome measures. If utilization and retention rates are found to be associated with patient demographics (age, sex, ethnicity, religion, geographical region, distance from treatment), then the program could consider limiting admissions to those with whom it works best (if utilization rates are high) or making modifications to retain the types of patients they generally lose (if utilization rates are low). To this end, it is desirable to maintain some record of patient characteristics. Also, patient demographics can be compared with those of the general population. It may be found that a certain type of patient is not represented in the treatment population and methods of attracting and serving them could be considered. Outcome measures are also important in guiding treatment programs and social policy, For example, optimum treatment can be determined only by outcome measures made some months or even years after treatment.

4.5. Influence of Treatment on Clinical Outcome

Programs that determine treatment objectives with the patient as well as with important members of the patient's social network generally achieve more favorable outcomes (i.e., higher retention rates, fewer treatment complications, more favorable long-term outcomes) than programs which do not.[3] Feedback requires prior agreement on the goals of treatment as well as observable measures of progress. For example, it would be helpful for a program to be able to show that patients had drug-free urines, or that the patients' medical complications had been resolved, or that patients had completed prescribed treatment plans by the time of discharge.

Most relapses occur within the first 3–6 months following treatment. Thus, evaluation of efficacy requires that follow-ups be conducted at least 6 months to a year after treatment. The key issue is whether the patient or the program is being evaluated. For programmatic evaluation, a 6–12-month follow-up would be adequate, while 5 years would be appropriate for assessing the course of individual patients. Data that are 2–3 years old may be irrelevant to current programmatic decision making. Also, a program's influence on a patient will wane as a function of time after treatment, since other host and environmental factors influence the outcome.

4.6. Methodological Issues in Studying Outcome

Low rates of success in locating former patients during follow-up introduce bias by limiting findings to only those patients who are easily found. This could result in adverse findings since patients who have not become self-sufficient could remain visible to the social system whereas those who do become self-sufficient no longer have their names and addresses on the rolls and thereby would be more difficult to locate. For other programs the bias could be reversed. That is, patients who remain active in alumni groups, or who contribute to alumni funds, would be the easiest to locate, whereas treatment failures are not likely to keep the agency informed of changes in address.

Illustrative of a follow-up study is Singer's[11] follow-up of Castle Peak Addiction Center, a government-operated program in Hong Kong. Following methadone detoxification, narcotic addicts volunteering for the 6-month residential program participated in individual and group psychotherapy, family counseling, and occupational and recreational therapy (inclusive of work assignments). Patients (sample size = 314) in good physical health and without disabling psychiatric conditions were followed up 7–9 years after entering treatment. Outcome measures included current abstinence, as well as an estimate of social adjustment based on combined ratings of personal satisfaction, employment, and interpersonal relations. The results were as follows:

- 44% abstinent (80% improved social adjustment, 10% unchanged, and 10% worse).
- 33% readdicted (5% improved social adjustment, 48% unchanged, and 47% worse).
- 9% dead.
- 14% lost to follow-up.

It is important to report both abstinence and improvement rates since (1) they are not identical and (2) improvement rates may be larger than abstinence rates alone and therefore may reflect favorably on the treatment process. Also, it is important to account for all patients in the sample. Had abstinence rates been based only on the patients who had been located, the abstinence rate would have been reported as 57%, which would have been misleading.

Laboratory or physical tests are often considered to have high reliability in follow-up studies, yet Suwanwela *et al.*[15] found only one opiate-dependent person who was missed by interview, but found by urinalysis. Urinalyses also generated several false positives among poppy farmers who may have ingested some alkaloids through household utensils or from poppy seeds. Also, since some users periodically abstain, false negatives can occur. Conversely, interviews and questionnaires can achieve high degrees of reliability and validity if anonymity, confidentiality, or protection from harm or prejudice for honest reporting is assured.[2,12–14] Similarly, there is little difference in accuracy between reports obtained from patients as opposed to family members or others with first-hand observation.[6] Other sources of data are official records, such as registries of admissions to hospitals, jails or prisons, social agencies, and morgues.

Who is best suited to conduct a follow-up? The answer is not clear. Many reliable studies have been initiated and carried out by program directors and staff members seriously interested in treatment outcome. By the same token, staff members of a program that provided the service may lose objectivity, depart from instructions, and be poorly motivated to accomplish acceptable follow-ups, especially when program funding or referrals depend on reporting high success rates.[7]

A common misunderstanding is the size of the sample. Some believe that the larger the sample, the more valid the results. However, validity (the close correlation between the data and the real world) is more a function of the quality of the effort than the quantity. Very large samples can improve the likelihood of obtaining a positive finding by demonstrating statistically significant results that are too small to be of practical significance.[5] For most follow-up studies the sample size need not exceed 100 cases per treatment group; often 30–50 subjects per treatment group are adequate to demonstrate significant results. The major risk with small samples (say, less than 30 subjects in a group) is that spurious relationships may result from sampling errors. It is important to ensure that the measures used are reliable (i.e., the observations would be similar if measured a second time or by a similar method).

4.7. Cost Benefit

Cost benefit refers to the monetary value of treatment compared to the monetary value of the resultant benefits. Twelve studies of the cost benefit of treatment for alcohol problems[4] present surprisingly consistent findings despite considerable differences in methodology. The studies are largely specific to employee-based programs, and the benefits are largely measured in terms of diminished costs of medical services, sick leave, or accident benefits. Still, on the average, they suggest that each monetary unit spent on alcohol rehabilitation results in a saving of 2.4 monetary units the next year, a 140% net gain. These figures, however, are primarily derived from programs in the workplace, which are known to use the least expensive services and to treat the patients with the best prognosis, so comparable cost/benefit ratios might not be expected for the more costly services or more severely impaired patients.

Cost-benefit analyses can be challenged on philosophical, as well as methodological, grounds. It can be argued that where human life is concerned, benefits are by definition infinite and the costs involved are therefore immaterial. Although it is impossible to put a price on human suffering or a human life, cost-benefit decisions become necessary when the cost of a service becomes a noticeable proportion of the average income, the annual revenues, or the gross national product of a population. Public policy makers have the responsibility to serve as stewards of collective resources and as arbitrators between contestants for commonly held resources. Treatment is often subsidized by other people's money, whether it be by means of prepaid group medical care plans or through governmental subsidization or control. Thus, it is valid to compare the relative cost of different treatment strategies that achieve comparable outcomes.

4.8. Cost Effectiveness

Cost effectiveness is easier to advocate than to measure. The simplest measure of cost effectiveness is cost per successful outcome. This figure is determined by dividing the total cost of a program by the number of successful outcomes. This formula does not penalize more costly programs if they produce superior outcomes than less costly programs. Total cost of treating the sample is determined by multiplying the cost of each treatment unit (day or visit) by the total number of patients in the sample and then multiplying the product by the average number of treatment days (or visits) for the sample. The determination of the denominator is more difficult. The question falls back on what is considered a valued outcome. As mentioned earlier, the general public would usually view greater productivity, less familial dysfunction, and diminished criminal activity as preferred outcomes. Yet service providers often emphasize diminished drug use, preferably total abstinence. Abstinence will be used as the first denominator, since it is the most commonly articulated treatment objective. The number of abstinent patients generated by each program is divided into the total cost for that sample to generate the cost per abstinent patient. The difficulty with using complete abstinence as a measure is that cost per successful abstinent outcome will be considerable. Since improvement rates generally are two times abstinence rates, the cost per improvement would be about half what the cost per full remission would be. For this reason, the cost per improved patient is usually calculated also.

Program administrators can argue that the magnitude of improvement is not addressed in these computations. For example, a drug-dependent patient who achieves abstinence after treatment has achieved a greater gain than a moderate problem user who continues using drugs at a lower dosage, yet each would be counted as a comparable improvement in the computation. It is worth it, they argue, to go to greater expense to achieve a larger improvement. It is a good argument but it does not bear out. Different treatment intensities do not usually generate different outcomes rates when severity of the drug problems is held constant. The resolution of the apparent inconsistency lies in the fact that the expensive, in contrast to the less expensive, programs have a greater proportion of severe cases. The apparent cost effectiveness of the inexpensive programs would probably not have occurred had patients been randomly assigned to the different treatment programs independent of the severity of their drug problem. When the cost per outcome is determined holding severity of problem constant, the difference dissipates.

Cost benefit requires that a monetary figure be assigned to benefits as well as cost. The employment figures, at best, are only indirect measures of income. Thus, the question remains "Will these patients pay back to society by increased productivity the costs of the services provided?" Such ultimate questions involve value judgments. Treatment planning and evaluation can help us explore our priorities to contribute to a just allocation of resources.

References

1. Action Committee Against Narcotics: *Hong Kong Narcotics Report 1975–76.* Hong Kong, Government Printer, 1976.
2. Ball JC: The reliability and validity of interview data obtained from 59 narcotic addicts. *Am J Sociol* 1967; 72:650–654.
3. Costello RM: Alcoholism treatment and evaluation: In search of methods I. *Int J Addict* 1975; 10:251–275.
4. Jones KR, Vishi TR: Impact of alcohol, drug abuse and mental health treatment on medical care utilization: A review of the research literature. *Med Care* 1979; 17(2)(12):1–26.

5. Meehl PE: *Clinical Versus Statistical Prediction: A Theoretical Analysis and a Review of the Evidence.* Minneapolis, University of Minnesota Press, 1954.
6. Polich JM, Armor DJ, Braiker HB: *The Course of Alcoholism: Four Years after Treatment.* Santa Monica, CA, Rand Corporation, 1979.
7. Poschyachinda V, Onthuam Y, Sitthi-Amorn C, Perugparn U: *Evaluation of Treatment Outcome: The Buddhist Temple Center, Tam Kraborg.* Mimeographed report. Bangkok, Chulalongkorn University, 1978.
8. Ross HL: *Deterring the Drinking Driver: Legal Policy and Social Control.* Lexington, MA, Lexington Books, 1982.
9. Siassir I, Fazoumi B: Dilemmas of Iran's opium maintenance program: An action research of evaluating goals, conflicts and policy changes. *Int J Addict* 1980; 15(8):1127–1140.
10. Simpson DD, Savage LJ, Lloyd MR, Sells SB: *Evaluation of Drug Abuse Treatment Based on First Year Follow-up.* DHEW Publication no. (ADM) 78-701. Washington, DC, NIDA, 1978.
11. Singer K: *Prognosis of Narcotic Addiction.* London, Butterworths, 1975.
12. Smart RG, Blair NI: Test–retest reliability and validity information for a high school drug use questionnaire. *Drug Alcohol Dependence* 1978; 3:265–271.
13. Sobell LC, Sobell MG: Outpatient alcoholics give valid self-reports. *J Nerv Ment Dis* 1975; 161:32:43.
14. Stephens R: The truthfulness of addict respondents in research projects. *Int J Addict* 1972; 7:549–558.
15. Suwanwela C, Poshyachinda V, Sitthi-Amorn C, Tasanapradit P, Dharmkrong-At A: *Overview of Drug Dependence in Thailand.* Mimeographed report. Bangkok, Chulalongkorn University, 1978.
16. Tims FM: *Effectiveness of Drug Abuse Treatment Programs.* NIDA Treatment Research Report. DHHS Publication no. (ADM) 81-1143. Washington, DC, NIDA, 1981.
17. Westermeyer J: The pro-heroin effects of anti-opium laws. *Arch Gen Psychiatry* 1976; 33:1135–1139.
18. World Health Organization: *Drug Dependence and Alcohol-Related Problems: A Manual for Community Health Workers, with Guidelines for Trainers.* Geneva, WHO, 1986.

Further Reading

Roemer R: *Legislative Action to Combat the World Smoking Epidemic.* Geneva, WHO, 1982.

World Health Organization: *Controlling the Smoking Epidemic.* World Health Organization Technical Report, no. 636, Geneva, WHO, 1979.

14

Prevention

1. Introduction

Prevention of drug dependence involves measures aimed at agent, host, and environment. Control of drug supply and drug demand are key features in these efforts. Health professionals are involved not only in the early diagnosis and timely treatment of individual patients, but also in prevention through health education, early intervention programs, and public policy. A special prevention opportunity for the medical profession lies in exerting great care in the prescription of dependence-producing drugs.

2. Public Health Approaches

Public health strategies are organized around three major factors—the drug (the agent), the environment in which drugs are used, and the person (the host) who uses drugs. The public health approach consists of strategies that affect two basic dimensions of drugs—supply and demand. Supply is affected by strategies that influence the agent and the environment. Demand is affected by strategies that affect the host. For example, moderate drinkers may encourage heavy drinkers to reduce their consumption. Advertising, strength of the dosage, cost of the drug, or attractiveness of the drug container can also influence usage levels.

In order to choose preventive approaches, it is necessary to understand the nature of drug consumption within the area and the roles drug use plays within the community. It is important to identify such key factors as the following:

1. The nature of harmful consumption.
2. The context in which the choice to use drugs is made.[60]

3. Indicators of drug problems that may be helpful for the development of a public policy on drugs.[51]
4. The natural sources of prevention within the cultural group, such as customs that may promote or inhibit harmful drug use.[1]

Establishing the levels of drug consumption through epidemiological surveys is a critical step. It is the base from which changes can be noted. Determining the extent of change is critical for ascertaining effective prevention. Changes in consumption often reflect policy changes or environmental factors within the country.[10,37,43]

The relative importance of various drug- or alcohol-related problems differs from country to country, as does the structure of institutions that lend themselves to epidemiological surveys. Assessment of problems can be done via means such as the following:

1. Use of instrumentation to measure blood or urine drug levels in a representative sample of vehicular accidents and fatalities.
2. Survey of the effects of drug dependence on productivity in various industries, the military, and civil service, including absenteeism, lateness, accidents, work errors, and excessive use of sick leave. (For example, a sample of employees displaying such patterns may be studied for drug dependence. Sick leaves and/or use of medical benefits may be analyzed for relationship to drug dependence.)
3. Studies of school problems, such as absence, truancy, vandalism, poor school work, excessive illness, and signs of abuse or neglect, may be undertaken. (For example, children involved may be living with parents who are drug dependent, and the children themselves may also be abusing drugs.[36,38,39])
4. Surveys of court systems: family court, juvenile court, and adult criminal court caseloads.[13]
5. Surveys of clinic, emergency medical service, and inpatient hospital populations for unidentified and untreated drug dependence. (A drug screening questionnaire, personal interview, or urine/blood tests may be used alone or in combination, and the results compared with routine hospital records.[8])
6. Studies of social agencies, jails, probation offices, health departments.[75]

3. Role of Public Policy

3.1. Public Policy toward Drugs

Overall public policy throughout the world is one of discouragement of excessive or inappropriate use of drugs. Epidemiological data on drug dependence that have accumulated in the past 30 years have clearly revealed enormous effects on individual health, as well as on crime and economics.[26,31] Hence, all countries have developed a variety of discouragement policies.

Conflicts and controversies in public policy often confront the health professional. For example, the agricultural production of tobacco, opium, alcohol, cocaine, and cannabis is condoned in some parts of the world for economic reasons, especially when these are exported to other countries. Some national governments have even stimulated tobacco or alcohol use among their own citizens as a source of tax revenues from tobacco or alcohol. In other instances, penalties for drug use may appear too lenient or harsh relative to the harmful effects of the drug. Mass media may be perceived to promote drug use, or to give erroneous information about drug effects. One culture may deem a certain drug use to be socially acceptable, while others may abhor it. Despite considerable national, regional, and religious differences, international cooperation in the field of drug dependence has been growing. International agencies involved in these problems are the United Nations (UN), World Health Organization, UN Narcotics Control Commission, UN Fund for Drug Abuse Cooperation, Interpol, European Economic Community, Southeast Asia Treaty Organization, and the Council of Europe.

A public controversy that embraces health professionals perhaps more frequently than any other is the public demand to know what level of drug use is safe (i.e., will not produce adverse health effects). Despite some ambiguities and conflicts in public policy, the health professionals' most important contribution must be to prevent drug use from harming health.

3.2. Standard Control Policies

Public methods to prevent drug dependence in various parts of the world include the following:

1. Laws to prohibit or control manufacture, transport, sale, and use of drugs (e.g., no sale of tobacco products to minors).[40,58]
2. Crop eradication (e.g., cannabis), crop replacement (e.g., to lessen dependence on opium poppy), and crop diversification (e.g., to reduce excessive tobacco production).
3. Criminal penalties for offenders.
4. Production and distribution quotas for drugs with medicinal value (e.g., opium).
5. Prescribing and dispensing restrictions on certain drugs (e.g., opioids, sedatives), including licensing of health professionals.
6. Public education (e.g., about alcohol, tobacco, prescription drugs, nonprescription or over-the-counter medication).
7. Establishment of treatment programs.

8. Public registration and community surveillance of known drug-dependent persons.
9. Early identification of drug-dependent persons in critical occupations (e.g., physicians, pilots) or at special risk (e.g., pregnant women, preoperative surgical patients).
10. Warning labels on abusable drugs that are sold commercially (e.g., alcohol content in cough remedies, tar and nicotine levels in tobacco).
11. Development of medications with less potential for drug dependence.

The oldest prevention strategies are generally those associated with laws that attempt to regulate the production, manufacture, transport, sale, and use of drugs by force of criminal sanctions. Many of the new prevention strategies, such as public education and early identification of drug-dependent persons, either affect or are implemented by health professionals.[15,45,53]

4. Classification of Prevention

Prevention has traditionally been classified as primary, secondary, or tertiary. This classification is useful in understanding the approaches to drug prevention. Primary prevention is any measure taken to prevent a disease from developing. Examples of primary prevention of drug dependence are eliminating illicit drug production and commerce, controlling drug access via prescribing laws, and rearing a child to reduce the tendency to begin drug use. Secondary prevention of a disease refers to its detection in the early phase so that intervention can keep the disease from becoming fully symptomatic. Screening of medical patients for pathogenic drug use or early drug problems during a routine checkup, followed by patient education, is an example of secondary prevention. Tertiary prevention refers to measures taken after a disease is established in order to retard further progression and to avoid complications of the disease. Examples of tertiary prevention include a patient who is given a safer maintenance drug, such as substituting oral methadone for heroin injection, or a patient with alcoholic cirrhosis who is treated in order to help achieve abstention from alcohol.

5. Primary Prevention

Despite historical and recent attention to primary prevention of drug dependence, it has been argued that chronic disorders such as drug dependence cannot be prevented because there is no one etiology. Thinking in terms of single causes, while sometimes useful for infectious or parasitic diseases, is not useful for chronic diseases, including drug dependence.

The dominance of an infectious-disease model in primary prevention schemes is understandable when one realizes that until recent decades infectious diseases were the leading cause of death. As total populations were at risk of developing an infectious disease, prevention strategies (such as immunization programs) evolved that dealt with identifying a single agent and isolating populations from the consequences of that agent.[5]

5.1. Populations at Risk

An infectious-disease approach to the primary prevention of chronic diseases ignores the special nuances characteristic of chronic diseases but not characteristic of infectious disease. For example, chronic diseases are not evenly distributed throughout the population. Everyone does not share the same risk of developing chronic disease. Thus special populations at risk to the chronic disease can often be identified. High-risk groups are subgroups of the general population who risk developing a specific disease, accident, or injury. Of course, many individuals who are at risk (even a majority of them in some cases) will not become drug dependent.

A second characteristic of chronic disease is multiple causation. That is, the causes of chronic disease typically include a variety of components—genetic, environmental, sociocultural, and behavioral. These components may be potential targets for preventive efforts. Chronic disease prevention may involve restricting the life-style of a symptomless individual in order to reduce the potential risk of developing a specific disease.

A number of antecedents and precursors of drug use have now been statistically determined to assist health professionals, educators, and families in the identification of persons at risk for subsequent drug dependence.[7,34,47,61,65,66,74] Once these factors are detected, they can be valuable in alerting potential victims to the risk of drug dependence. Some of the risk factors that have been reported are as follows:

1. Family history of drug, alcohol, and tobacco dependence.[7,61]
2. Broken home (e.g., parents divorced).[74]
3. Low income.[74]
4. Lack of religious training.[66]
5. Lack of discipline in home.[67]
6. Cigarette smoking before age 12 years.[62,65]
7. Association with peers who are drug dependent.[38,39]
8. Poor work conditions.[59,61]

It is emphasized that these risk factors are only antecedents or precursors that are statistically associated with higher-than-expected levels of drug dependence, including tobacco dependence. They do not necessarily imply a cause-and-effect relationship. In addition, it is unknown whether correction of any risk factors will prevent drug dependence. There may also be wide differences from culture to culture regarding the potential risk associated with these factors.

High-risk groups can be divided into two types:

1. Due to a genetic characteristic, familial pattern, or long-term behavioral pattern, an individual has greater potential for the development of a drug-related illness, disease, accident, injury, or consequence. This risk may be termed longitudinal or chronic. For example, children of alcoholic parents have a risk of alcoholism three to four times greater than others, even if reared apart from their alcoholic parents.

2. Due to a temporary or short-term occurrence, an individual is considered to have a greater potential for the development of acute drug-related problems, such as an injury or other negative consequence. This risk may be termed transitional or situational. The results of this transitional risk status can itself be a long-term event, such as a chronic injury sustained in a drug-related car accident.[57] The time during which accident victims are at risk is short (e.g., the time they are in the car), but the consequences can be lifelong (e.g., paraplegia, brain damage).

A number of techniques have been attempted with individuals, particularly children and adolescents, who possess high-risk characteristics. Health professionals have participated by educating parents and teachers of the child and by encouraging them to modify their child-rearing methods and the behavior of the child in a manner that best addresses the risk factor.[67] For example, parents of a group of adolescents who socialize together might meet together and collectively set curfews, rules, and other guidelines for their children. These curfews, rules, and policies may reduce the risk of exposure to drug dependence.

5.2. Education

Educational strategies must be integrated within an overall primary prevention plan. Unless a clear prevention policy exists, education efforts may produce conflicting messages which will only confuse the target audience.[6]

Education has been a major effort in primary prevention, especially for tobacco dependence.[54,68,70,73] In addition to didactic learning about the health and social consequences of drug and alcohol use, such education programs often convey social values. Techniques have included written literature, radio and television programs, group discussions, and class teaching (including teaching by specially trained students as well as teachers).

Systematic evaluation of such classes given to children have shown positive results under specific circumstances.[46,69] Long-term benefits of drug education are largely unknown.[61] For example, even if a primary-school youngster is educated and has no intention of smoking tobacco or using other drugs, drug use may begin when he reaches teenage years.[38,39,62] Initial studies of brief drug education among students showed little effect,[30] but recent evaluations of tobacco smoking reveal that a series of classes will significantly reduce tobacco-smoking behavior.[46,70]

Certain curricula have been shown to be effective for high-risk students, as well as students in general. Such curricula undertake the following objectives and techniques:

1. The curricula are designed to reflect the norms of the community; they can therefore be supported by the community.
2. Teachers are trained to be comfortable with teaching about drugs. This involves reviewing their own attitudes, values, and behaviors and feeling at ease discussing the conflicts that the raising of this topic in a classroom is likely to uncover.
3. Teachers are trained to teach objectively about drugs rather than to display a specific bias.
4. Curricula are designed to cover more basic topics such as clarification of values, self-control, self-care, and improving self-concept. They also utilize specific information concerning drug use.
5. Each curriculum covers multiple grades, some beginning early in preschool years and continuing through secondary school. There are even special curricula designed for college students.
6. Integration through the curriculum links teaching about drugs and drug use with other school subjects, including language, music, history, and health.
7. Curricula usually involve some education for the community. This is done so that the parents and community leaders have input into the school process and so they can support the content of the information covered in the classroom.[21]

Public education also can be of value to a primary prevention effort. For public education programs to be effective they must be designed much like advertising. Such programs are developed with the following factors in mind:

1. The target audience: for example, young pregnant women living in a densely populated city.
2. The immediate relevance of the information to the target audience.
3. Conveying the action being suggested for the target audience: for example, not to drink if pregnant.
4. The mode in which the message is to be presented. (This is important because if a message is presented only at times when the target audience may not be watching or listening, it will not have an impact. The medium for transmission of a message to an audience can vary from placing a

warning label on the containers of alcoholic beverages, to making pamphlets available at food stores and in health clinics and doctors' offices, to presenting messages on television and radio.)

5. The need for repetition of the message. (This is crucial to the success of a public information effort, for if a message is seen only once, or only for a week, it is not likely to affect the target audience. What is needed is repetition of the message to the audience. This is similar to advertising any product or service to an audience.)

There is some consensus on what constitutes safe drug-use levels. For example, most experts in the drug field believe that any use of certain drugs (e.g., phencyclidine, D-lysergic acid, volatile inhalants) carries unacceptable risks. While medical use of certain drugs (e.g., opioids, diazepines, barbiturates) is warranted, their social or recreational use is highly likely to lead to drug dependence and/or major medical problems. Some drugs (e.g., alcohol, tobacco) may be consumed with relative safety if use is infrequent and socially controlled. Still other drugs (e.g., caffeine) have low dependence potential, but can occasionally lead to medical problems. There may be little or no safe drug use possible under certain circumstances, such as pregnancy,[17,22,23,48] certain occupational activities, certain sports or recreational activities, and use of certain compounds (such as industrial solvents).

Beyond such a general consensus, however, more specific data on safe levels are lacking. Perhaps most attention has been focused on safe levels of alcohol use. There is considerable individual variability, with smaller or lighter persons being at risk from lower doses. Women are at greater risk from drugs that distribute through total body water (such as alcohol). The unborn fetus may be sensitive to extremely small doses. Even large males appear at risk to eventual organ damage if they consume more than 8 or 10 standard drinks per day, regardless of whether their blood alcohol concentration reaches intoxicating levels (e.g., 100 mg%).[18] Even regular daily consumption of five standard drinks per day (perhaps four in a small person) increases the risk of contracting cirrhosis after a decade or two. Of interest, a nineteenth-century British physician, Anstie, proposer of the so-called Anstie's limit, suggested that daily drinking be limited to half a bottle of table wine or 3 pints of beer.[3] A special committee of the Royal College of Psychiatrists has suggested that no one should exceed an intake in 1 day of 1900 ml (4 pints) of beer, 120 ml (4 oz) of spirits, or 750 ml of wine. Further, they advised that it is unwise to make a habit of regular drinking even at these levels, and that anyone driving a vehicle should not drink at all before driving.[18]

5.3. Strategies Utilizing the Agent

Control over the consumption of drugs through the use of laws has a long history. As early as 4000 years ago, the Code of Hammurabi contained four articles on the regulation of alcohol. Similarly, the Aztecs closely regulated the use of alcohol.[41] It has been only recently that codes have moved away from the regulation of use to controls over availability, obtaining revenue for the state, and standardizing selling practices. Regulatory codes are now being viewed as tools for the prevention of drug-related problems.[35] Codes regulating the following areas are currently seen as a preventive focus for licit drugs (e.g., tobacco, alcohol, khat in certain countries):

1. The density of sales outlets (e.g., number and location).
2. Hours and days of sale.
3. Pricing and taxation of licit drugs.
4. Local option—allowing local governments to determine whether or not drugs are sold.
5. Advertising restrictions.
6. Regulations that state conditions of sale—i.e., not near a school or a house of worship, only with food, not to persons under a certain age, not to intoxicated persons.
7. Prescribing regulations for dangerous drugs by physicians, in order to prevent casual, prolonged, or excessive use.

Different regulatory policies have been found to produce different effects. Implicit within this strategy is the existence of a centralized government authority with the power to regulate drug sales.[5,10]

5.4. Strategies Utilizing Host Factors

Persons suffering from illnesses and injuries leading to chronic pain have been known to become drug dependent. Those with psychosis, depression, anxiety, and other mental disorders may also become drug dependent in an effort to self-medicate. This is particularly true in the manic phase of manic–depressive illness, in some recurrent depressions, and perhaps in panic disorders. Long-term treatment in all mental illnesses should involve close attention to the drug-use patterns of each patient. Preventive counseling should also include a discussion of the interactions between drugs and various prescribed medications.[4,27]

Case histories of individuals who become drug dependent regularly reveal their early psychological dependence on the ability of drugs to relieve unpleasant feelings such as shyness, anxiety, anger, boredom, or loneliness. Some drug-dependent patients entering treatment are able to identify stressful situations during which their drug use began. People with unusual life stresses are appropriate target groups for primary prevention efforts. Examples include people undergoing divorce, recent bereavement, adjustments to a physical disability, or separation from family and/or a social support group through military service, migration, or work assignment.[21,38,61] Individual and group counseling, education about drugs, recreation, and social support complement restrictions on drug availability.

All patients should be considered potential candidates for drug dependence. A physician's recommendation for drug use can overcome social controls and cultural protections against dependence on drugs as a remedy for insomnia, tension, or chronic pain. Since the first duty of a physician is to do no harm, primary prevention of drug dependence should include the avoidance of prescribing dependence-producing drugs in cases where their use may cause more harm than benefit.[9] For cases in which such drugs are warranted, the doses and duration of drug prescription must be carefully considered.

5.5. Strategies Utilizing Environmental Factors

Environmental factors include a society's norms regarding drug use. Social norms influence not only the type of drug problems a society possesses, but also the locus of the problems. Norms may change, and this will influence not only the manifestation of the drug problem but also the definition of a drug problem. For example, in many countries, new norms have emerged which encourage cigarette smoking, cannabis smoking, alcohol drinking, or heroin smoking.

Attempts to control the physical environment aim at minimizing rather than preventing drug-related problems. These attempts reduce the seriousness of drug-related problems and make the environment safer for drug users. Examples of safety devices that can reduce drug-related injuries include the following:

- Seatbelts or airbags to reduce serious injury in automobile crashes.
- Fire-retardant upholstery and bedding (home fires are often due to tobacco, cannabis, or opiate smoking in bed).
- Devices to prevent falls in the home and injuries in the workplace due to drug use.

Sound policies designed to discourage dangerous drug use can reduce injuries, loss of productivity, and death.[50]

6. Secondary Prevention

Case finding for all types of diseases is a traditional responsibility of health professionals. Secondary prevention for drug dependence, therefore, should be routine in health-care settings.

Studies of the outcome of treatment for drug problems show that both the presence of social stability (e.g., job, family ties, intact social network) and the absence of late-stage, irreversible physical and mental damage are positive prognostic indicators.[24,72] Early-intervention programs focus on populations that have a high incidence of drug-related problems. Populations at risk include convicted drinking drivers, medical and surgical hospital patients, and populations in whom early indications of such problems may be systematically detected, such as employees in the workplace. These programs characteristically take advantage of special motivational opportunities provided by the setting in which they operate.

Common factors of early intervention programs include the following:

1. An overall policy statement, indicating that drug dependence is a disease which can be successfully treated.
2. Definition of a population at risk for drug problems, such as persons showing deteriorating work or school performance or persons convicted for offenses involving drugs.
3. Specific screening of such individuals for drug dependence, using reviews of records, personal interviews, talks with family members, supervisors, or others, and/or questionnaires or other screening methods.
4. A counselor links the drug-use patterns with negative life consequences; the overall situation is interpreted as one which can be rectified through treatment.
5. Development of a treatment plan, including the element of choice, but with special motivation. (For example, a restricted driver's license may be returned to a convicted drinking driver who agrees to enter a rehabilitation program, or disciplinary action may be deferred if a drug-dependent employee enters treatment. The individual may choose not to be treated and will then be handled on the basis of past and continuing performance.)
6. Follow-up monitoring and encouragement of the patient to follow through with the treatment plan. (Deferred penalties may be applied if the individual is uncooperative or fails to improve.)

6.1. Screening for Drug Dependence

Screening for drug dependence is a time-honored procedure. Common practices include testing motorists for breath alcohol, assaying blood of comatose patients for barbiturates, and narcotic-antagonist challenges for heroin detection. Modern-day clinical screening can be traced to the development of chromatographic and immunoassay techniques which can detect drugs of dependence. This screening has been used on a mass scale in specific populations, including the military, persons arrested, and specific occupation groups, such as pilots and machine operators who might endanger others if they are under the influence of drugs. Owing to its relative high cost, blood testing for drugs generally has been restricted to diagnostic problems caused by overdoses.[33] Urine screening of persons arrested for a variety of criminal offenses is now commonplace in many jurisdictions. Identified drug-dependent persons then receive some special intervention, education, or treatment designed to prevent further drug dependence.

6.2. Case Finding in the Clinical Setting

Detection methods for early drug-dependence problems are of two types. First, one can elicit clinical findings that occur before physical dependence or gross tissue damage is established. These problems can be recognized in either ambulatory or inpatient settings. Second, there are problems associated with chronic use and dependence but which have been previously concealed and remained undetected. These findings are more often recognized in the inpatient location.

The clinical findings that may alert the physician to the possibility of drug dependence are not usually specific for drug dependence. However, their occurrence should raise the index of suspicion that this is a possible cause of the problem. The competent and sensitive clinician will pursue a course of action that can prove or disprove the clinical suspicion. For example, one cause of insomnia is the use of sedative drugs, including alcohol, but other disorders (e.g., anxiety, depression, nocturnal cardiac insufficiency) may cause insomnia.

Health admission forms or questionnaires can include routine questions on drug use; these are effective screening methods.[20,64] In research surveys, subjects usually give more honest answers when asked by written questionnaire than when asked person to person.[32] Clinicians do not, however, rely only on written information alone. They take a drug history regarding the type of drug used, frequency of use, dosage, and possible impairment. Health professionals must respect confidentiality of patient communications. Drug- and alcohol-dependent persons often have multiple poor health behaviors, and the presence of certain health problems should raise the index of suspicion in the clinician's mind. These include a history of suicide attempt, smoking, accidents, and acts of violence.[56] Insomnia, irritability, depression, and anxiety occur frequently among drug dependents. Relatives of drug dependents may present with allergies, psychosomatic problems (e.g., irritable bowel syndrome, dyspareunia, migraine), or as victims of physical abuse or neglect, due to family stress brought about by drug-related behavior.[52]

Social changes that may be caused by drug use are often related to work or occupational problems, such as declining productivity. Absenteeism, particularly if it seems to occur after a weekend, holiday, or vacation, should arouse the suspicion of the clinician. Adolescents whose school performance declines, who engage in acting-out behavior, who withdraw from their usual activities, or who choose new friends who are also in difficulty at school or with their parents may be engaging in more than an occasional experiment with chemicals and sliding into dependency. Occasionally the first difficulty with drug use is apprehension by the police. This sometimes motivates the law-abiding person to seek professional help.

Affective disorders may be another clinical lead early in the course of drug dependence. It is necessary to determine whether the depression is a primary disorder or secondary to the use of chemicals. Major mental disorders may occur early in the course of stimulant or hallucinogen dependence, and late in alcoholism and sedative dependence.

Patients should be routinely examined for common physical signs of undetected drug dependence. Physical signs do not by themselves indicate a drug-dependence problem, but they do call for further inquiry about its possibility. Early medical complaints are commonly multiple and vague.

Occasionally, and often dramatically, the first clinical evidence of a drug-dependence problem may occur when the patient is being treated for some other complaint. Concealment of the problem by the patient, denial by both the patient and the family, or failure of the clinician to uncover the problem may be reasons for the late recognition of drug dependence. An example of such an event would be a first seizure due to sedative withdrawal.

Drug use may interfere with medical and surgical treatment. Commonly occurring alcohol–drug interactions include the synergistic effect with CNS depressant drugs, increase in the anticoagulant levels in persons taking coumadin, upper gastrointestinal bleeding with salicylates, and disulfiramlike effect from sulfonylurea class of oral hypoglycemics. Polydrug dependence (e.g., alcohol and marijuana, opium and sedatives, sedatives and cocaine) has the ever-present potential of producing a serious or even life-threatening drug interaction.

Urine testing for drugs of dependence and breathalyzer testing for alcohol may be routinely indicated in some clinical populations. Pregnant women, persons desiring clearance for driving a vehicle, those with complaints that have no obvious cause, and those seeking employment that involves mechanical precision are commonly screened today.

Some of the most exciting data to emerge in drug dependence has been the ability of health professionals in clinic or office practice to effectively treat drug dependents who are early in their course. Clinical visits that emphasize health advantages of abstinence can be effective in motivating many persons with drug dependence.[11,42] Health professionals should begin counseling the patient as soon as drug dependence is detected and then follow the patient until abstinence or some other desired behavior change is achieved. For example, the health professional may not be able to bring about complete drug abstinence, but may be successful in getting the patient to reduce intake to a level where problems no longer result.

6.3. Prescribing to Prevent Dependence

Dependence on prescription drugs may occur with analgesics, muscle relaxants, anorexiants, sedatives, and anxiolytic drugs.[44,63] Antihistamines also may be abused, but they, like tricyclic antidepressants, are usually abused in combination with alcohol, opioids, or sedatives. Most physicians learn treatment techniques to avoid overuse of prescription drugs since the patient may be harmed, and the physician may suffer legal consequences.

The physician should attempt not to prescribe drugs with dependence potential to a patient who exhibits drug dependence tendencies as evidenced by history of alcohol-related problems or tobacco dependence. Drugs with dependence potential should be given only to reliable patients who keep regular appointments and take medication as prescribed. Only small amounts of drug should be prescribed at one time, and the patient should visit the physician regularly. On each visit, any patient who takes a drug with dependence potential should be carefully assessed for motor function, reflexes, pupil size, nystagmus, quality of speech, and mental impairment. Any abnormality of these signs may indicate overmedication, dependence, or other inappropriate consumption. If there are questions about the patient's compliance, a blood level of the prescription drug may give the clinician a true picture of drug intake. If a patient is found becoming dependent on prescription drugs, the physician should not hesitate to change drugs and refer the patient for drug-dependence treatment.[19]

A hospital, clinic, or community record system can allow monitoring and identification of patients who receive frequent prescriptions of drugs with dependence potential.[29] These systems require the cooperation of pharmacists and physicians. If properly done, they can be very effective in reducing the number of prescriptions issued to dependence-prone patients. Pharmacists should stock only small quantities of drugs with dependence potential, and patients should be required to wait 1 or 2 days for delivery.[14]

The most important thing the physician can do with sedative drugs is avoid doing harm. Many drug-dependent patients ask for them. They are seldom helpful over the long term and may be very harmful, developing into an additional dependence problem or precipitating a relapse of drug dependence. Since sedative drugs show cross-tolerance and cross-dependence with alcohol, prescribing them to a sober alcoholic is similar to giving one cigarette a day to a formerly tobacco-dependent person. This should be avoided unless the clinical circumstances are extraordinary.[76]

A recovered alcoholic undergoing general anesthesia should be instructed that the body has experienced the equivalent of being intoxicated. The patient may have some symptoms of early alcohol recovery, such as an increased impulse to drink, emotional lability, or confusion. This postoperative patient should be helped to increase social supports and behavioral controls for a few weeks or months afterward.

6.4. Early Case Finding in Nonclinical Settings

Perhaps the most successful programs in demonstrating the cost effectiveness of early intervention have been those based in the workplace, often called employee assistance programs.[12,28] The earliest programs focused primarily on identifying drug problems in employees, with training for job supervisors to detect specific signs of drug dependence. Recently, a more general approach has been employed.[49,77] The work supervisor in this type of program need not make a diagnosis, but must merely identify problems in job performance and refer the employee to a counselor. Such programs must be prepared to identify a range of personal problems, including family dysfunction, compulsive gambling, and mental disorder. Similar programs may be established for professionals such as physicians, attorneys, teachers, military personnel, or others through their professional societies or governmental licensing boards.

Monitoring requirements differ depending on the nature of the industry. For example, airline pilots require different monitoring criteria compared to clerical workers. Some programs also provide help to family members. The program may employ treatment professionals, but more often outside facilities are needed for definitive diagnosis and treatment. Some companies conduct self-help group meetings at the workplace or sponsor recreational/mutual support clubs for recovering alcoholic workers and their families. Work supervisors must be trained to understand and utilize the program appropriately.

Early intervention programs may be developed in schools.[36] Teachers and other school personnel refer students based on school performance and also encourage self-referrals. Trained clinicians assess the problem. Individual or group counseling may take place in school, or a treatment referral to an outside agency may be made. Family involvement is desirable, and counselors must be prepared to work with drug problems in the students' families.

Court-based early-intervention programs have been established for driving offenses, domestic violence, juvenile delinquency, and other antisocial behavior.

7. Tertiary Prevention

7.1. Prevention of Medical Complications

The ideal outcome for most drug-dependent patients is abstinence with full rehabilitation. However, clinicians sometimes encounter drug-dependent patients who cannot or will not completely stop use or can only cease use for short periods of time.[42,46] In these cases, the major goal may be to prevent or reduce medical complications.[55] This can be done in many cases by encouraging cessation for intermittent, short periods, or reducing the dosage, even in patients unable to sustain lifelong abstinence. For example, to be at high risk for lung cancer, a person must smoke about 30 pack-years, which is one pack (20 cigarettes) per day for 30 years, or two packs per day for 15 years. Chronic bronchitis and emphysema begin to occur after about 20 pack-years. By using the pack-year model, one can appreciate the preventive value of intermittent cessation to prevent 20 or 30 pack-years of cigarette smoking. Even after 20 or 30 pack-years, cessation may produce an improvement in morbidity and mortality.

Health professionals need to be cognizant that drug dependence is frequently a chronic, relapsing condition. Prevention of drug-dependence complications depends on recurrent treatment episodes for some patients.

7.2. Patient Registration and Community Surveillance

Some countries have established systems in which identified drug-dependent persons are required to register with government agencies.[25] There are several potential advantages of these systems, such as preventing drug dependents from patronizing multiple sources of drug supply, or early identification if relapse occurs. Special prescription forms for highly dependence-producing prescription drugs have also been developed to monitor prescribing.

One form of tertiary prevention that has been very effective in many geographical areas of the world has been community surveillance of known drug dependents who have entered the criminal justice system.[16] Drug-dependent persons who have been arrested and identified enter a surveillance system referred to as parole or probation. In this system, the drug dependents are regularly monitored for relapse. In addition to monitoring, they may also receive assistance in obtaining health care, job placement, and counseling. Monitoring may take the form of needlemark inspection, breath or urine testing, or opioid-antagonist challenges. If relapse does occur, the surveillance system may have the option of incarceration. A long-term study of chronic opioid-dependent patients suggests that community surveillance, when combined with appropriate medical treatment, provides the best outcome.[2,71]

Case registration has been effectively employed in several metropolitan areas, such as New York, Hong Kong, and Singapore. Malaysia, Iran, and Burma have also implemented similar systems. Ideally, these systems should be confidential; otherwise, many patients will demur from seeking treatment.

References

1. Akcasu A: A survey on the factors preventing opium use by poppy growing peasants in Turkey. *Bull Narcotics* 1976; 28(2):13–17.
2. Anderson GS, Nutter RW: Clients and outcomes of methadone treatment program. *Int J Addict* 1975; 10(6):937–948.
3. Baldwin AD: Anstie's alcohol limit. *J Public Health* 1977; 67:679–681.
4. Bayer I: The abuse of psychotropic drugs. *Bull Narcotics* 1973; 25:11–25.
5. Beauchamp D: *Beyond Alcoholism: Alcohol and Public Health Policy*. Philadelphia, Temple University Press, 1980.
6. Bergeret J: Prevention primaire en matiere de toxicomanies: Perspectives, erreurs et illusions. *Drug Alcohol Dependence* 1983; 11:71–75.
7. Bewley BR, Bland JM, Harris R: Factors associated with the starting of cigarette smoking by primary school children. *Br J Prev Soc Med* 1974; 28:37–44.
8. Bliding G, Bliding A, Fex G, Törnqvist C: The appropriateness of laboratory tests in tracing young heavy drinkers. *Drug Alcohol Dependence* 1982; 10:153–158.

9. Blume S: Iatrogenic alcoholism. *Q J Stud Alcohol* 1973; 34:1348–1352.
10. Bruun K, Edwards G, Lumio M, Makela K, Osterberg E, Pan L, Popham RE, Room R, Schmidt W, Skog OJ, Sulkenen P: *Alcohol Control Policies in Public Health Perspective,* Publication no. 25. Helsinki, Finnish Foundation for Alcohol Studies, 1975.
11. Burnum JF: Outlook for treating patients with self-destructive habits. *Ann Intern Med* 1974; 81:387–393.
12. Cahill MH, Volicer BJ: Male and female differences in severity of problems with alcohol at the workplace. *Drug Alcohol Dependence* 1981; 8:143–156.
13. Coid J: Alcoholism and violence. *Drug Alcohol Dependence* 1982; 9:1–13.
14. Council on Scientific Affairs: Drug abuse related to prescribing practices. *JAMA* 1982; 247:864–866.
15. Cudal A: Educational programmes on the prevention and control drug abuse in the Philippines. *Bull Narcotics* 1976; 28(3):1–9.
16. Desmond DP, Maddux JF: The effect of probation on behavior of chronic opioid drug users. *Contemporary Drug Prob* 1977; 6:41–58.
17. Dumars KW: Parental drug usage: Effect upon chromosomes of progeny. *Pediatrics* 1971; 47(6):1037–1041.
18. Edwards G: *Alcohol and Alcoholism: The Report of a Special Committee of the Royal College of Psychiatrists.* New York, Free Press, 1979.
19. Ehrhardt HE, Schroder O: The effect of prescription orders on the control of narcotic drugs. *Bull Narcotics* 1977; 29(2):1–7.
20. Favazza AR, Cannell B: Failure to diagnose alcoholism and drug abuse. *Drug Alcohol Dependence* 1979; 4:499–501.
21. Finn P, O'Gorman P: *Teaching about Alcohol.* Newton, MA, Allyn and Bacon, 1981.
22. Finnegan LP: Pathophysiological and behavioural effects of the transplacental transfer of narcotic drugs to the foetuses and neonates of narcotic dependent mothers. *Bull Narcotics* 1979; 31(3,4):1–58.
23. Fried PA: Marihuana use by pregnant women: Neurobehavioural effects in neonates. *Drug Alcohol Dependence* 1980; 6:415–424.
24. Gerard DL, Saenger G: *Out-patient Treatment of Alcoholism.* Brookside Monograph no. 4. Toronto, Ontario, Canada, Addiction Research Foundation, 1966.
25. Glaser FB, Ball JC: The British narcotic "Register" in 1970: A factual review. *JAMA* 1971; 216:1177–1182.
26. Goar GB, Richter BJ: Macroeconomics of disease prevention in the United States. *Science* 1978; 200:1124–1130.
27. Granier-Doyeux M: Influence of certain social factors on the development of drug dependence. *Bull Narcotics* 1973; 25(1):1–8.
28. Jones K, Vischi T: Impact of alcohol, drug abuse, and mental health treatment on medical care utilization: A review of the research literature. *Med Care* 1979; 17(2)(12):1–26.
29. Kaufman A, Brickner PW, Varner R, Mashburn W: Tranquilizer control. *JAMA* 1972; 221:1504–1506.
30. Kinder BN, Pape NE, Walfish S: Drug and alcohol education programs: A review of outcome studies. *Int J Addict* 1980; 15:1035–1054.
31. Luce BR, Schweitzer SO: Smoking and alcohol abuse: A comparison of their economic consequences. *N Engl J Med* 1978; 298:569–571.
32. Luetgert MJ, Armstrong AH: Methodological issues in drug usage surveys: Anonymity, recency, and frequency. *Int J Addict* 1973; 8:683–689.
33. McCarron MM, Schulze BW, Walberg CB, Thompson GA, Ansari A: Short-acting barbiturate overdosage: Correlation of intoxication score with serum barbiturate concentration. *JAMA* 1982; 248:55–61.
34. Malkin SA, Allen DL: Differential characteristics of adolescent smokers and non-smokers. *J Family Pract* 1980; 10:437–440.

35. Moore MH, Gerstein DR: *Alcohol and Public Policy: Beyond the Shadow of Prohibition.* Washington, DC, National Academy Press, 1981.
36. Morehouse ER: Working in the schools with children of alcoholic parents. *Health Social Work* 1979; 4(4):144–162.
37. Moser J: *Prevention of Alcohol-Related Problems: An International Review of Preventive Measure, Policies Programmes.* Toronto, Ontario, Canada, Alcohol and Drug Addiction Research Foundation, 1980.
38. Murad JE: Drug abuse among students in the State of Minas Gerais, Brazil. *Bull Narcotics* 1979; 31:49–58.
39. Navaratnam V, Aun LB, Spencer CP: Extent and patterns of drug abuse among children in Malaysia. *Bull Narcotics* 1979; 31:59–68.
40. Noll A: Drug abuse and its prevention as seen by the international legal profession. *Bull Narcotics* 1975; 27(1):37–47.
41. Paredes A: Social control of drinking among the Aztec Indians of Mesoamerica. *Q J Stud Alcohol* 1975; 36:1139–1153.
42. Pederson LL: Compliance with physician advice to quit smoking: A review of the literature. *Prev Med* 1982; 11:71–84.
43. Pela OA, Ebie JC: Drug abuse in Nigeria: A review of epidemiological studies. *Bull Narcotics* 1982; 34(3,4):91–99.
44. Petursson H, Lader MH: Benzodiazepine dependence. *Br J Addict* 1981; 76:133–145.
45. Popham RE, Schmidt W, deLint J: The prevention of alcoholism: Epidemiological studies of the effects of government control measures. *Br J Addict* 1975; 70:125–144.
46. Powell DR, McCann BS: The effects of a multiple treatment program and maintenance procedures on smoking cessation. *Prev Med* 1981; 10:94–104.
47. Pratt C: Child rearing methods and children's health behavior. *J Health Soc Behav* 1973; 14:61–64.
48. Pratt O, Path FRC: Alcohol and the women of childbearing age: A public health problem. *Br J Addict* 1981; 76:383–390.
49. Presnall LF: *Occupational Counseling and Referral Systems.* Salt Lake City, Utah, Utah Alcoholism Foundation, 1981.
50. Redfield JT: Drugs in the workplace-substituting sense for sensationalism. *Am J Public Health* 1973; 63(12):1064–1070.
51. Richman A, Rootman I: Epidemiologic field units on narcotic-related problems. *Bull Narcotics* 1982; 34(2):17–28.
52. Rydelius PA: Children of alcoholic fathers: Their social adjustment and health status after twenty years. *Acta Pediatr Scand* 1981; suppl 286:1–89.
53. Schankula H: *Alcohol: Public Education and Social Policy.* Toronto, Ontario, Canada, Addiction Research Foundation, 1981.
54. Schioler P: Information, teaching and education in the primary prevention of drug abuse among youth in Denmark. *Bull Narcotics* 1981; 33(4):57–65.
55. Schmidt W, Popham RE: Alcohol consumption and ischemic heart disease: Some evidence from population studies. *Br J Addict* 1981; 76:407–417.
56. Seltzer CC, Friedman GO, Siegelaub AB: Smoking and drug consumption in white, black, and Oriental men and women. *Am J Public Health* 1974; 64:466–473.
57. Simpson HM, Mayhew DR, Warren RA: Epidemiology of road accidents involving young adults: Alcohol, drugs and other factors. *Drug Alcohol Dependence* 1982; 10:35–63.
58. Smart RG: Legislation restrictive et usage de la drogue: Analyse d'etudes empiriques. *Bull Stupefiants* 1976; 28(1):55–66.
59. Souief MI: The use of cannabis in Egypt: A behavioural study. *Bull Narcotics* 1971; 23:17–28.
60. Soueif MI: Cannabis ideology: A study of opinions and beliefs centering around cannabis consumption. *Bull Narcotics* 1973; 25:33–38.

61. Soueif MI: Some issues of major importance for prevention of drug dependence. *Natl Rev Social Sci* 1974; 11:39–61.
62. Soueif MI, El-Sayed AM, Darweesh ZA, Hamoura MA: The extent of non-medical use of psychoactive substances among secondary school students in Greater Cairo. *Drug Alcohol Dependence* 1982; 9:15–41.
63. Swanson DW, Weddige RL, Morse RM: Abuse of prescription drugs. *Mayo Clin Proc* 1973; 48:359–367.
64. Tennant FS Jr, Day CM, Ungerleider JT: Screening for drug and alcohol abuse in a general medical population. *JAMA* 1979; 242:533–535.
65. Tennant FS Jr, Detels R: Relationship of alcohol, cigarette, and drug abuse in adulthood with alcohol, cigarette, and coffee consumption in childhood. *Prev Med* 1976; 5:70–77.
66. Tennant FS Jr, Detels R, Clark V: Some childhood antecedents of drug and alcohol abuse. *Am J Epidemiol* 1975; 102:377–385.
67. Tennant FS Jr, La Cour JL: Children at high risk for addiction and alcoholism: Identification and intervention. *Pediatr Nurs* 1980; 6 (Jan-Feb):26–27.
68. Tennant FS JR, Mohler PJ, Drachler DH: Effectiveness of drug education classes. *Am J Public Health* 1974; 64:422–426.
69. Tennant FS Jr, Weaver SC, Lewis CE: Outcomes of drug education: Four case studies. *Pediatrics* 1973; 52:246–252.
70. Thompson EL: Smoking education program 1960–1976. *Am J Public Health* 1978; 68:250–257.
71. Vaillant GE: A 20-year follow-up of New York narcotic addicts. *Arch Gen Psychiatry* 1973; 29:237–241.
72. Vaillant GE: *The Natural History of Alcoholism.* Cambridge, MA, Harvard University Press, 1983.
73. Warner KE: Cigarette smoking in the 1970's: The impact of the antismoking campaign on consumption. *Science* 1981; 211:729–730.
74. Weppner RS, Agar MH: Immediate precursors to heroin addiction. *J Health Soc Behav* 1971; 12:10–18.
75. Westermeyer J, Berman J: A proposed social indicator system for alcohol-related problems. *Prev Med* 1973; 2:438–444.
76. Woody GE, O'Brien CP, Greenstein R: Misuse and abuse diazepam: An increasingly common medical problem. *Int J Addict* 1975; 10(5):843–848.
77. Wrich JT: *The Employee Assistance Program.* Center City, MN, Hazeldon, 1980.

Glossary

Agent Any power or substance capable of acting on the organism, whether curative, morbific, or other.

Altered state of consciousness A change in the usual state of consciousness, which may be accompanied by such effects as reduced or enhanced awareness of environmental stimuli or of various emotional or feeling states; it can be induced by drugs, fatigue, meditation, various mental exercises.

Apathy Lack of feeling or emotion; indifference.

Binge use Periodic heavy use of drugs or alcohol.

Blackout The alcoholic's amnesia for his behavior during drinking episodes. Such blackouts are indicative of beginning, but still reversible, brain damage.

Bolus Administration of a drug such that blood concentration level of the drug rapidly increases and then gradually decreases; the "bolus" phenomenon occurs with intravenous injection, sniffing, or smoking.

Booster sessions Episodic readministration of a treatment, particularly in the case of aversive conditioning.

Breathalyzer An apparatus for testing a person's breath for body alcohol content.

Career hypothesis A poorly defined model of drug dependence that implies a natural history, with waxing and waning of the disorder over time, with eventual deterioration in some patients and recovery or "maturing out" in other patients.

Central nervous system Those parts of the nervous system in the cranium and vertebrae (i.e., brain, spinal cord).

Cold-turkey withdrawal No medication or other somatotherapy is prescribed during withdrawal; the term is derived from the piloerection or "turkey skin" which occurs with unmedicated opioid withdrawal.

Contingency The predetermined consequence that ensues from a patient's behavior; either the clinician or another person may administer the contingency.

Controlled double-blind study A clinical research study in which (1) two or more treatment conditions are administered to different groups of patients randomly assigned to regimens Tx, Tx, . . . Tx and (2) both the patients and the treating clinicians do not know (i.e., are "blind" to) each patient's treatment regimen.

Craving Longing for or desiring strongly the effects of drug or alcohol; there is an obsessional quality to this phenomenon, often accompanied by dysphoria.

Cross-tolerance One drug will ameliorate the withdrawal effects of another drug (e.g., alcohol and benzodiazepines).

Delirium A mental disturbance marked by illusions, hallucinations, short unsystematized delusions, cerebral excitement, physical restlessness and incoherence, and having a comparatively short course.

Delirium tremens A variety of acute mental disturbances marked by delirium with trembling, sweating, agitation, confusion, and hallucinations (often visual); it occurs after withdrawal of alcohol or sedatives in addicted persons.

Delusion A false belief that cannot be corrected by reason; it is illogically founded and cannot be corrected by argument or persuasion or even by the evidence of the patient's own senses.

Depersonalization Loss of the sense of personal identity or of personal ownership of the parts of one's body.

Derealization The feeling of changed reality; the feeling that one's surroundings have changed.

Diaphoresis Perspiration, especially profuse perspiration.

Distractibility A morbid or abnormal variation of attention; inability to fix attention on any subject.

Drug abuse Problem-producing use of a drug, but without tolerance or withdrawal.

Drug dependence Increased tolerance or withdrawal syndrome associated with chronic heavy use of a chemical substance.

Emergency intoxicants Substitute drugs used when the person's drug of choice is not available; these are often inexpensive or readily available drugs (e.g., household or industrial hydrocarbons).

Enabling Providing the means or opportunity for doing or accomplishing something; with regard to drug dependence, friends or relatives are said to engage in "enabling" behavior when they assist the person in ways which support drug dependence (e.g., providing money, rescuing the person from consequences of drug-related behavior).

Enterohepatic circulation Drugs absorbed from the intestine travel to the liver before entering the general circulation; much of an ingested drug may be metabolized in this process—sometimes referred to as "first-pass effect."

Enterohepatic recirculation Some drugs removed by the liver are secreted in the bile and then reabsorbed through the intestine; this can result in a prolonged effect from the drug.

Environment The external surroundings and influences.

Enzyme An organic compound, frequently a protein, capable of accelerating or producing by catalytic action some change in its substrate for which it is often specific.

Epidemiology The field of science dealing with the relationships of the various factors which determine the frequencies and distributions of an infectious process, a disease, or a physiological state in a human community.

Ethos The distinguishing character or time of a racial, religious, social, or other group.

Extended family A group of relatives greater than a nuclear family, usually tracing common relationship to a common grandparent or more distant ancestor.

Fervor therapeuticus Being overly enthusiastic about a treatment, so that emotion beclouds judgment.

First-pass effect Removal by the liver of ingested drugs, as they pass from the intestine through the portal vein to the liver; due to first-pass effect, an ingested drug—even if completely absorbed—may have less effect than an injected drug without the first-pass effect.

Hallucination A sense perception not founded on objective reality (e.g., hearing, seeing, smelling, feeling things that others do not perceive).

Hangover The aftereffect syndrome following ingestion of alcohol or other sedatives, such as barbiturates; symptoms include bad taste, nausea, vomiting, tachypnea, pallor, irritability, sweating, conjunctival injection, headache.

Homeostasis A dynamic condition of balance in living organisms, which usually refers to physiological phenomena, but may also apply to some psychological phenomena.

Host In infectious disease terminology, an animal or plant that harbors or nourishes another organism.

Illusion A false or misinterpreted sensory impression; a false interpretation of a real sensory image (e.g., seeing window curtains blowing at night and interpreting them to be a ghost).

Incidence In epidemiology, the number of new cases appearing in a population over a specific time, such as a year.

Indigent An unemployed person with no permanent residence.

Loading dose A higher initial dose, followed by lower subsequent doses.

Mainlining A slang expression for taking narcotics by intravenous injection.

Medication Substances taken into or rubbed on the body to sustain health, or to return the diseased body to a healthy state.

Microsome One of the minute granules found in protoplasm.

Modality Any method or technique of treatment; a class or group within the therapeutic armamentarium.

Mores The traditions and habits generally regarded as conducive to social welfare.

Myelotoxic Destructive to bone marrow.

Naloxone challenge test Administration of naloxone precipitates a withdrawal state if physical dependence is present; used to establish the presence of addiction.

Nodding off Brief slumber during opioid intoxication, often while sitting or slumped in an apparently uncomfortable position.

Nuclear family A two-generation family consisting of parents and their children.

Objective Perceptible to the senses; pertaining to things that are the objects of the external senses.

On the nod *see* Nodding off.

Operant conditioning Form of learning in which a particular response is reinforced and becomes likely to occur.

Opiate Alkaloids derived from opium which have morphinelike properties.

Opioid Any drug, whether synthetic or obtained from opium, which has morphinelike properties.

Outreach programs Programs that extend from the clinical setting to the patient's social setting, for purposes of early treatment, follow-up treatment, or crisis intervention.

Over-the-counter drug A drug that is sold without need of a prescription.

Panic attack An attack of overwhelming and unreasoning fear and anxiety, associated with a sense of imminent death or impending doom.

Pathoplastic Diverse forms of a disease as distinct from the particular cause of a disease.

Pavlovian conditioning An unconditioned stimulus (such as meat with a hungry dog) is joined with a conditioned stimulus (such as a bell) so that either stimulus produces the unconditioned response (such as salivation in a hungry dog).

Phases (of treatment) Any one of the varying aspects or stages through which a disease or recovery process may pass.

Piloerection Erection of the hair; it often occurs in opiate withdrawal.

Polydrug abuse Abuse of two or more drugs, simultaneously or sequentially.

Prevalence The number of cases of a disease or disorder existing in a population at a particular point in time.

Primary prevention Efforts to ensure that a disease or disorder does not occur.

Prognosis A forecast as to the probable result or outcome of a disorder or disease; the prospect as to recovery from a disease as indicated by the nature and symptoms of the case.

Program In treatment, the sum total of scheduled activities, treatment modalities, and skills available through staff members.

Prospective study A study begun before an event occurs to explore possible outcomes of various approaches.

Psychedelic Mind-manifesting; sometimes used to describe certain pharmacological agents that have an effect on mental processes.

Psychoactive substance Any drug (stimulant, depressant, or tranquilizer) with an effect on mental processes.

Psychosis A mental disorder characterized by delusions and hallucinations; it is often accompanied by bizarre or maladaptive behavior.

Public inebriate An individual who displays intoxicated behavior (e.g., ataxia, disorientation, inappropriate speech) in public.

Refractory Not readily yielding to treatment.

Reinforcing drug In certain animal models for assessing drugs, animals repeat a behavior (such as pressing a bar) in order to obtain the drug; the drug is then said to "reinforce" or reward the behavior.

Rescuing In the jargon of drug dependence, this refers to the tendency of friends and relatives to "rescue" the drug-dependent person from the consequences of drug-related behaviors, rather than to allow the person to experience these consequences.

Retrospective study A study begun after an event has occurred to assess the impact of the event.

Scapegoat The person or object who is blamed for the actions of others; the object of projection.

Secondary prevention Preventive techniques focusing on early detection and correction of maladaptive patterns within the context of the individual's present life situation.

Sequencing (of education) Having continuity, connection, and often uniformity, i.e., united by a single theme.

Sign An indication of the existence of something; an objective evidence of a disease.

Skid row A slang expression to denote a place where the persons who are not succeeding in their lives congregate; persons most often referred to as residing in this area are persons with alcohol or mental problems.

Skin popping A street term for subcutaneous injection of a drug.

Social network The family, relatives, friends, co-workers and other associates with whom a person is affiliated.

Stage (in the course of a disease) A period or distinct phase in the course of a disease.

Status epilepticus A series of rapidly repeated epileptic convulsions without any periods of consciousness between them.

Symptom Any functional evidence of disease or of a patient's condition; a change in a patient's condition indicative of some bodily or mental state; these tend to be subjective, as compared to the more objective signs of a disease.

Synesthesia A secondary sensation accompanying an actual perception; the experience of a sensation in one place, due to stimulation applied to another place (e.g., feeling pain, then seeing red).

Tertiary prevention Preventive techniques focusing on short-term hospitalization and intensive aftercare when an emotional breakdown has occurred, with the aim of returning the individual to the family or community setting as soon as possible.

Titer use Many heavy drug or alcohol users consume a fairly consistent dosage of the drug each day, often consuming the drug through the day, so that blood levels remain within specific limits; since this use of drug resembles chemical titration to some extent, it is sometimes referred to as titer use.

Tolerance A physiological condition in which increased dosage of an addictive drug is needed to obtain effects previously produced by smaller dose.

Tough love A lay term referring to the fact that a relative or friend may have to undertake "tough" actions (e.g., refusing to pay for more drugs, not rescuing the drug-dependent person from the consequences of drug use) in order to help or express "love" for the drug-dependent person; this is a difficult, often complex process in which the family members may benefit from professional guidance and support.

Tracks The slang expression used to refer to the marks left after numerous intravenous drug injections.

Treatment approach The management and care of a patient for the purpose of combining appropriate treatment with a particular disease or disorder.

Treatment program *see* Program.

Treatment modality *see* Modality.

Triage The sorting out, classification, and disposition of patients who have been brought to a hospital.

Index